# Imaging of Lymphoma

*Guest Editor*

Jürgen Rademaker, MD

## RADIOLOGIC
## CLINICS OF NORTH AMERICA

www.radiologic.theclinics.com

March 2008 • Volume 46 • Number 2

SAUNDERS an imprint of ELSEVIER, Inc.

**W.B. SAUNDERS COMPANY**
*A Division of Elsevier Inc.*

1600 John F. Kennedy Boulevard ● Suite 1800 ● Philadelphia, Pennsylvania 19103-2899

http://www.theclinics.com

**RADIOLOGIC CLINICS OF NORTH AMERICA Volume 46, Number 2**
**March 2008 ISSN 0033-8389, ISBN 13: 978-1-4160-6347-6, ISBN 10: 1-4160-6347-1**

*Editor:* Barton Dudlick

*Radiologic Clinics of North America* (ISSN 0033-8389) is published bimonthly in January, March, May, July, September, and November by Elsevier Inc., 360 Park Avenue South, New York, NY 10010-1710. Business and Editorial Offices: 1600 John F. Kennedy Boulevard., Suite 1800, Philadelphia, PA 19103-2899. Customer Service Office: 6277 Sea Harbor Drive, Orlando, FL 32887-4800. Periodicals postage paid at New York, NY and additional mailing offices. Subscription prices are USD 290 per year for US individuals, USD 431 per year for US institutions, USD 142 per year for US students and residents, USD 339 per year for Canadian individuals, USD 530 per year for Canadian institutions, USD 394 per year for international individuals, USD 530 per year for international institutions, and USD 192 per year for Canadian and foreign students/residents. To receive student and resident rate, orders must be accompanied by name of affiliated institution, date of term and the signature of program/residency coordinatior on institution letterhead. Orders will be billed at individual rate until proof of status is received. Foreign  air speed delivery is included in all *Clinics* subscription prices. All prices are subject to change without notice. **POSTMASTER:** Send address changes to *Radiologic Clinics of North America*, Elsevier Journals Customer Service, 6277 Sea Harbor Drive, Orlando, FL 32887-4800. **Customer Service: 1-800-654-2452 (US). From outside of the United States, call (+1) 407-563-6020. Fax: 407-363-9661. E-mail: JournalsCustomerService-usa@elsevier.com.**

*Reprints.* For copies of 100 or more of articles in this publication, please contact the Commercial Reprints Department, Elsevier Inc., 360 Park Avenue South, New York, New York 10010-1710. Tel.: (+1) 212-633-3812; Fax: (+1) 212-462-1935; E-mail: reprints@elsevier.com.

*Radiologic Clinics of North America* also published in Greek Paschalidis Medical Publications, Athens, Greece.

*Radiologic Clinics of North America* is covered in *MEDLINE/PubMed (Index Medicus), EMBASE/Excerpta Medica, Current Contents/Life Sciences, Current Contents/Clinical Medicine, RSNA Index to Imaging Literature, BIOSIS, Science Citation Index,* and *ISI/BIOMED.*

Printed in the United States of America.

# Contributors

## GUEST EDITOR

**JÜRGEN RADEMAKER, MD**
Assistant Attending Radiologist, Department of
Radiology, Memorial Sloan-Kettering Cancer
Center; and Assistant Professor of Radiology,
Weill Medical College of Cornell University,
New York, New York

## AUTHORS

**SARA J. ABRAMSON, MD, FACR**
Professor of Clinical Radiology and Attending
Radiologist, Department of Radiology, Memorial
Sloan-Kettering Cancer Center, Weill Medical
College of Cornell University, New York, New York

**LAUREN E. ABREY, MD**
Vice-Chairman and Director of Clinical Research,
Department of Neurology, Memorial Sloan-
Kettering Cancer Center; and Associate Professor
of Neurology, New York Presbyterian Hospital/
Weill Cornell Medical College, New York,
New York

**ASHLEY H. AIKEN, MD**
Assistant Professor of Radiology, Department
of Radiology, San Francisco General Hospital,
University of California San Francisco, San
Francisco, California

**MARTIN ALLEN-AUERBACH, MD**
Assistant Clinical Professor, Department
of Molecular and Medical Pharmacology,
Ahmanson Biological Imaging Center/Nuclear
Medicine, David Geffen School of Medicine,
University of California Los Angeles,
Los Angeles, California

**EDWIN PASCAL ALYEA III, MD**
Associate Professor of Medicine, Division of
Medical Oncology, Dana Farber Cancer Institute;
and Department of Medicine, Brigham and
Women's Hospital, Boston, Massachusetts

**MUNAZZA ANIS, MD**
Assistant Professor, Department of Radiology,
Medical University of South Carolina, Charleston,
South Carolina

**YOUNG A BAE, MD**
Clinical Assistant Professor of Radiology and
Attending Radiologist, Department of Radiology,
Center for Imaging Science, Samsung Medical
Center, Sungkyunkwan University School of
Medicine, Seoul; and Department of Radiology,
Hallym University College of Medicine,
Kyungki-do, Republic of Korea

**SANDRA BRENNAN, MD, FFR RCSI, FRCR (UK)**
Assistant Attending, Department of Radiology,
Memorial Sloan-Kettering Cancer Center, New
York, New York

**BRUCE D. CHESON, MD**
Professor of Medicine and Head of Hematology,
Georgetown University Hospital, Lombardi
Comprehensive Cancer Center,
Washington, DC

**JOHANNES CZERNIN, MD**
Professor, Department of Molecular and Medical
Pharmacology, Ahmanson Biological Imaging
Center/Nuclear Medicine, David Geffen School of
Medicine, University of California Los Angeles, Los
Angeles, California

**SVEN de VOS, MD, PhD**
Assistant Professor, Department of Medicine, Division of Hematology/Oncology, David Geffen School of Medicine, University of California Los Angeles, Los Angeles, California

**SANJIV SAM GAMBHIR, MD, PhD**
Professor, Departments of Medicine and Bioengineering, Molecular Imaging Program at Stanford, Stanford University School of Medicine, Stanford, California

**RITU R. GILL, MBBS**
Instructor, Department of Radiology, Brigham and Women's Hospital, Boston, Massachusetts

**CHRISTINE GLASTONBURY, MBBS**
Associate Professor of Radiology, Department of Radiology, University of California San Francisco, San Francisco, California

**MARC J. GOLLUB, MD**
Associate Professor of Radiology, Weill Medical College of Cornell University; and Director of CT and Gastrointestinal Radiology, Department of Radiology, Memorial Sloan-Kettering Cancer Center, New York, New York

**MICHAEL L. GORIS, MD, PhD**
Professor, Department of Radiology, Division of Nuclear Medicine, Stanford University Medical Center, Stanford, California

**LUCY E. HANN, MD**
Assistant Attending, Department of Radiology, Memorial Sloan-Kettering Cancer Center; and Professor of Radiology, Weill Medical College of Cornell University, New York, New York

**SOFIA HAQUE, MD**
Assistant Attending, Department of Radiology, Memorial Sloan-Kettering Cancer Center; and Assistant Professor of Radiology, New York Presbyterian Hospital/Weill Cornell Medical College, New York, New York

**SINCHUN HWANG, MD**
Assistant Professor , Weill Medical College of Cornell University; and Assistant Attending Radiologist, Department of Radiology, Memorial Sloan-Kettering Cancer Center, New York, New York

**ANDREI IAGARU, MD**
Instructor, Department of Radiology, Division of Nuclear Medicine, Stanford University Medical Center, Stanford, California

**ABID IRSHAD, MD**
Assistant Professor, Department of Radiology, Medical University of South Carolina, Charleston, South Carolina

**JYOTHI P. JAGANNATHAN, MD**
Instructor, Department of Radiology, Harvard Medical School; and Staff Radiologist, Dana Farber Cancer Institute, Brigham and Women's Hospital, Boston, Massachusetts

**MENG LAW, MD**
Associate Professor, Departments of Radiology and Neurosurgery, Mount Sinai Medical Center, New York, New York

**KYUNG SOO LEE, MD**
Professor of Radiology and Section Director of Thoracic Radiology, Department of Radiology, Center for Imaging Science, Samsung Medical Center, Sungkyunkwan University School of Medicine, Seoul, Republic of Korea

**MATTHEW J. MATASAR, MD, MS**
Fellow, Medical Oncology/Hematology, Memorial Sloan-Kettering Cancer Center, New York, New York

**CRAIG MOSKOWITZ, MD**
Associate Attending Physician and Associate Member, Lymphoma Service, Department of Medicine, Memorial Sloan-Kettering Cancer Center; and Associate Professor of Medicine, Weill Cornell Medical College, New York, New York

**KEVIN C. OEFFINGER, MD**
Attending, Departments of Pediatrics and Medicine, Memorial Sloan-Kettering Cancer Center, New York, New York

**ANITA P. PRICE, MD, FACR**
Attending, Department of Radiology, Memorial Sloan-Kettering Cancer Center, New York, New York

**JÜRGEN RADEMAKER, MD**
Assistant Attending Radiologist, Department of Radiology, Memorial Sloan-Kettering Cancer Center; and Assistant Professor of Radiology, Weill Medical College of Cornell University, New York, New York

**NIKHIL RAMAIYA, MD**
Director of MRI, Department of Radiology, Dana
Farber Cancer Institute; and Instructor in
Radiology, Brigham and Women's Hospital,
Harvard Medical School, Boston, Massachusetts

**PABLO ROS, MD, MPH**
Professor, Department of Radiology, Harvard
Medical School; and Staff Radiologist, Dana
Farber Cancer Institute, Brigham and Women's
Hospital, Boston, Massachusetts

**HEIKO SCHÖDER, MD**
Associate Attending Physician and Associate
Member, Nuclear Medicine Service, Department
of Radiology, Memorial Sloan-Kettering Cancer
Center; and Associate Professor of Radiology,
Weill Cornell Medical College, New York,
New York

**JOACHIM YAHALOM, MD**
Professor of Radiation Oncology in Medicine,
Weill Medical College of Cornell University;
and Attending and Member of Department of
Radiation Oncology, Memorial Sloan-Kettering
Cancer Center, New York, New York

**ROBERT J. YOUNG, MD**
Assistant Attending, Department of Radiology,
Memorial Sloan-Kettering Cancer Center; and
Assistant Professor of Radiology, New York
Presbyterian Hospital/Weill Cornell Medical
College, New York, New York

**ANDREW D. ZELENETZ, MD, PhD**
Chief, Lymphoma Service, Memorial
Sloan-Kettering Cancer Center, New York,
New York

# Contents

The malignant lymphomas, including both Hodgkin lymphoma (HL) and non-Hodg-kin lymphoma (NHL), represent a diverse group of diseases that arise from a clonal proliferation of lymphocytes. Each of the more than 30 unique types of lymphoma is a disease with a distinct natural history. This biologic heterogeneity gives rise to marked differences among the lymphomas with respect to epidemiology, pathologic characteristics, clinical presentation, and optimal management. This article empha-sizes the principles of diagnosis, including appropriate pathologic evaluation and staging considerations, and focuses on the clinical presentation, staging, and opti-mal management strategies for the most common types of lymphoma.

Fully diagnostic positron emission tomography (PET)/CT scans acquired during oral and intravenous contrast can be provided to patients and referring physicians in a single imaging session. Although FDG uptake varies, most low-grade lymphomas exhibit sufficient FDG avidity to also be staged reliably with FDG PET/CT. PET/CT imaging is more accurate for lymphoma staging than PET or CT alone and has sub-stantial impact on patient management. This accurate whole-body glucose meta-bolic survey should serve as the baseline for subsequent treatment response evaluations. PET/CT has evolved to become the modality of choice for staging of nodal and extranodal lymphoma, for assessing therapeutic response, and for estab-lishing patient prognosis.

The International Harmonization Project developed recommendations for the use of positron emission tomography (PET) in managing patients who have lymphoma. It provided guidance as to the interpretation of fluorodeoxyglucose (FDG) PET and generated response definitions, incorporating metabolic imaging with the goal of im-proving interpretation of response and comparability among studies, leading to ac-celerated new agent development, more rapid availability of more effective therapies, and the enhancement of outcome for patients with lymphoma.

Fluorodeoxyglucose positron emission tomography (FDG-PET) is now considered the most accurate tool for the assessment of treatment response and prognosis in patients with Hodgkin lymphoma and aggressive non-Hodgkin lymphoma. This article discusses the potential and limitations of FDG-PET for response assessment in malignant lymphoma during chemotherapy (interim PET) and at the end of chemotherapy. Interim PET is used to predict the likelihood for a complete response at the end of such therapy. End-of-treatment PET aims to establish the completeness of response or the presence of residual viable tumor tissue. Until the results of ongoing clinical trials emerge over the next 5 years, interim PET should be considered investigational and should not be used for patient management outside of study protocols.

Successful treatment of Hodgkin lymphomas and non-Hodgkin lymphomas depends on accurate staging and prognostic estimations, as well as evaluation of response to therapy as early after initiation as possible. We focus on several aspects of molecular imaging and therapy that affect the management of patients who have lymphoma. First, we review prior use of gallium-67 citrate for evaluation of lymphoma patients, mainly from a historical perspective, since it was the mainstream lymphoma functional imaging tracer for decades. Next, we review current clinical uses of 18F Fluoro-2-Deoxyglucose (18F FDG) PET and PET/CT for evaluation of lymphoma patients and use of radioimmunotherapy in lymphoma. Finally, we discuss advances in molecular imaging that may herald the next generation of PET radiotracers after 18F FDG.

In patients who have lymphoma, the presence and distribution of thoracic involvement is important in both tumor staging and treatment. Thoracic involvement in Hodgkin lymphoma (HL) is more common than in non-Hodgkin lymphoma (NHL). In HL, mediastinal lymphadenopathy with contiguous spread is a hallmark, and lung parenchymal involvement at the initial presentation is almost always associated with mediastinal lymphadenopathy. NHL is more heterogeneous and generally presents at a more advanced stage than HL. Most often, mediastinal involvement occurs as a disseminated or recurrent form of extrathoracic lymphoma. Bulky mediastinal disease with compression of adjacent structures can occur, particularly with high-grade subtypes of NHL and isolated lung disease without mediastinal lymphadenopathy can occur in contrast to HL.

This article discusses the radiologic appearances of solid organ involvement with Hodgkin and non-Hodgkin lymphoma in the abdominopelvic region. The most common radiologic patterns of involvement are illustrated. The imaging characteristics of lymphomatous involvement of abdominal organs overlap with several other disorders and the specific features pertaining to lymphoma are highlighted. In patients who have known lymphomas, other important management considerations, such as staging, response to therapy, malignant transformation, and identification of recurrent disease, are also discussed. The emerging role of fluorodeoxyglucose positron emission tomography is briefly outlined.

The gastrointestinal (GI) tract contains the largest collection of lymphocytes anywhere in the body. GI lymphoma may arise at any site in the GI tract but typically involves the stomach and small bowel in cases of systemic disease. Most cases are non-Hodgkin B-cell type. Enteropathy-associated T cell lymphoma can complicate celiac disease. Less commonly, lymphoma may originate in the GI tract without systemic involvement. This sometimes occurs in response to chronic infections. This article discusses the role of imaging in detecting and staging GI tract lymphomas, using fluoroscopy and cross-sectional imaging, primarily CT.

Hodgkin lymphoma (HL) and non-Hodgkin lymphoma (NHL) represent 10% to 15% of all malignancies occurring in children younger than 20 years of age. Advances in cross-sectional imaging and the availability of positron emission tomography (PET) and PET-CT have had a major impact on imaging and management of pediatric patients. This article reviews the clinical features of lymphoma, focusing on the spectrum of imaging findings seen in diagnosis, staging, and follow-up of HL and NHL. Pediatric NHL has four major histologic subtypes: Burkitt lymphoma, diffuse large B-cell lymphoma, anaplastic large cell lymphoma, and lymphoblastic lymphoma. The most important subtype of HL is nodular sclerosis.

Lymphomas of the central nervous system, spine, and orbit consist of both systemic lymphomas and primary central nervous system lymphomas. This article addresses the typical imaging findings of lymphoma in both immunocompetent and immunocompromised patients, discusses the differential possibilities, and reviews the response criteria being used in clinical trials. Also described are metabolic imaging techniques with nuclear medicine and advanced MR imaging and how they can help improve the understanding of tumor biology.

Hodgkin (HL) and non-Hodgkin lymphoma (NHL) involving the head and neck have many overlapping imaging features. Definitive diagnosis depends on histology, but imaging trends may help distinguish lymphoma from other common pathologic entities in the head and neck. CT is useful for staging and assessing bony involvement, whereas MR imaging is performed for soft tissue detail in extranodal disease, especially when there is transpatial disease or intracranial or intraspinal extension. Positron emission tomography has become an important part of staging and surveillance imaging and is particularly useful to distinguish posttreatment fibrosis and residual tumor.

Imaging plays a crucial role in staging and the assessment of treatment response in patients who have lymphoma of the musculoskeletal system. This article reviews imaging features of lymphoma of bone, muscles, cutaneous, and subcutaneous tissue. At radiography, lymphoma of the bone is most commonly lytic, but the affected bone also can appear deceivingly normal, even when a large tumor is present. At CT, lymphoma of muscle can be homogenous in attenuation, and it may not show contrast enhancement, making tumor detection more difficult. Post-treatment changes often are encountered at MR imaging and positron emission tomography, and when considered in light of the patient's therapy regimen (eg, radiation therapy and granulocyte-colony stimulating factor), they usually can be differentiated from tumor. Post-treatment changes include diffuse FDG uptake in marrow after chemotherapy, indicating rebound of normal marrow, and MR imaging signal abnormalities that may persist for anywhere from a few months to years after treatment.

Hematopoietic stem cell transplantation is increasingly used for treatment of malignant and nonmalignant disorders, genetic and immunologic disorders, and solid tumors. Although advances in immunosuppressive therapy and management of infections have improved long-term survival, transplant recipients remain at risk for a multitude of complications, many of which are serious and life threatening. Posttransplant complications may be classified either according to the organ system or according to the timeframe following transplantation. Complications may involve the chest, abdominopelvic organs, the central nervous system, or musculoskeletal tissues. This article reviews the various clinical and radiologic findings of key complications following hematopoietic stem cell transplantation and the pertinent differentiating factors.

Hodgkin lymphoma is one of the most curable cancers because of its sensitivity to both radiation and several chemotherapy agents. Radical radiotherapy alone provided curative therapy for patients who had Hodgkin lymphoma as early as six decades ago. Yet, the radiation field included normal organs, such as breast tissue, thyroid, and coronary arteries, which were at risk for long-term complications. Dedicated imaging approaches have been developed to evaluate late radiation effects on these structures.

# Radiologic Clinics of North America

## THE CLINICS ARE NOW AVAILABLE ONLINE!

Access your subscription at:
**www.theclinics.com**

## GOAL STATEMENT

The goal of *Radiologic Clinics of North America* is to keep practicing radiologists and radiology residents up to date with current clinical practice by providing timely articles reviewing the state of the art in patient care.

## ACCREDITATION

The *Radiologic Clinics of North America* is planned and implemented in accordance with the Essential Areas and Policies of the Accreditation Council for Continuing Medical Education (ACCME) through the joint sponsorship of the University of Virginia School of Medicine and Elsevier. The University of Virginia School of Medicine is accredited by the ACCME to provide continuing medical education for physicians.

The University of Virginia School of Medicine designates this educational activity for a maximum of 15 *AMA PRA Category 1 Credits*™. Physicians should only claim credit commensurate with the extent of their participation in the activity.

The American Medical Association has determined that physicians not licensed in the US who participate in this CME activity are eligible for 15 *AMA PRA Category 1 Credits*™.

Credit can be earned by reading the text material, taking the CME examination online at: http://www.theclinics.com/home/cme, and completing the evaluation. After taking the test, you will be required to review any and all incorrect answers. Following completion of the test and evaluation, your credit will be awarded and you may print your certificate.

## FACULTY DISCLOSURE/CONFLICT OF INTEREST

The University of Virginia School of Medicine, as an ACCME accredited provider, endorses and strives to comply with the Accreditation Council for Continuing Medical Education (ACCME) Standards of Commercial Support, Commonwealth of Virginia statutes, University of Virginia policies and procedures, and associated federal and private regulations and guidelines on the need for disclosure and monitoring of proprietary and financial interests that may affect the scientific integrity and balance of content delivered in continuing medical education activities under our auspices.

The University of Virginia School of Medicine requires that all CME activities accredited through this institution be developed independently and be scientifically rigorous, balanced and objective in the presentation/discussion of its content, theories and practices.

All authors/editors participating in an accredited CME activity are expected to disclose to the readers relevant financial relationships with commercial entities occurring within the past 12 months (such as grants or research support, employee, consultant, stock holder, member of speakers bureau, etc.). The University of Virginia School of Medicine will employ appropriate mechanisms to resolve potential conflicts of interest to maintain the standards of fair and balanced education to the reader. Questions about specific strategies can be directed to the Office of Continuing Medical Education, University of Virginia School of Medicine, Charlottesville, Virginia.

**The authors/editors listed below have identified no financial or professional relationships for themselves or their spouse/partner:**

Sara J. Abramson, MD, FACR; Lauren E. Abrey, MD; Ashley H. Aiken, MD; Martin Allen-Auerbach, MD; Edwin Pascal Alyea III, MD; Munazza Anis, MD; Young A Bae, MD; Sandra Brennan, MD, FFR, RCSI, FRCR (UK); Bruce D. Cheson, MD;  Sven de Vos, MD, PhD; Barton Dudlick (Acquisitions Editor); Ritu R. Gill, MBBS; Marc J. Gollub, MD; Michael L. Goris, MD, PhD; Lucy E. Hann, MD; Sofia Haque, MD; Sinchin Hwang, MD; Abid Irshad, MD; Jyothi P. Jagannathan, MD; Theodore E. Keats, MD (Test  Author); Kyung Soo Lee, MD; Matthew J. Matasar, MD, MS; Craig Moskowitz, MD; Kevin C. Oeffinger, MD; Anita P. Price, MD, FACR; Jürgen Rademaker, MD (Guest Editor); Nikhil Ramaiya, MD; Pablo Ros, MD, MPH; Heiko Schöder, MD; Joachim Yahalom, MD: Robert J. Young, MD; and Andrew D. Zelenetz, MD, PhD.

**The authors/editors listed below identified the following financial or professional relationships for themselves or their spouse/partner:**

**Johannes Czernin, MD** is a consultant for Siemens and Eli Lily.

**Sanjiv Sam Gambhir, MD, PhD** serves on the Vivo Imaging Subcommittee, Tumor Biology Section and Program Committee for AACR, serves on the Board of Directors for the Academy for Molecular Imaging, serves on the Diagnostic Imaging Committee for ACOSOG, serves on the Advisory Board for ADAC, Chiron, CTI/PetNet Pharmaceutical, Inc., Endra, Enlight, GE, GSK, Henry Ford Health Systems, Lumen Therapeutics, MediCene, Inc., Memorial Sloan Kettering, Philips Medical Systems, Plexera, Varian Medical, Inc., and VisualSonics, has received a grant from Alza, Bayer Schering, the Department of Energy, GE, and Pfizer, serves on the Neural Disorders and Gene therapy Committee for Amgen and ASGT, serves on and is the chair for the Committee on Biomarkers and Imaging for ASCO, serves on the Advisory Committee for Centella, the Center for Molecular Imaging, Clirical and Translational Technologies and Resources, the Doris Duke Distinguished Clinical EMIL, and the Society of Nuclear Medicine, owns stock in Endra, Enlight, Pfizer, Spectrum Dynamics, and VisualSonics, has received royalties from Elsevier, serves on the Industrial Scientific Board for Genentech, has received Industrial Research Collaboration from GSK, NOVA R&D, Inc., Pfizer, and RMD, Inc., is the President of the Board for the Institute for Molecular Imaging, is a consultant for MediGene, Inc., Millenium, Philips Medical Systems, and Spectrum Dynamics, serves on the Molecular Imaging Abstract Review Committee for RSNA, has received an honorarium from Siemens, is a board member for the Society of Molecular Imaging, and the Society of Nuclear Medicine, is the Vice President, Publications Committee member, Task Force member, Bio-X Leadership Council member for the Society of Nuclear Medicine, and is employed by, is the director for, and serves on the IPS Cancer Center Executive Committee for Stanford University.

**Christine M. Glastonbury, MBBS** is a consultant and owns stock in Amirsys.

**Andrei H. Iagaru, MD** is a consultant for MediGene AG and has received funding from Genentech.

**Meng Law, MD** serves on the Speakers Burear for Siemens and the Advisory Committee for Prism Clinical Imaging, and is a consultant for Bayer and Bracco.

***Disclosure of Discussion of Non-FDA Approved Uses for Pharmaceutical and/or Medical Devices:***
**The University of Virginia School of Medicine, as an ACCME provider, requires that all authors identify and disclose any "off label" uses for pharmaceutical and medical device products. The University of Virginia School of Medicine recommends that each physician fully review all the available data on new products or procedures prior to clinical use.**

## TO ENROLL

To enroll in the *Radiologic Clinics of North America* Continuing Medical Education program, call customer service at 1-800-654-2452 or sign up online at http://www.theclinics.com/home/cme. The CME program is available to subscribers for an additional annual fee USD 205.

# Preface

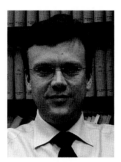

Jürgen Rademaker, MD
*Guest Editor*

The diagnosis and management of lymphoma have undergone significant changes in the past 10 years. These changes are linked with higher expectations for imaging, such as the detection of more subtle lymphoma manifestations, the evaluation of residual changes, and the better assessment of early response. This issue of *Radiologic Clinics of North America* presents a wide spectrum of topics related to imaging of lymphoma. It includes a clinical update, a discussion of positron emission tomography (PET) imaging in lymphoma, and a review of the imaging features of lymphoma in the different anatomic regions. Also reviewed are the late complications from mantle field radiation in lymphoma patients and the imaging of complications from hematopoietic stem cell transplantation.

I would like to thank all of the authors for their outstanding efforts toward the assembly of this issue of the *Radiologic Clinics of North America*. In addition, I would like to thank Barton Dudlick and the remainder of the staff at Elsevier for their assistance on this issue. I hope that readers will find it a valuable resource in their clinical practice.

Jürgen Rademaker, MD
Department of Radiology
Memorial Sloan-Kettering Cancer Center
1275 York Avenue
New York, NY 10021, USA

E-mail address:
Rademakj@mskcc.org

doi:10.1016/j.rcl.2008.06.001
0033-8389/08/$ – see front matter

# Overview of Lymphoma Diagnosis and Management

Matthew J. Matasar, MD, MS[a],*, Andrew D. Zelenetz, MD, PhD[b]

**KEYWORDS**

- Lymphoma • Hodgkin lymphoma
- Non-Hodgkin lymphoma

The appropriate classification of the malignant lymphomas was a subject of contention since the first attempts to define distinct subtypes of lymphoma. From the original report by Thomas Hodgkin in 1832 through the early twentieth century, a multitude of clinical entities were named and described with variable and imprecise language, ranging from reticulum cell sarcoma to lymphosarcoma. The earliest attempts at systematic classification of the lymphomas emerged in the 1930s and 1940s, based on either morphology alone or in combination with clinicopathologic considerations. These efforts led in part to the Rappaport classification, which was the first system to incorporate prognosis in a lymphoma classification system.[1]

## PATHOLOGY

Since that time, an expansion of understanding of immunology has led to a similar blossoming in number and variety of classification systems for the lymphomas, although the two that were the first to be widely adopted were the Kiel classification (generally favored in Europe) and the Lukes and Collins classification (more popular in North America). These systems coexisted and competed with other proposed modifications of the Rappaport classification, including Dorfman's working classification and the British National Lymphoma Investigation classification. Driven by a desire to adopt a common language, in part to facilitate the conduct and comparison of clinical research, unification was attempted in 1982, when Rosenberg, DeVita, and Kaplan, under the auspices of the United States National Cancer Institute (NCI), brought together experts with the intent of identifying one of the extant classification systems as the most prognostically powerful. No single system emerged victorious, however, and instead an "international working formulation" (IWF) was put forward to allow clinicians to interpret findings reported within the context of classification systems with which they were potentially unfamiliar.[2] The IWF soon was adopted in North America for classifying lymphomas, although the Kiel classification and subsequent modifications retained prominence in Europe.[3] However, by the 1990s even the modifications to the Kiel classification were felt to have become outdated, and the most obvious flaw of the IWF—its strict emphasis on morphology and natural history at the expense of excluding the growing body of knowledge of lymphoma biology—made the need for a modern classification system all the more apparent. A second attempt at unification was attempted under the aegis of the International Lymphoma Study Group, an effort charged with incorporating all of the then-available understanding of morphology, genetics, and molecular science in creating a classification system that could be broadly adopted and allow for consistent language and reproducible diagnosis. The report of their efforts was published in 1994 as the Revised European-American Lymphoma (REAL) classification.[4] The REAL was updated and refined with the World Health

[a] Medical Oncology/Hematology, Memorial Sloan-Kettering Cancer Center, 1275 York Avenue, New York, NY 10065, USA
[b] Lymphoma Service, Memorial Sloan-Kettering Cancer Center, 1275 York Avenue, New York, NY 10065, USA
* Corresponding author.
*E-mail address:* matasarm@mskcc.org (M. Matasar).

Radiol Clin N Am 46 (2008) 175–198
doi:10.1016/j.rcl.2008.03.005
0033-8389/08/$ – see front matter © 2008 Elsevier Inc. All rights reserved.

Organization (WHO) classification, maintaining the structure of the REAL and sharing its focus on morphology and immunophenotype over clinical outcomes. The resulting WHO classification remains the currently accepted worldwide classification system for lymphoma.

Within the WHO classification, there exist 27 distinct types of lymphoma, not including acknowledged subtypes and subcategories that were also recognized. The major diagnostic entities are listed in **Box 1**. In addition to characteristic architectural morphology, different types of lymphoma often possess stereotypical immunophenotypic and molecular lesions that can aid in accurate classification (**Table 1**).

## EPIDEMIOLOGY

In the WHO classification, the initial major distinction is the putative cell of origin: B cell, T cell, or natural killer (NK) cell. The lymphomas are next classified as derived from either precursor or mature lymphocytes. More than 30 types of lymphoma are recognized, with clinical behavior spanning from remarkably indolent to profoundly aggressive. In the United States in 2007, there are expected to have been 8200 new diagnoses of Hodgkin lymphoma (HL) and 63,200 new diagnoses of NHL.[5] Distribution of the subtypes of non-Hodgkin lymphoma (NHL) vary worldwide by geographic region (**Table 2**). In the United States, more than half of newly diagnosed NHL consists of either diffuse large B-cell lymphoma (DLBCL), an aggressive B-cell lymphoma, or follicular lymphoma (FL), an indolent B cell lymphoma, comprising 31% and 22%, respectively. Several other subtypes are relatively common (>5% of newly diagnosed NHL), including marginal zone B-cell lymphoma of mucosa-associated lymphoid tissue (MALT), 5%; small lymphocytic lymphoma (chronic lymphocytic leukemia type), 6%; peripheral T-cell lymphoma, unspecified (PTCLu), 6%; and mantle cell lymphoma (MCL) 6%. The 12 most common subtypes of lymphoma (treating Burkitt and Burkitt-like lymphoma as a single disease entity, as in the WHO classification) account for 88% of new diagnoses of NHL in the United States.[6,7]

Epidemiologic associations for many of the common types of lymphoma remain incompletely understood. Risk factors for certain types of lymphoma can include chronic infection, immunosuppression, and hereditary traits. It is clear that chronic infection can lead to lymphomagenesis, either through direct viral effects (eg, Epstein-Barr virus [EBV] in HL, post-transplantation lymphoproliferative disorder [LPD], and endemic Burkitt lymphoma [BL]; human T lymphotropic

virus type 1 [HTLV-1] in adult T-cell leukemia/lymphoma; human herpesvirus 8 [HHV8] and primary effusion lymphoma),[8–12] or due to chronic stimulation of the immune system (eg, *Helicobacter pylori* gastritis in gastric mucosa-associated lymphoid tissue [MALT] lymphoma; hepatitis C virus in splenic and extranodal marginal zone lymphomas).[13,14] Autoimmune diseases may similarly increase the risk of lymphoma through chronic stimulation of the immune system, potentially giving rise to a dysregulated clone of B cells. Specific associations include rheumatoid arthritis and Sjögren's syndrome with both DLBCL and marginal zone lymphomas, and celiac sprue with enteropathy-associated T-cell lymphoma.[15] Immunosuppression clearly confers an increased risk of both HL and NHL, as can be seen in the increased incidence of lymphomas in patients infected by human immunodeficiency virus (HIV) as well as patients on immunosuppressive treatment following solid-organ transplantation.[16–18] Additional risk is associated with environmental stressors such as ionizing radiation (including sunlight), agricultural pesticides, and dark hair dyes before 1980.[19–21]

Clearly, stressors, be they infectious, inflammatory, or toxic, interact with the host genetic makeup in a complex fashion to lead to lymphomagenesis. It has been established that hereditary risk of lymphoma, while apparently a lesser element epidemiologically, does exist. Odds of developing Hodgkin lymphoma are increased for first-degree relatives of probands, and further increased for siblings of probands.[22] Risks of all types of NHL are increased in first-degree family members of probands, although patterns of apparent heritability vary by subtype.[23–25] At this time, however, no specific genetic testing is available, and screening for family members is not routine.

## DIAGNOSIS

Appropriate management of lymphoma begins with an accurate and precise diagnosis. Traditionally, this has necessitated a surgical (either excisional or incisional) biopsy specimen to obtain adequate tissue. However, as discussed earlier, the WHO classification is built not only on morphologic criteria but also incorporates immunophenotypic and, in some instances, genetic data in establishing a diagnosis. To obtain tissue of greatest diagnostic quality, a new diagnosis of lymphoma will ideally be based on an excisional lymph node biopsy. Although fine needle aspiration (FNA) can be accurate and cost-effective in the diagnosis of certain types of lymphoma, and

Box 1
**World Health Organization classification scheme for lymphoma**

B-cell lymphoma/leukemias

Precursor B-cell lymphoblastic leukemia/lymphoma

Chronic lymphocytic leukemia/small lymphocytic lymphoma

B-cell prolymphocytic leukemia

Lymphoplasmacytic lymphoma/Waldenström macroglobulinemia

Splenic marginal zone lymphoma

Hairy cell leukemia

Plasma cell myeloma/plasmocytoma

Extranodal marginal zone lymphoma of mucosa-associated lymphoid tissue (MALT)

Nodal marginal zone lymphoma

Follicular lymphoma

Mantle-cell lymphoma

Diffuse large B-cell lymphoma

Mediastinal (thymic) large B-cell lymphoma

Primary effusion lymphoma

Burkitt lymphoma/leukemia

T-cell and NK-cell lymphomas/Leukemias

Pre-T-cell lymphoblastic leukemia/lymphoma

T-cell prolymphocytic leukemia

Blastic NK-cell lymphoma

T-cell large granular lymphocytic leukemia

Aggressive NK-cell leukemia

Adult T-cell leukemia/lymphoma (human T-lymphotropic virus type1 -positive)

Extranodal NK-cell/T-cell lymphoma, nasal type

Enteropathy-type T-cell lymphoma

Hepatosplenic T-cell lymphoma

Subcutaneous panniculitis-like T-cell lymphoma

Mycosis fungoides/Sézary's syndrome

Primary cutaneous anaplastic large cell lymphoma

Angioimmunoblastic T-cell lymphoma

Peripheral T-cell lymphoma, unspecified

Primary systemic

Anaplastic large cell lymphoma

Box 1
**(continued)**

Hodgkin lymphoma

Nodular lymphocyte-predominance

Classical Hodgkin lymphoma

Nodular sclerosis

Mixed cellularity

Lymphocyte depleted

Lymphocyte rich

*Data from* Jaffe ES, Harris NL, Stein H, et al. World Health Organization classification of tumors. Pathology and genetics of tumors of hematopoietic and lymphoid tissues. Lyon (France): IARC Press; 2001.

is accurate in the setting of relapsed disease,[26] excisional biopsy remains the standard of care for initial diagnosis and for clinical scenarios in which cellular morphology and nodal architecture are relevant to the diagnosis (eg, transformation of low-grade lymphoma, as is discussed later).[27,28]

## STAGING

The clinical staging of both HL and NHL derive form the Ann Arbor (AA) staging system originally developed for HL alone, as subsequently modified at the Cotswolds meeting in 1989 (**Box 2**).[29] The modification retained the previous four-stage system, adding the modifier "X" for bulk, defined as greater than 10 cm in long axis or for a mediastinal mass as measuring greater than one third of the internal transverse thoracic diameter of a standard posteroanterior chest radiograph at the level of the fifth or sixth thoracic vertebral body. The staging system is based on the extent of involvement of nodal groups: stage I is a single lymph node group; stage II is multiple lymph node groups ipsilateral to the diaphragm; stage III is involvement of lymph node groups both above and below the diaphragm; and stage IV includes noncontiguous extranodal involvement (eg, lung nodules or involvement of bone marrow). The "E" modifier qualifies direct extension to an extranodal site or, for stage IE disease, isolated involvement of a single extranodal site without evidence of nodally based disease (eg, primary lymphoma of bone or thyroid). The "B" modifier refers to the presence of one or more of a set of symptoms associated with lymphoma that have been associated with more aggressive disease or worse prognosis: unexplained recurrent or persistent fever, drenching night sweats, or unexplained loss of 10% or more of body weight.

**Table 1**
**Characteristics of common lymphomas**

| Subtype | Immunophenotype | Molecular Lesions |
|---|---|---|
| Classical Hodgkin lymphoma (HL) | CD15+ CD30+ | Variable |
| Nodular lymphocyte-predominant HL | CD20+ CD15- CD30- | Variable |
| Diffuse large B-cell | CD20+ | BCL2, BCL6, CMYC |
| Follicular | CD20+ CD10+ CD5- | BCL2 |
| Small B-cell (CLL type) | CD20+ CD5+ CD23+ | V gene, p53, +12, 11q- |
| Peripheral T-cell unspecified | CD20- CD3+ | Variable |
| Mantle cell | CD20+ CD5+ CD23- | Cyclin D1 |
| Marginal zone, MALT type | CD20+ CD5- CD23- | BCL10, MALT1 |
| Primary mediastinal large B-cell | CD20+ | Variable |
| Anaplastic large cell, T/null | CD20- CD3+ CD30+ CD15- EMA+ | ALK |
| Lymphoblastic (T/B) | T cell: CD3+ | TCL1-3 |
|  | B cell: CD19+ | Variable |
| Marginal zone, nodal type | CD20+ CD5- CD23- | +3, +18 |
| Burkitt lymphoma | CD20+ CD10+ CD5- | CMYC |

Staging is characterized as either clinical stage if it is based on physical examination, routine radiographic evaluation, including cross-sectional imaging of relevant anatomic regions and in select cases functional imaging such as [18]F fluoro-2-deoxyglucose positron emission tomography (18-FDG PET) and bone marrow biopsy, or pathologic stage if confirmed by one or more additional surgical staging procedures, such as staging laparoscopy or gastrointestinal endoscopy. Many types of lymphoma, particularly the indolent B-cell NHLs, routinely involve marrow, resulting in clinical stage IV disease being the norm rather than the exception. However, marrow involvement has not been demonstrated to independently confer worse prognosis, and grouping by limited stage (Ann Arbor stage I/II) and advanced stage (AA stage III/IV) is more clinically relevant in NHL. Given the limited predictive power of AA stage for both HL and NHL, clinical prognostic models (incorporating characteristics of both the patient and the malignancy) have been developed to aid clinical trial interpretation and to assist clinicians in conveying prognostic information to patients. Several models have subsequently been developed for common lymphoma subtypes, including the Hodgkin Lymphoma International Prognostic Score (**Table 3**), the International Prognostic Index (IPI) for diffuse large B-cell lymphoma (**Table 4**), and the Follicular Lymphoma International Prognostic Index (FLIPI) for follicular lymphoma (**Table 5**).

The following discussion addresses specific features of eight common types of lymphoma, which collectively account for more than 80% of lymphoma diagnosed in Western countries.

## HODGKIN LYMPHOMA

Approximately 8200 new cases of Hodgkin lymphoma (HL) will have been diagnosed in 2007 in the United States.[5] There is a modest male predominance (1.4:1), and in Western countries there is a bimodal age distribution, with the first peak in the third decade of life and a second smaller and broader peak after age 50.[30] Heritable characteristics may contribute to risk, as siblings have a two-fold to ninefold increased risk, and as first-degree relatives have a less striking but nonetheless greater risk than age-matched controls.[22,31] Investigations have identified risk associations with certain HLA antigens, lending further support to a genetic contribution to risk.[32] Infection with Epstein-Barr virus (EBV) resulting in infectious mononucleosis has been associated with an increased incidence of HL in a large Danish study, and evidence of EBV early RNA can frequently be detected in the classic Reed-Sternberg cells.[8,33] Other contributors to risk of HL have not been fully elucidated. While an increased incidence of HL has been noted in patients infected by HIV, there is no evidence of virally mediated oncogenesis from HIV (unlike EBV), and the observation that rates of HL in HIV have increased despite the advent of highly active anti-retroviral therapy (HAART) offers circumstantial evidence against direct viral pathogenesis.[17,18,34]

**Table 2**
Distribution of the major non-Hodgkin lymphoma subtypes by geographic region

| Major NHL Subtypes | Omaha (n = 200) | Vancouver (n = 200) | Capetown (n = 188) | London (n = 119) | Würzburg/ Göttingen (n = 203) | Lyon (n = 192) | Locarno/ Bellinzona (n = 79) | Hong Kong (n = 197) |
|---|---|---|---|---|---|---|---|---|
| Small B-lymphocytic | 7% | 1% | 8% | 8% | 11% | 8% | 5% | 3% |
| Mantle cell | 7% | 7% | 1% | 7% | 8% | 7% | 14% | 3% |
| Follicular | 32% | 31% | 33% | 28% | 18% | 17% | 11% | 8% |
| Marginal zone B-cell, MALT type | 6% | 7% | 4% | 3% | 9% | 13% | 9% | 10% |
| Diffuse large B-cell | 28% | 29% | 28% | 27% | 30% | 25% | 36% | 36% |
| Primary mediastinal large B-cell | 0% | 2% | 3% | 2% | 0% | 4% | 9% | 3% |
| Peripheral T-cell unspecified | 3% | 1% | 8% | 8% | 4% | 4% | 6% | 10% |
| Anaplastic large T/null cell | 2% | 3% | 3% | 2% | 1% | 3% | 0% | 3% |
| Angiocentric nasal T/NK cell | 0% | 0% | 0% | 0% | 0% | 2% | 0% | 8% |
| Other | 15% | 19% | 12% | 15% | 19% | 17% | 10% | 16% |

*Data from* Anderson JR, Armitage JO, Weisenberger DD, et al. Epidemiology of the non-Hodgkin's lymphomas: distributions of the major subtypes differ by geographic locations. Non-Hodgkin's Lymphoma Classification Project. Ann Oncol 1998;9:717–20.

**Box 2**
**Cotswolds modification of Ann Arbor staging classification**

Stage I

Involvement of a single lymph-node region or lymphoid structure (eg, spleen, thymus, Waldeyer's ring) or involvement of a single extralymphatic site (IE)

Stage II

Involvement of two or more lymph-node regions on the same site of the diaphragm (II) or localized contiguous involvement of only one extranodal organ or side and its regional lymph-nodes with or without other lymph node regions on the same side of the diaphragm (IIE)

Note: The number of anatomic regions involved may be indicated by a subscript (eg, II3)

Stage III

Involvement of lymph-node regions on both sides of the diaphragm (III), which may also be accompanied by involvement of the spleen (IIIS) or by localized contiguous involvement of only one extranodal organ side (IIIE) or both (IIISE)

Stage IV

Disseminated (multifocal) involvement of one or more extranodal organs or tissues, with or without associated lymph-node involvement or isolated extralymphatic organ involvement with distant (non-regional) nodal involvement

Designations Applicable to Any Disease Stage

A

No symptoms

B

Fever (temperature > 38° C), drenching night sweats, unexplained loss of more than 10% of body weight during the previous 6 months.

X

Bulky disease

E

Involvement of an extranodal site that is contiguous or proximal to the known nodal site

**Box 2**
**(continued)**

Remarks

- Involvement of hilar nodes on both sides constitutes stage II disease.
- Bulky mediastinal disease has been defined as a thoracic ratio of maximum transverse mass diameter greater than or equal to one third of the internal transverse thoracic diameter measured at the T5/6 intervertebral disk level on chest radiography. Other authors have designated a lymph node mass measuring 10 cm or more in greatest dimension as bulky disease.
- Evidence of invasion of adjacent structures such as bone, chest wall, or lung is an important consideration as this may influence management. For example, a mediastinal or hilar mass that invades the adjacent lung is classified as II E, whereas pulmonary involvement separate from adenopathy represents stage IV. A mass may have multiple E lesions, such as a mediastinal mass involving lung and sternum.

*Adapted from* Lister TA, Crowther DM, Sutcliffe SB, et al. Report of a committee convened to discuss the evaluation and staging of patients with Hodgkin's disease: Cotswolds meeting. J Clin Oncol 1989;7:1630–6. Reprinted with permission of the American Society of Clinical Oncology.

Historically, Hodgkin lymphoma was subdivided into five histologic variants: nodular sclerosis, mixed cellularity, lymphocyte-rich, lymphocyte-depleted, and nodular lymphocyte-predominant. With modern therapy the differences in prognosis between subtypes have largely vanished; as a result, nodular sclerosis, mixed cellularity, lymphocyte-rich, and lymphocyte-depleted HL have been collectively grouped under the unified diagnosis of "classical HL" in the WHO classification. Nodular lymphocyte-predominant HL (NLPHL) remains a clinically distinct entity, with different natural history and immunophenotype (see earlier). Classical HL (hereon, HL) and NLPHL will be addressed separately as follows.

*Classical Hodgkin Lymphoma*

Classical Hodgkin lymphoma (HL) is pathologically defined by the presence of Reed-Sternberg cells and their variants that are seen against a background of nodular sclerosis, mixed cellularity, lymphocyte-depleted, or a lymphocyte-rich stroma. HL is a distinct entity both pathologically and clinically, with a unique natural history and disease-specific management strategies.

**Table 3**
**Hodgkin lymphoma international prognostic scoring system**

| Factors |
| --- |
| Serum albumin, <4 g/dL |
| Hemoglobin, <10.5 g/dL |
| Male gender |
| Stage IV disease |
| Age ≥45 years |
| White blood cell count, ≥15,000/mm$^3$ |
| Lymphocyte count, <600/mm$^3$ or <8% of white blood cells |

**Rates of freedom from freedom from progression and overall survival by number of factors**

| Number of Factors | 5-year Progression-Free Survival | 5-year Overall Survival |
| --- | --- | --- |
| 0 | 84 | 89 |
| 1 | 77 | 90 |
| 2 | 67 | 81 |
| 3 | 60 | 78 |
| 4 | 51 | 61 |
| ≥5 | 42 | 56 |

*Data from* Hasenclever D, Diehl V. A prognostic score for advanced Hodgkin's disease. N Eng J Med 1998;339: 1506–14.

## Clinical presentation

The most typical presentation of HL is painless, enlarged superficial lymphadenopathy that on investigation involves contiguous nodal chains in a predictable and orderly fashion as the disease progresses; only late in disease progression does vascular invasion occur, permitting hematogenous dissemination. Most patients will present with supradiaphragmatic disease; in most large series, isolated infradiaphragmatic disease occurs in only 3% to 7% of cases.[35–37] Between 60% and 80% of patients will present with cervical and/or supraclavicular adenopathy, and approximately 30% with axillary disease. Mediastinal involvement is common at presentation (50%–60%), and frequently large masses can be found with routine radiography in the absence of symptoms. Infradiaphragmatic disease tends to develop after involvement of para-aortic lymph nodes, but involvement of abdominal viscera is an infrequent event. Indeed, only 10% to 15% of patients with HL will harbor extranodal disease, with the most frequent sites being bone, bone marrow, lung, and liver. Central nervous system (CNS) involvement is extremely rare, although extension into the epidural space from contiguous para-aortic adenopathy can lead to neurologic symptoms at time of presentation.

A significant proportion of patients with undiagnosed HL will develop one or more systemic symptoms before discovery of adenopathy. "B" symptoms are present in 25% of patients with newly diagnosed HL, although this proportion is greater in patients presenting with advanced disease, and the presence of these symptoms independently predicts a worse prognosis in both early- and advanced-stage disease. Other systemic symptoms that are often present with, or

**Table 4**
**International Prognostic Index for aggressive lymphoma**

| Factor | Adverse Feature |
| --- | --- |
| Age | >60 years |
| Performance status | ≥3 (limited in self-care) |
| LDH | >upper limit normal |
| Extranodal disease | ≥2 sites |
| Stage (Ann Arbor) | III or IV |

| Risk Group | No. Adverse Factors | 5-year Disease-Free Survival, % | 5-year Overall Survival, % |
| --- | --- | --- | --- |
| Low | 0 or 1 | 70 | 73 |
| Low-intermediate | 2 | 50 | 51 |
| High-intermediate | 3 | 49 | 43 |
| High | 4 or 5 | 40 | 26 |

*Data from* Shipp MA, Harrington DP, Anderson JR, et al. International Non-Hodgkin's Lymphoma Prognostic Factors Project. N Engl J Med 1993:329(14);987–94.

**Table 5**
**Follicular Lymphoma International Prognostic Index**

| Factor | Adverse Feature |
|--------|-----------------|
| Age | >60 years |
| Hgb | <12 g/dL |
| LDH | >upper limit normal |
| Number of nodal sites | ≥5 |
| Stage (Ann Arbor) | III or IV |

| Risk Group | No. Factors | % Patients | 5-year Overall Survival, % | 10-year Overall Survival, % |
|------------|-------------|------------|----------------------------|------------------------------|
| Low | 0 or 1 | 36 | 90.6 | 70.7 |
| Intermediate | 2 | 37 | 77.6 | 50.9 |
| High | 3 to 5 | 27 | 52.5 | 35.5 |

*Data from* Solal-Seligny P, Roy P, Colombat P, et al. Follicular lymphoma international prognostic index. Blood 2004;104:1258–65.

even antedate, the diagnosis of HL include pruritus, which can be severe, and alcohol-induced pain occurring minutes after ingestion and localizing to regions of involved adenopathy. While uncommon (reported in fewer than 10% of patients), it is felt to be pathognomonic for HL.[38] Rare neurologic paraneoplastic syndromes, including cerebellar degeneration and the stiff-person syndrome, have been reported and interestingly can be present in early-stage disease, persist despite curative therapy, or even develop following curative therapy.[39]

### Staging

Clinical staging of HL according to the Cotswolds modification of the Ann Arbor staging system remains standard now almost 20 years after its introduction. Currently recommended approaches for determining clinical stage consist of routine physical examination, laboratory analysis including assessment of renal and hepatic function, chest x-ray; CT scans of the chest, abdomen, and pelvis; and bone marrow biopsy for any extent of disease beyond clinical stage (CS) IA. 18-FDG PET is included in the most recent National Comprehensive Cancer Network (NCCN) staging recommendations for pretreatment evaluation, particularly in the setting of equivocal CT scan results.[27] However, given the near universal pretreatment FDG-avidity of HL, a baseline 18-FDG PET may not be necessary when CT imaging establishes minimal CS III disease. However, even in this scenario, 18-FDG PET can be beneficial for restaging, and response by PET criteria is emerging as a powerful prognostic tool.[40,41]

### Management

The advent first of effective radiotherapy and later of combined-modality therapy and chemotherapy-only regimens has made HL a highly curable malignancy. Management of HL is currently tailored according to the stage of disease, clinical features including prognostic factors, and considerations of potential long-term toxicities of therapy. Attempts to advance the management of early-stage HL (ESHL) have been driven by the observation that, despite variability in rates of disease control among different treatments, overall outcome is excellent even for patients who relapse, resulting in similar overall survival rates. Furthermore, treatment of HL, while effective, has significant short-term and long-term toxicity (**Box 3**), and in long-term survivors, treatment-related toxicity surpasses HL as the greatest contributor to overall mortality (**Fig. 1**). Poor prognostic factors in ESHL were identified, including male sex, age greater than 40 years, "B" symptoms, erythrocyte sedimentation rate greater than 50, large mediastinal mass, extranodal disease, infradiaphragmatic disease, and involvement of three or four lymph node stations. Historically, good-risk ESHL was managed with extended field radiotherapy, whereas poor-risk ESHL received full-course combined-modality therapy (CMT) (chemotherapy and radiotherapy), but CMT has become standard for both groups on the basis of progression-free survival benefits seen in trials performed in Europe and the United States.[42,43] The optimal multiagent chemotherapy program has also evolved over time, from alkylator-based therapy (MOPP) to anthracycline-based therapy (ABVD). Efforts in advancing the treatment of ESHL have focused

Box 3
**Toxicities associated with treatment of Hodgkin lymphoma**

Acute toxicity

  Alopecia

  Anemia

  Antabuse-like reaction to alcohol (procarbazine)

  Leukopenia

  Mucositis

  Nausea/vomiting

  Neuropathy

  Pneumonitis (bleomycin)

  Thrombocytopenia

Second primary malignancy

  Acute myelogenous leukemia (chemotherapy)

  Acute lymphoblastic leukemia (chemotherapy)

  Breast (radiotherapy)

  Gastric

  Lung (radiotherapy)

  Melanoma

  Non-Hodgkin lymphoma

  Sarcoma (radiotherapy)

  Thyroid (radiotherapy)

Late cardiovascular toxicity

  Accelerated atherosclerosis

  Non-ischemic cardiomyopathy

  Pericardial fibrosis (radiotherapy)

Endocrine toxicities

  Hypothyroidism (radiotherapy)

  Premature ovarian failure (chemotherapy)

  Azoospermia (chemotherapy)

risk of breast cancer are an important clinical consideration.

For advanced-stage HL (ASHL), treatment is also based in part on clinical features. The HL international prognostic scoring system identifies seven poor prognostic features: age older than 45 years, male gender, serum albumin less than 4, hemoglobin less than 10.5, white blood cell (WBC) count greater than 15,000, absolute lymphopenia (<600), and stage IV disease. Whereas the standard of care has been full-course ABVD, with treatment given every 2 weeks for 24 weeks, patients with high-risk disease, defined by the presence of four or more of these poor prognostic features, have unacceptably poor outcomes. Intensified treatment with the dose-intensified regimen escalated-BEACOPP and post-treatment radiation therapy to residual nodal masses of 2 cm or larger has been shown to improve survival when compared with a regimen clinically equivalent to standard ABVD.[44] Investigation of a CMT regimen of an eight-drug weekly chemotherapy program (the Stanford V regimen) and more intensive radiotherapy for any nodal mass measuring larger than 5 cm before treatment has demonstrated excellent activity in single-institution experiences,[45] and is currently being compared with ABVD in ASHL, but mature data are not yet available.

While most patients with HL are cured with chemotherapy, radiation therapy, or CMT, patients who relapse after achieving complete remission or demonstrate refractory disease have poor outcomes when treated with routine salvage therapy. However, for those patients who demonstrate chemotherapy-sensitive disease when treated with second-line systemic therapy, consolidation of second-line therapy with high-dose chemotherapy and autologous stem cell rescue (HDT/ASCR) has been shown to achieve durable remission in between 45% and 60% of patients.[46–52] The role of allogeneic stem-cell transplantation, particularly nonmyeloablative transplantation of HLA-identical siblings, in the treatment of patients not cured with second-line therapy and consolidative HDT/ASCR is a subject of ongoing investigation and is a clinical consideration in select cases.[53,54]

### Nodular Lymphocyte-Predominant Hodgkin Lymphoma

The epidemiology of NLPHL differs from that of HL, with a bimodal age distribution peaking in childhood and the fourth decade of life, and with a 3:1 male predominance.[55,56] It is an uncommon disease, with only approximately 500 newly diagnosed cases annually in the United States.

on testing whether reduction of dose and volume of radiotherapy, decreasing the number of cycles of chemotherapy or eliminating bleomycin (and avoiding its well-characterized pulmonary toxicity), or even replacing CMT with chemotherapy-only programs. At the present time, however, CMT with four cycles of ABVD and subsequent radiation of involved fields (involved field radiation therapy [IFRT]) remains a standard of care in the treatment of ESHL in all patients except young women who would receive radiation to breast tissue. For such patients, chemotherapy-only programs that can spare the recognized increased

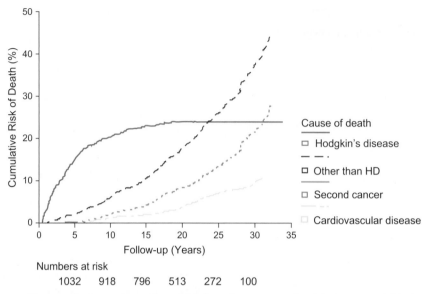

**Fig. 1.** Cause-specific mortality in survivors of Hodgkin lymphoma. Mortality risk due to Hodgkin lymphoma plateaus after 10 years, whereas risks due to second malignancy, cardiovascular disease, and other causes increase continually following treatment. By 25 years, more patients in the cohort had died from other causes than from their Hodgkin lymphoma. (*From* Aleman BMPP, van den Belt-Dusebout AW, Klokman WJ, et al. Long-term cause-specific mortality of patients treated for Hodgkin's disease. J Clin Oncol 2003;21(18):3431–9. Reprinted with permission of the American Society of Clinical Oncology.)

Evidence now exists to implicate the germinal center lymphocyte as the putative cell of origin of the characteristic lymphocytic and histiocytic (L&H) cell of NLPHL.[57,58] The natural history of NLPHL is often quite distinct from that of HL. More than 75% of patients will present with early-stage (clinical stage I or II) disease, and both extranodal disease and systemic symptoms are rare.[56,59] Staging of NLPHL routinely includes physical examination, laboratory analyses, and CT of the chest, abdomen, and pelvis; bone marrow biopsy is of limited yield. The utility of 18-FDG PET in staging of NLPHL has yet to be fully elucidated; the theoretic ability to upstage disease is of questionable clinical benefit in NLPHL, and the specificity of 18-FDG-PET in NLPHL has been called into question, as the disease can coexist with a benign disease of lymph nodes, progressive transformation of germinal centers (PTGC), which can also be 18-FDG avid.[60]

Historically, NLPHL was treated in a fashion identical to HL, and many of the largest clinical trials in the management of HL have included small subsets of NLPHL. However, the natural history of NLPHL is quite distinct from HL; whereas HL is typically an aggressive disease that, when not cured, will lead to significantly shorter survival, NLPHL is responsive to many therapies but tends to follow a relapsing pattern more similar to indolent B-cell NHL. Accordingly, aggressive treatment programs such as combination chemotherapy or CMT have in many cases been replaced by more conservative management strategies.

For limited stage disease that is considered amenable to radiation (disease within a single reasonable involved field radiation port), IFRT is often favored in patients and disease locations amenable to such therapy. Systemic chemotherapy for limited disease is now typically reserved for patients who are not suitable for radiation therapy (RT) and for whom observation would be inappropriate due to clinical features. For advanced stage (stages III/IV) disease, treatment has largely consisted of regimens with activity in HL, including anthracycline-based regimens such as ABVD. Unlike early-stage NLPHL, it is not clear that advanced stage NLPHL has a natural history drastically different from HL.[59]

Given that NLPHL is generally recognized as an incurable malignancy, and one with which patients can live for many years, concerns about cumulative toxicity of therapy are particularly relevant. In modern cohorts, cause of death for patients with NLPHL has been more likely to be due to second primary malignancies (including secondary leukemia), cardiac disease, or other conditions than due to the lymphoma itself.[59,61] Given concerns about the cumulative toxicity of chemotherapy, there is significant interest in the potential use of rituximab, a monoclonal antibody against CD20 that was first approved by the Food and Drug Administration (FDA) in 1997 and has become a component of the treatment of many B cell lymphomas. Experience using rituximab in the treatment of NLPHL continues to develop, but its optimal role in the management of the disease, both alone and in combination, has yet to be firmly established.[62,63]

## NON-HODGKIN LYMPHOMA
### Diffuse Large B-Cell Lymphoma

Diffuse large B cell lymphoma (DLBCL) is a clinically aggressive non-Hodgkin lymphoma (NHL) and is the single most common type of lymphoma in Western countries, accounting for over 30% of new diagnoses.[6] Although a pathologically heterogeneous set of disorders, the diagnosis DLBCL is understood to include routine centroblastic large B-cell lymphoma, immunoblastic lymphoma, T-cell/histocyte-rich B-cell lymphoma, and B-cell anaplastic large cell lymphoma.

Some insight into the clinical significance of the pathologic heterogeneity of DLBCL has been shed by profiling of differential gene expression. Using DNA microarrays, individual cases of lymphoma can be classified based on gene expression patterns into one of three categories of putative cell of origin: germinal-center B-cell-like (GCB, favorable), activated B-cell-like (ABC, unfavorable), and type 3 (also unfavorable).[64–66] Others have attempted to simplify the full DNA microarray classification to either assessment of expression of a small group of genes or, even more practical, commonly available immunohistochemistry.[67,68] The determination of gene expression pattern was found to be strongly predictive of outcome with cyclophosphamide, doxorubicin, vincristine, and prednisone (CHOP) chemotherapy, leading some to begin to approach these subsets as clinically distinct entities. However, it is unclear if the gene expression pattern continues to offer important prognostic information, as there are conflicting data regarding the prognostic impact of cell of origin for patients treated with CHOP and rituximab, as has become standard (see later in this article).[69–73]

### Clinical presentation
The most typical presenting complaint in newly diagnosed DLBCL is a symptomatic enlarging nodal mass, either centrally or peripherally located. Approximately 20% of patients will present with stage I or stage IE disease, and approximately 40% of patients will present with disease limited to one side of the diaphragm (stage II).[74] An additional 20% of patients will present with nodal involvement above and below the diaphragm, and 40% of patients have disseminated disease with extranodal involvement at presentation. Common sites of extranodal dissemination include liver, kidney, bone, lung, and bone marrow. This stands in contrast to common primary extranodal sites of origin of DLBCL (representing approximately 30% of all DLBCL), which include the gastrointestinal tract, thyroid, bone, brain, testis, soft tissue, kidney, liver, breast, and skin.[75] When extranodal disease is present with no or minimal nodal involvement, the disease is typically considered primary extranodal DLBCL, whereas when both nodal and extranodal disease are present, the disease is typically considered nodal lymphoma. Symptomatically, in addition to those symptoms directly referable to locally invasive or extranodal disease, patients will often experience systemic symptoms before diagnosis. Approximately 30% of patients will report "B" symptoms, whereas less specific symptoms of malaise and fatigue are more common yet.

The range of clinical presentations of DLBCL is made all the more diverse when transformation of low-grade lymphoma is considered. Low-grade B-cell lymphomas, including follicular lymphoma, small lymphocytic lymphoma, marginal zone lymphoma, and lymphoplasmacytic lymphoma can all develop high-grade transformation of disease into DLBCL, an event believed to be typically triggered by acquisition and accumulation of additional transforming mutations.[76] Transformation of low-grade lymphoma is a common event, occurring at a rate of 3% per year in patients with FL with a cumulative risk of approximately 50% after 15 years.[77–79] It can occur in patients without a known clinical history of the original indolent disease (de novo transformation), or at any point during the clinical course of illness, although patients without transformation after living with a low-grade B cell lymphoma for more than 15 years are unlikely ever to experience transformaton.[77] Staging and management of transformed low-grade lymphoma mirrors that of DLBCL, with the exception of post-treatment follow-up, as the nontransformed component of the low-grade lymphoma will continue to follow its own natural history, "unaware" that transformation had occurred.

### Staging
In addition to the routine application of body imaging with CT and 18-FDG PET and bone marrow biopsy, lumbar puncture for both diagnostic and therapeutic purposes (with administration into the cerebrospinal fluid [CSF] of chemotherapy, either methotrexate or cytarabine) is indicated in select cases. Analyses of patterns of failure in DLBCL

have shown a predilection for CNS recurrence when the original disease arises in the testis, paranasal sinuses, or when disease involves the bone marrow or epidural space.[80,81] Primary breast DLBCL may also present an increased risk of CNS recurrence, prompting consideration of CNS prophylaxis, although data are conflicting.[82–84] Accordingly, such patients must undergo diagnostic lumbar puncture to rule out primary leptomeningeal disease, and when involvement of the CSF is not present, are believed to benefit from CNS prophylaxis, as the typical chemotherapeutic programs for DLBCL have poor CNS penetrance.

## Management

Patients with newly diagnosed DLBCL are treated with curative intent. Indeed, many patients can achieve a long-term disease-free status with aggressive combination chemotherapy or CMT. Treatment with CHOP emerged as the preferred chemotherapeutic regimen when compared with even more intensive chemotherapy regimens in the National High-Priority Lymphoma Study.[85] The addition of rituximab to CHOP (R-CHOP) has been shown to further improve survival regardless of age, stage, or IPI score based on the results of 4 randomized clinical studies.[86–89] For patients presenting with favorable early-stage, nonbulky disease, shortened chemotherapy with only three to four cycles of R-CHOP and consolidative IFRT is associated with excellent outcomes, as is a full six cycles of R-CHOP without radiation therapy.[87,90] Bulky early-stage disease is often treated in a manner similar to advanced-stage disease, with treatment consisting of six cycles of R-CHOP chemotherapy, although there is no well-established standard of care, and one study did find an aggressive chemotherapy regimen without radiation to be superior to three cycles of CHOP and RT.[91]

Recurrent or refractory disease, however, continues to represent a clinical challenge. Ongoing research to improve first-line therapy has focused on shortening time intervals between cycles, administering medicines by continuous infusion, or including sequential non–cross-reactive regimens.[72,86,92] Following relapse, or in the face of disease that persists despite first-line chemotherapy, optimal management involves administration of second-line chemotherapy to attempt to achieve remission, followed by stem cell mobilization and administration of high-dose therapy, either chemotherapy alone or CMT, with administration of banked stem-cells to rescue the patient from supralethal therapy. High-dose therapy and autologous stem cell rescue (HDT/ASCR), or "autologous bone marrow transplantation," for patients responding to second-line therapy, offers the potential of cure in a substantial fraction of patients.[93] Patients ineligible for HDT/ASCR or whose disease is not chemotherapy sensitive have poor outcomes.

Two clinical variants of DLBCL merit brief discussion, given differences in natural history and outcomes from typical DLBCL: Primary mediastinal large B cell lymphoma and intravascular large B cell lymphoma.

### Primary mediastinal large B-cell lymphoma

Primary mediastinal large B cell lymphoma (PMLBCL) is a distinct clinicopathological entity that has been shown by gene expression profiling studies to share more genetic features with HL than with DLBCL.[94,95] Unlike DLBCL, PMLBCL is typically diagnosed in the fourth decade of life and shows a mild female predominance. It will most often present with a locally advanced anterior mediastinal mass, and patients will show clinically overt signs of superior vena cava (SVC) syndrome in more than 50% of cases and radiographic evidence of SVC compromise in as many as 80% of cases.[96] Management typically consists of full-course anthracycline-based chemotherapy (eg, R-CHOP) and consolidative IFRT or with more aggressive sequential chemotherapy programs.[97–99]

### Intravascular large B-cell lymphoma

Intravascular large B-cell lymphoma (IVLBCL) is an uncommon variant of DLBCL, presenting with systemic complaints and end-organ dysfunction due to vascular insufficiency. Organ infiltration can be seen, but nodal disease is the exception. It appears that there are two clinical variants of this disease, with the European form frequently presenting with neurologic symptoms and CNS involvement, while the Asian form more frequently presents with marrow failure, "B" symptoms, and hemophagocytosis. Although the rarity of IVLBCL makes it difficult to draw conclusions regarding optimal management, long-term remission seems achievable with timely initiation of anthracycline-based chemotherapy such as R-CHOP.[100,101]

## Follicular Lymphoma

Follicular lymphoma (FL) is the most common indolent B-cell NHL, and is defined as a lymphoma of follicle center cells (centrocytes and centroblasts) with a partially or completely follicular morphologic pattern. There is significant morphologic variability among cases of FL, with the presence of large-cell centroblasts varying from minimal with grade 1 FL to significant with grade 3 FL.

## Clinical presentation

FL has a median age of diagnosis of approximately 60 years, and a slight male predominance exists; the disease is more common among Caucasians than those of African descent, and FL is rare in Asia (but less so in the descendants of Asian immigrants to Western countries).[30] The most typical clinical presentation is that of subacute or chronic asymptomatic peripheral adenopathy, sometimes having persisted or waxed and waned for years. Abdominal, pelvic, or retroperitoneal adenopathy can often be bulky without leading to gastrointestinal or genitourinary symptoms, and nodal masses tend not to be locally invasive or destructive. There tends not to be an orderly progression of lymph node station involvement, and early hematogenous dissemination is common. When sensitive assays are applied, blood or bone marrow involvement by FL can be detected in 80% of patients,[102] but other sites of extranodal disease are uncommon at presentation. "B" symptoms are also uncommon, seen in fewer than 20% of patients presenting with FL, and should prompt consideration of transformed lymphoma (see earlier in this article).

## Staging

Staging of FL routinely consists of physical examination; routine laboratory evaluation including a serum lactate dehydrogenase (LDH); and CT imaging of the chest, abdomen, and pelvis. Bone marrow biopsy is required before initiation of therapy to complete staging as well as to determine whether repeat bone marrow biopsy (to evaluate response to therapy) will subsequently be required. 18-FDG PET scanning is useful in select cases, particularly either to confirm a clinical impression of early-stage disease amenable to RT with curative intent or to help guide diagnostic evaluation for possible transformation to large cell lymphoma (see later in this article).

## Management

Many of the basic principles of management of FL apply, at least in part, to the other types of indolent B-cell NHL discussed later in this article. Appropriate staging of FL includes physical examination; routine laboratory analyses; and CT imaging of the chest, abdomen, and pelvis. While not universally necessary at time of diagnosis, bone marrow biopsy and aspiration are required in the evaluation of cytopenias and of completion of staging before initiation of therapy. 18-FDG PET is a useful adjunct to CT and physical examination, and is of particular utility when there is a clinical suspicion of transformed lymphoma; when feasible, diagnostic surgical biopsy of the most 18-FDG-avid

site of disease should be performed in such instances.

When the results of a complete staging evaluation for newly diagnosed FL determine that the disease is localized (stage I or II within a single radiation port), IFRT has the potential of eradicating the disease. Long-term follow-up of patients receiving radiation for early stage FL have reported that between 20% and 60% of patients remain free of recurrence 10 or more years following treatment.[103–105] Although the vast majority of relapses occur outside the radiation field, more extensive nodal radiation has not been associated with improved overall survival. Similarly, the addition of chemotherapy to radiation therapy in the treatment of early-stage irradiable FL does not appear to improve overall survival, although this question has not been readdressed during the rituximab era.[104]

In the setting of advanced-stage disease, the goals of treatment are considered palliative in nature, as routine therapies are not expected to be curative; indeed, only allogeneic stem-cell transplantation has been consistently associated with long-term disease-free survival for patients with advanced stage disease. Furthermore, treatment of low-bulk asymptomatic patients with systemic therapy has not been associated with a firm survival advantage. A widely accepted set of criteria for treatment (**Box 4**) emphasizes the principle of treating only patients who have symptomatic or progressive disease. Thus, many patients can be

---

**Box 4**
**Criteria for initiation of therapy for advanced stage indolent lymphoma**

Involvement of ≥3 nodal sites, each with a diameter (long axis) of ≥3 cm

Any nodal or extranodal tumor mass with a diameter (long axis) of ≥7 cm

B symptoms

Symptomatic splenomegaly

Pleural effusions or abdominal ascites

Cytopenias (leukocytes $<1 \times 10^9/L$ and/or platelets $<100 \times 10^9/L$)

Leukemic phase ($>5 \times 10^9/L$ malignant cells in peripheral blood)

Patient insistence

*Data from* Solal-Celigny P, Lepage E, Brousse N, et al. Recombinant interferon alfa-2b combined with a regimen containing doxorubicin in patients with advanced follicular lymphoma. Groupe d'Etude des Lymphomes de l'Adulte. N Eng J Med 1993;329: 1608–14.

observed following initial diagnosis, with a median time from initial diagnosis to requiring systemic therapy of 2 to 3 years.[106] When treatment is required, the most frequently used regimens combine immunotherapy (such as rituximab) and chemotherapy, with alkylating agents, anthracyclines, and purine analogs the most frequently used and the best studied in the disease. Radiation therapy is reserved for locoregional palliation, although the radiolabeled anti-CD20 antibodies 90-Y-ibritumomab tiuxetan and 131-I-tositumomab are administered systemically and deliver radiation to microscopic sites of disease. Autologous stem cell transplantation can be considered to consolidate responses in relapsed disease, and allogeneic stem cell transplantation is associated with a long-term disease-free survival in patients with multiply relapsed FL of between 40% and 50%.[107,108]

## Marginal Zone Lymphomas

Marginal zone lymphoma (MZL) consists of three clinically and genetically distinct subtypes: extranodal MZL of mucosa-associated lymphoid tissue (MALT), splenic MZL, and nodal MZL. They are uncommon diseases, both individually and collectively. MALT lymphoma comprises approximately 5% of new diagnoses of NHL, and collectively the MZLs account for fewer than 10% of new diagnoses.[6] Although each is considered an indolent B-cell NHL, there is little clinical overlap among the three diseases despite shared morphologic and immunophenotypic characteristics.[109]

### Clinical presentation

MALT lymphoma is the most common of the three MZLs, and accounts for 5% of newly diagnosed lymphomas. Common sites of MALT lymphoma include stomach, lung, and the ocular-adnexa; although less common in other sites, MALT is the most common low-grade lymphoma of the breast, thyroid, bowel, skin and soft tissue, and dura. No strong age or gender predominance exists in MALT lymphoma. In the case of gastric MALT lymphoma, the predominant force behind lymphomagenesis is felt to be chronic stimulation of activated T cells by *Helicobacter pylori*. Associations with other infections, including *Chlamydia psittaci* in ocular-adnexal MALT lymphoma and chronic infection with hepatitis C virus and MALT lymphoma of various sites, are more controversial. Dissemination to other sites typical of MALT can occur, and approximately one third of patients have evidence of bone marrow involvement at time of initial presentation.[110] Presenting signs and symptoms relate to the site or sites of involvement; here as well, "B" symptoms are rare and

should raise the clinical consideration of transformed lymphoma.

Nodal MZL has significant clinical overlap with FL (see earlier in this article) and small lymphocytic lymphoma of chronic lymphocytic leukemia-type (SLL/CLL) (see later in this article). Its immunophenotype readily distinguishes it from these entities, as it does not express the germinal center antigen CD10 seen in FL or CD5 or CD23, antigens typically present in SLL/CLL.

Splenic MZL is largely a disease of the elderly, with a median age at diagnosis of 65 to 70 and with few diagnoses made in patients before the sixth decade of life. The most typical presentation is an older patient with significant or even massive splenomegaly, potentially resulting in symptomatic early satiety or cytopenias due to hypersplenism. Adenopathy tends to be minimal and involvement of the bone marrow by disease is the norm, seen in greater than 90% of patients when sensitive assays are applied.[111,112] An association with chronic hepatitis C virus (HCV) infection has been reported, although there appears to be geographic variability in the interaction between HCV and lymphomagenesis, and may be due more to associated cryoglobulinemia than to viral infection itself.[14,113–116]

### Staging

The appropriate pretreatment evaluation of each type of MZL follows from its unique natural history. For extranodal MZL, evaluation will routinely include endoscopic evaluation of the gastrointestinal tract for gastrointestinal MALT lymphoma (or bronchial mucosa–associated lymphoid tissue [BALT] lymphoma, which is frequently associated with gastrointestinal involvement), pulmonary function testing for BALT lymphoma, or imaging of other relevant anatomic regions (eg, MR imaging of orbits for ocular-adnexal MALT lymphoma). For nodal MZL, added to this is evaluation of relevant regional extranodal sites that could be the subclinical site of dissemination of the nodal disease (eg, gastrointestinal tract for abdominal adenopathy, lungs for hilar or mediastinal adenopathy, thyroid and ocular adnexa for neck adenopathy). For splenic MZL, routine physical examination; laboratory analyses; CT of the chest, abdomen, and pelvis; and bone marrow biopsy complete the requisite evaluation. 18-FDG PET scan will be positive in between 65% and 80% of patients with MALT lymphoma, but may be more sensitive in splenic and nodal MZL.[117–119]

### Management

While in many circumstances the management of the marginal zone lymphomas is substantively similar to that of FL, there are specific clinical scenarios where management diverges significantly. For early-stage gastric MALT lymphoma, eradication of *H. pylori* in patients with favorable cytogenetics leads to regression or remission in 50% to 80% of patients.[120] Patients with limited disease for whom *H. pylori* eradication is ineffective are still frequently cured, with a 70% to 90% long-term disease-free survival with definitive radiotherapy.[121,122] Another important divergence from routine management of FL exists for splenic MZL. For patients with symptomatic splenomegaly and associated cytopenias, surgical splenectomy can lead to normalization of peripheral blood counts, and also can help achieve disease stabilization or regression systemically; splenectomy in MZL is perhaps the only setting in the management of the lymphoma in which "surgical debulking" is a routine consideration.[112]

## Small Lymphocytic Lymphoma of Chronic Lymphocytic Leukemia Type

Chronic lymphocytic leukemia (CLL) and small lymphocytic lymphoma of CLL type (SLL/CLL) are felt to represent one underlying pathophysiologic process with a spectrum of phenotypic presentation ranging from purely bone marrow and blood disease (CLL) to almost completely extramedullary disease (SLL). The distinction between leukemia and lymphoma is more semantic than pathophysiologic in nature, although the presence of adenopathy can in certain cases influence management decisions.

### Clinical presentation

While CLL is a relatively common disease, only 10% of patients with the disease present as predominantly nodal disease; as such, SLL accounts for fewer than 5% of new diagnoses of NHL in the United States. Furthermore, even when presenting as a nodal disease, the majority of patients will go on to have clinically detectible marrow involvement during the course of their illness. SLL is an aging-associated disease, with no apparent plateau in adjusted incidence rates by age, and in the United States is more common in Caucasians than in individuals of African descent or Hispanic ethnicity.[123] Common presenting signs and symptoms include painless peripheral adenopathy, often chronic in nature, asymptomatic lymphocytosis with persistence of absolute lymphocyte counts greater than (and at times markedly greater than) 5,000 cells/mm[3], or symptoms attributable to cytopenias due either to bone marrow infiltration or autoimmune processes associated with the disease. A monoclonal antibody can be detected in 20% of cases, and hypogammaglobulinemia with recurrent infections may be present in up to 40% of cases. This stands in contrast to lymphoplasmacytic lymphoma (LPL), in which the malignant lymphocytes share morphologic characteristics with mature plasma cells, and the immunophenotype is more consistent with MZL. When a significant IgM paraprotein is detectable with an underlying LPL, the disease is typically referred to as Waldenström's macroglobulinemia; such patients can present with coronary, cerebral, or ophthalmic insufficiency due to hyperviscosity caused by marked elevation in circulating IgM. Either SLL or LPL can present with cryoglobulinemia, often also in the context of coinfection with hepatitis C. Richter's transformation, the transformation of small lymphocytic lymphoma to DLBCL that was the first description of transformed lymphoma, occurs less frequently than transformation of the other indolent lymphomas, with lifetime risk estimates for patients with SLL between 2% and 8%, and is typically heralded by rapidly progressive signs and symptomatology.[124]

### Staging

Routine evaluation before initiation of treatment for SLL includes routine physical examination; laboratory analyses; CT scan of the chest, abdomen, and pelvis; and bone marrow biopsy and aspiration. 18-FDG PET is useful in select situations, including patients presenting for treatment with a clinical suspicion of Richter's transformation, as standard uptake velocities (SUVs) can help inform the clinician on which site of disease to which a biopsy should be directed to rule *out* transformation, as sites of transformed lymphoma tend to have SUVs greater than sites without transformation. It should be emphasized that although measurement of SUVs can be useful for the clinician, they cannot replace a surgical biopsy in treatment planning.

The extremely variable natural history of patients with SLL (and CLL), even within given Rai stages, has prompted investigators to attempt to delineate predictors of more aggressive disease. Certain karyotypic abnormalities have been found to be associated with shorter survival, including deletion of chromosome 17p (the locus of the *p53* tumor suppressor gene) and deletion of chromosome 11q (the locus of the *ATM* gene), whereas in patients who have a deletion of chromosome 13q as the only cytogenetic abnormality, survival has been reported to be superior to those patients without detectable mutations.[125] Of additional prognostic importance is whether the malignant clone has undergone somatic mutation of the immunoglobulin $V_H$ (Ig $V_H$) gene, an event in the maturation of the lymphocyte when it is exposed to a germinal center. Prognosis for patients with SLL that has not undergone Ig $V_H$ somatic mutation is significantly worse, independent of other cytogenetic features of the disease; patients with unmutated Ig $V_H$ have a median survival from the time of diagnosis of 117 months, compared with 293 months for patients with mutated Ig $V_H$.[126]

## Management

Treatment paradigms for SLL (and LPL) reflect the chronic, remitting, and relapsing nature of these diseases. However, the natural history of SLL is extremely heterogeneous, with subsets of patients stratified by cytogenetic and molecular features having median survivals despite treatment ranging from 32 months to 310 months.[125–127] When indicated, initial therapy often consists of a combination of rituximab and purine analog-based chemotherapy, with reservation of anthracycline or anthracenedione for use in the event of clinical transformation or resistant/refractory disease. The presence of high-risk cytogenetic abnormalities, particularly loss of the tumor suppressor p53 from a 17p deletion, predicts a worse response to purine analog-based therapy, however, and although no standard of care for such patients yet exists, alternative strategies that incorporate alemtuzumab, a monoclonal antibody targeting CD52, are an evolving consideration, particularly in patients without bulky nodal disease. Allogeneic stem cell transplantation has traditionally been reserved for relapsed or refractory high-risk disease, and (as in other indolent B-cell NHL) can potentially be curative therapy.

## Mantle Cell Lymphoma

Mantle cell lymphoma (MCL) comprises approximately 7% of new diagnoses of NHL. It is a mature B-cell lymphoma that historically has been considered an indolent B-cell NHL, although its clinical behavior often tends to be more aggressive. It can be difficult to distinguish morphologically from SLL, and the distinction is made on the basis of differences in genetic and immunophenotype findings (see **Table 1**).

### Clinical presentation

MCL has a median age at diagnosis of approximately 65, and between 70% and 90% of patients will present with detectable stage IV disease. Involvement of the bone marrow is frequently observed, and a leukemic phase is seen in as frequently as 75% of cases in some series.[128] Gastrointestinal involvement is frequently identified, and can present along a spectrum from diffuse lymphomatous polyposis to a normal lumen with microscopic disease detected on blind biopsy. Other sites of common involvement include the spleen and Waldeyer's ring. In 20% to 30% of patients, MCL will at some time during the course of illness undergo transformation to a blastoid variant, an event associated with rapid progression of disease, resistance to therapy, and a median survival of 4 months.[129,130]

### Staging

Stemming from this understanding of the clinical presentation of MCL, appropriate pretreatment evaluation includes routine physical examination and laboratory analyses; CT imaging of the chest, abdomen, and pelvis; bone marrow biopsy; and upper and lower endoscopy with, if no evident abnormalities, blind luminal biopsies. 18-FDG PET is not recommended as routine, although it does have utility in evaluation response to therapy, which itself can help guide management (see the following section). Sites of original disease involvement are routinely reevaluated during or after completion of therapy to evaluate the degree of response to the prescribed regimen.

### Management

No single standard of care exists for the initial therapeutic approach to a patient with newly diagnosed MCL. For patients with early-stage MCL, careful evaluation of bone marrow and both upper and lower gastrointestinal tracts for evidence of subclinical involvement by lymphoma are required before administering radiation therapy with curative intent. For patients with distinct evidence of having experienced an indolent course or with low-bulk and low-risk disease, initial observation can be appropriate. However, most patients will require treatment at time of presentation. Historically, outcomes with first-line treatment with alkylator, purine analog, or anthracycline-based regimens with or without rituximab were disappointing; for instance, R-CHOP alone leads to infrequent complete responses (<50%) and a brief duration of treatment benefit (<2 years).[131]

More aggressive treatment programs have been associated with improved outcomes in previously untreated MCL. Regimens including either alternating or sequential non-crossreactive chemotherapy regimens have led to complete remission rates in excess of 90%. Consolidation of such treatment with high-dose chemotherapy and autologous stem cell transplantation is associated with 5-year disease-free survival rates of between 40% and 65%.[132,133] Management of relapsed disease frequently will incorporate previously unused classes of cytotoxic chemotherapy and novel agents such as bortezomib, an inhibitor of the cellular proteosome that has been approved by the Food and Drug Administration for the treatment of relapsed MCL. Selected patients may be considered for consolidative allogeneic stem cell transplantation in second or later remission, or in first remission of blastoid MCL.

## Burkitt Lymphoma

BL is a highly aggressive mature B-cell NHL characterized by a stereotypical morphology, an extremely high rate of cellular proliferation, with mitotic indices approaching 100%, and dysregulation of the c-myc due to translocations of chromosome 8. It is a rare form of lymphoma, with fewer than 1% of newly diagnosed NHL in Western countries diagnosed as BL, and demonstrates a strong male preponderance of disease. Nonetheless, its unique clinical features make BL an important disease entity.

### Clinical presentation

There are three forms of BL with distinct clinical and epidemiologic features: endemic (African), sporadic (American), and immunodeficiency-related. Endemic BL classically presents in children as a tumor of the jaw or facial bones, and tends to disseminate hematogenously early in the course of illness to extranodal sites, including testis or ovary, kidney, CNS, and meninges. Sporadic BL typically presents as bulky abdominal disease involving cecum, small bowel, or stomach, with associated ascites. Renal, testicular or ovarian, and CNS or meningeal involvement is common as well. Immunodeficiency-related BL more frequently presents as nodally based disease, although it can involve bone marrow, CNS, or meninges, and rarely may present with a leukemic phase. Interestingly, although patients with HIV infection are at increased risk of developing BL, patients affected typically have adequate CD4+ T-cell reserves and frequently have no history of opportunistic infection.[134] Each form shares the typical presentation of rapidly growing disease, elevated lactate dehydrogenase (LDH), and both systemic symptoms as well as symptoms directly attributable to disease infiltration.

### Staging

Routine pretreatment evaluation of patients with BL includes routine physical examination; laboratory analyses (including the LDH); and CT scan of the chest, abdomen, and pelvis. BL tends to be markedly 18-FDG avid on PET scan, making 18-FDG PET a potentially useful modality in following response to therapy. Given the propensity for early hematogenous spread and early involvement of the CNS, bone marrow biopsy and diagnostic lumbar puncture are routine elements in the pretreatment evaluation.

### Management

The treatment of BL is based on rapid institution of intensive combination chemotherapy, frequently adapting regimens developed for the treatment of pediatric acute lymphoblastic leukemia. These regimens incorporate agents with known CNS penetrance, and additional multi-agent intrathecal prophylaxis is considered obligatory given otherwise high risks of CNS recurrence. These intensive regimens are associated with complete remission rates of approximately 80% to 90% and 5-year disease-free survival rates of 50% to 75%.[135,136] Although some data suggest that HIV infection confers a worse prognosis in the treatment of BL, selection of chemotherapy does not differ by HIV status. For patients with relapsed or refractory BL, outcomes are poor, although one third of patients with chemosensitive relapsed disease may enjoy long-term disease-free survival with consolidation of a second remission with high-dose therapy and autologous stem cell rescue.[137]

## Peripheral T-Cell Lymphoma

The peripheral T-cell lymphomas (PTCLs) are a heterogeneous group of diseases that collectively comprise between 5% and 10% of newly diagnosed NHL in the United States, although they are more common in other regions. These diseases differ morphologically, immunophenotypically, and clinically, spanning the spectrum from indolent mild disease to moderately aggressive (and frequently curable) to aggressive and incurable. And while some subtypes are now managed in a tailored fashion, our ability to treat many of these diseases in a specific and evidence-based fashion remains limited.

The PTCLs can be broadly classified as diseases with predominantly leukemic, nodal, or extranodal distributions. A subset of the peripheral T-cell lymphomas frequently presents with a leukemic phase, including T-cell prolymphocytic leukemia, T-cell large granular lymphocytic (LGL), natural killer/T (NK/T)-cell leukemia, and adult T-cell leukemia/lymphoma (ATLL).[138] A second set of T-cell lymphomas typically present with adenopathy, including angioimmunoblastic T-cell lymphoma (AITL), systemic anaplastic large cell lymphoma (ALCL), and peripheral T-cell lymphoma, unspecified (PTCLu).

The extranodal PTCLs include mycosis fungoides (MF) and cutaneous ALCL; these can have a chronic and indolent natural history, enjoying long remissions, and patients with early stage and nonprogressive disease have actuarial life expectancies that do not differ from the general population.[139–144] Sézary syndrome represents a leukemic progression of MF, presenting with abnormal circulating lymphocytes (Sézary cells), adenopathy, and erythrodermia, and carries a worse prognosis.[145] Extranodal NK/T-cell lymphoma, nasal type (nasal NK/T lymphoma) is an aggressive lymphoma that is the most common cause of the "lethal midline granuloma" syndrome. Pathophysiologically, it is strongly associated with EBV infection, and although rare in the United States is seen more frequently in East Asia and among indigenous peoples in Peru. It can affect children or adults, and typically presents as a locally invasive disease presenting with nasal obstruction and destruction of nasal passages, hard palate, and sinuses.

For many types of PTCL, there exists no consensus approach to treatment. Indolent cutaneous T-cell lymphomas, including early-stage MF and cutaneous ALCL, can often be observed or treated with skin-directed therapies (topical medications, ultraviolet or electron radiation, or involved-field radiotherapy) or mild systemic treatments such as retinoids. 18-FDG PET scanning can be useful in selected cases, and can be particularly relevant in the evaluation of a patient with cutaneous T-cell lymphoma, as identification of extracutaneous disease can fundamentally alter both prognosis and therapeutic approach. For the aggressive PTCLs, multi-agent chemotherapy is often attempted, such as CHOP, although with the exception of Alk-1–positive ALCL, it is frequently associated with brief progression-free durations. For nasal NK/T lymphoma, early incorporation of radiation therapy into a combined modality therapy program has been shown to improve outcomes.[146–150] The roles of autologous and allogeneic stem cell transplantation continue to be explored in the settings of consolidation of first remission as well as treatment of relapsed or refractory disease.[151,152]

## SUMMARY

The malignant lymphomas, each arising from a different stage in lymphocyte ontogeny, are extremely varied in epidemiology, clinical presentation, and optimal management. The range includes diseases that routinely present as early-stage or late-stage disease; require staging that ranges from cross-sectional imaging alone to inclusion of functional imaging and evaluation of bone marrow, cerebrospinal fluid, or gastrointestinal tracts; and are managed with strategies ranging from observation to intensive combined-modality therapy or consolidative high-dose therapy with either autologous or allogeneic stem cell transplantation. An understanding of the principles of lymphoma, including the importance of a thorough diagnostic evaluation and the relevance of staging to treatment planning, and an appreciation of the unique elements of the natural history of specific types of lymphoma, are prerequisites to the appropriate management of patients with these challenging diseases.

## REFERENCES

1. Sheehan WW, Rappaport H. Morphological criteria in the classification of the malignant lymphomas. Proc Natl Cancer Conf 1970;6:59–71.
2. The Non-Hodgkin's Lymphoma Pathologic Classification Project. National Cancer Institute sponsored study of classifications of non-Hodgkin's lymphomas: summary and description of a working formulation for clinical usage. Cancer 1982;49:2112–35.
3. Nabholtz JM, Friedman S, Collin F, et al. Modification of Kiel and working formulation classifications for improved survival prediction in non-Hodgkin's lymphoma. J Clin Oncol 1987;5:1634–9.
4. Harris N, Jaffe E, Stein H. A revised European-American classification of lymphoid neoplasms: a proposal from the International Lymphoma Study Group. Blood 1994;84:1631–92.
5. Jemal A, Siegel R, Ward E, et al. Cancer statistics, 2007. CA Cancer J Clin 2007;57:43–66.
6. Armitage JO, Weisenburger DD. New approach to classifying non-Hodgkin's lymphomas: clinical features of the major histologic subtypes. Non-Hodgkin's Lymphoma Classification Project. J Clin Oncol 1998;16:2780–95.
7. The Non-Hodgkin's Lymphoma Classification Project. A clinical evaluation of the International Lymphoma Study Group Classification of Non-Hodgkin's Lymphoma. Blood 1997;89:3909–18.
8. Hjalgrim H, Askling J, Rostgaard K, et al. Characteristics of Hodgkin's lymphoma after infectious mononucleosis. N Engl J Med 2003;349:1324–32.
9. Randhawa PS, Jaffe R, Demetris AJ, et al. Expression of Epstein-Barr virus-encoded small RNA (by the EBER-1 gene) in liver specimens from transplant recipients with post-transplantation lymphoproliferative disease. N Engl J Med 1992;327:1710–4.
10. Gunven P, Klein G, Henle G, et al. Epstein-Barr virus in Burkitt's lymphoma and nasopharyngeal carcinoma. Antibodies to EBV associated membrane and viral capsid antigens in Burkitt lymphoma patients. Nature 1970;228:1053–6.
11. Blayney DW, Jaffe ES, Blattner WA, et al. The human T-cell leukemia/lymphoma virus associated

with American adult T-cell leukemia/lymphoma. Blood 1983;62:401–5.

12. Said W, Chien K, Takeuchi S, et al. Kaposi's sarcoma-associated herpesvirus (KSHV or HHV8) in primary effusion lymphoma: ultrastructural demonstration of herpesvirus in lymphoma cells. Blood 1996;87:4937–43.

13. Wotherspoon AC, Ortiz-Hidalgo C, Falzon MR, et al. *Helicobacter pylori*-associated gastritis and primary B-cell gastric lymphoma. Lancet 1991; 338:1175–6.

14. Arcaini L, Paulli M, Boveri E, et al. Splenic and nodal marginal zone lymphomas are indolent disorders at high hepatitis C virus seroprevalence with distinct presenting features but similar morphologic and phenotypic profiles. Cancer 2004;100:107–15.

15. Smedby KE, Baecklund E, Askling J. Malignant lymphomas in autoimmunity and inflammation: a review of risks, risk factors, and lymphoma characteristics. Cancer Epidemiol Biomarkers Prev 2006;15: 2069–77.

16. Biggar RJ, Jaffe ES, Goedert JJ, et al. Hodgkin lymphoma and immunodeficiency in persons with HIV/AIDS. Blood 2006;108:3786–91.

17. Hooper WC, Holman RC, Clarke MJ, et al. Trends in non-Hodgkin lymphoma (NHL) and HIV-associated NHL deaths in the United States. Am J Hematol 2001;66:159–66.

18. Tirelli U, Spina M, Gaidano G, et al. Epidemiological, biological and clinical features of HIV-related lymphomas in the era of highly active antiretroviral therapy. AIDS 2000;14:1675–88.

19. Cartwright R, McNally R, Staines A. The increasing incidence of non-Hodgkin's lymphoma (NHL): the possible role of sunlight. Leuk Lymphoma 1994; 14:387–94.

20. Chiu BCH, Weisenburger DD, Zahm SH, et al. Agricultural pesticide use, familial cancer, and risk of non-Hodgkin lymphoma. Cancer Epidemiol Biomarkers Prev 2004;13:525–31.

21. Zahm SH, Weisenburger DD, Babbitt PA, et al. Use of hair coloring products and the risk of lymphoma, multiple myeloma, and chronic lymphocytic leukemia. Am J Public Health 1992;82:990–7.

22. Shugart YY, Hemminki K, Vaittinen P, et al. A genetic study of Hodgkin's lymphoma: an estimate of heritability and anticipation based on the familial cancer database in Sweden. Hum Genet 2000;106: 553–6.

23. Wang SS, Slager SL, Brennan P, et al. Family history of hematopoietic malignancies and risk of non-Hodgkin lymphoma (NHL): a pooled analysis of 10 211 cases and 11 905 controls from the International Lymphoma Epidemiology Consortium (InterLymph). Blood 2007;109:3479–88.

24. Zhu K, Levine RS, Brann EA, et al. Risk factors for non-Hodgkin's lymphoma according to family history of haematolymphoproliferative malignancies. Int J Epidemiol 2001;30:818–24.

25. Altieri A, Bermejo JL, Hemminki K. Familial risk for non-Hodgkin lymphoma and other lymphoproliferative malignancies by histopathologic subtype: the Swedish Family-Cancer Database. Blood 2005; 106:668–72.

26. Mourad W, Tulbah A, Shoukri M. Primary diagnosis and REAL/WHO classification of non-Hodgkin's lymphoma by fine-needle aspiration: cytomorphologic and immunophenotypic approach. Diagn Cytopathol 2003;28:191–5.

27. Zelenetz AD, Hoppe RT. NCCN: Non-Hodgkin's lymphoma. Cancer Control 2001;8:102–13.

28. NCCN practice guidelines for Hodgkin's disease. National Comprehensive Cancer Network. Oncology (Williston Park) 1999;13:78–110.

29. Lister TA, Crowther D, Sutcliffe SB, et al. Report of a committee convened to discuss the evaluation and staging of patients with Hodgkin's disease: Cotswolds meeting. J Clin Oncol 1989;7:1630–6 [published erratum appears in J Clin Oncol 1990 Sep;8(9):1602].

30. Morton LM, Wang SS, Devesa SS, et al. Lymphoma incidence patterns by WHO subtype in the United States, 1992–2001. Blood 2006;107: 265–76.

31. Siebert R, Louie D, Lacher M, et al. Familial Hodgkin's and non-Hodgkin's lymphoma: different patterns in first-degree relatives. Leuk Lymphoma 1997;27:503–7.

32. Harty LC, Lin AY, Goldstein AM, et al. HLA-DR, HLA-DQ, and TAP genes in familial Hodgkin disease. Blood 2002;99:690–3.

33. Brousset P, Knecht H, Rubin B, et al. Demonstration of Epstein-Barr virus replication in Reed-Sternberg cells of Hodgkin's disease. Blood 1993;82: 872–6.

34. International Collaboration on HIV and Cancer. Highly active antiretroviral therapy and incidence of cancer in human immunodeficiency virus-infected adults. J Natl Cancer Inst 2000;92: 1823–30.

35. Vassilakopoulos TP, Angelopoulou MK, Siakantaris MP, et al. Pure infradiaphragmatic Hodgkin's lymphoma. Clinical features, prognostic factor and comparison with supradiaphragmatic disease. Haematologica 2006;91:32–9.

36. Kalkner KM, Enblad G, Gustavsson A, et al. Infradiaphragmatic Hodgkin's disease: the Swedish National Care Programme experience. The Swedish Lymphoma Study Group. Eur J Haematol 1997; 59:31–7.

37. Ifrah N, Hunault M, Jais JP, et al. Infradiaphragmatic Hodgkin's disease: long-term results of combined modality therapy. Leuk Lymphoma 1996;21: 79–84.

38. Atkinson K, Austin DE, McElwain TJ, et al. Alcohol pain in Hodgkin's disease. Cancer 1976;37: 895–9.

39. Hammack J, Kotanides H, Rosenblum MK, et al. Paraneoplastic cerebellar degeneration. II. Clinical and immunologic findings in 21 patients with Hodgkin's disease. Neurology 1992;42:1938–43.

40. Gallamini A, Hutchings M, Rigacci L, et al. Early interim 2-[18F]fluoro-2-deoxy-D-glucose positron emission tomography is prognostically superior to international prognostic score in advanced-stage Hodgkin's lymphoma: a report from a joint Italian-Danish study. J Clin Oncol 2007;25:3746–52.

41. Zinzani PL, Tani M, Fanti S, et al. Early positron emission tomography (PET) restaging: a predictive final response in Hodgkin's disease patients. Ann Oncol 2006;17:1296–300.

42. Press OW, LeBlanc M, Lichter AS, et al. Phase III randomized intergroup trial of subtotal lymphoid irradiation versus doxorubicin, vinblastine, and subtotal lymphoid irradiation for stage IA to IIA Hodgkin's disease. J Clin Oncol 2001;19:4238–44.

43. Noordijk EM, Carde P, Dupouy N, et al. Combined-modality therapy for clinical stage I or II Hodgkin's lymphoma: long-term results of the European Organisation for Research and Treatment of Cancer H7 randomized controlled trials. J Clin Oncol 2006;24:3128–35.

44. Diehl V, Franklin J, Pfreundschuh M, et al. Standard and increased-dose BEACOPP chemotherapy compared with COPP-ABVD for advanced Hodgkin's disease. N Engl J Med 2003;348:2386–95.

45. Horning SJ, Hoppe RT, Breslin S, et al. Stanford V and radiotherapy for locally extensive and advanced Hodgkin's disease: mature results of a prospective clinical trial. J Clin Oncol 2002;20:630–7.

46. Jagannath S, Armitage JO, Dicke KA, et al. Prognostic factors for response and survival after high-dose cyclophosphamide, carmustine, and etoposide with autologous bone marrow transplantation for relapsed Hodgkin's disease. J Clin Oncol 1989;7:179–85.

47. Linch DC, Winfield D, Goldstone AH, et al. Dose intensification with autologous bone-marrow transplantation in relapsed and resistant Hodgkin's disease: results of a BNLI randomised trial. Lancet 1993;341:1051–4.

48. Reece DE, Connors JM, Spinelli JJ, et al. Intensive therapy with cyclophosphamide, carmustine, etoposide +/− cisplatin, and autologous bone marrow transplantation for Hodgkin's disease in first relapse after combination chemotherapy. Blood 1994;83:1193–9.

49. Horning SJ, Chao NJ, Negrin RS, et al. High-dose therapy and autologous hematopoietic progenitor cell transplantation for recurrent or refractory Hodgkin's disease: analysis of the Stanford University results and prognostic indices. Blood 1997;89:801–13.

50. Moskowitz CH, Nimer SD, Zelenetz AD, et al. A 2-step comprehensive high-dose chemoradiotherapy second-line program for relapsed and refractory Hodgkin disease: analysis by intent to treat and development of a prognostic model. Blood 2001;97:616–23.

51. Schmitz N, Pfistner B, Sextro M, et al. Aggressive conventional chemotherapy compared with high-dose chemotherapy with autologous haemopoietic stem-cell transplantation for relapsed chemosensitive Hodgkin's disease: a randomised trial. Lancet 2002;359:2065–71.

52. Moskowitz CH, Kewalramani T, Nimer SD, et al. Effectiveness of high dose chemoradiotherapy and autologous stem cell transplantation for patients with biopsy-proven primary refractory Hodgkin's disease. Br J Haematol 2004;124:645–52.

53. Peggs KS, Hunter A, Chopra R, et al. Clinical evidence of a graft-versus-Hodgkin's-lymphoma effect after reduced-intensity allogeneic transplantation. Lancet 2005;365:1934–41.

54. Anderlini P, Saliba R, Acholonu S, et al. Reduced-intensity allogeneic stem cell transplantation in relapsed and refractory Hodgkin's disease: low transplant-related mortality and impact of intensity of conditioning regimen. Bone Marrow Transplant 2005;35:943–51.

55. Mauch PM, Kalish LA, Kadin M, et al. Patterns of presentation of Hodgkin disease. Implications for etiology and pathogenesis. Cancer 1993;71: 2062–71.

56. Regula DP, Hoppe RT, Weiss LM. Nodular and diffuse types of lymphocyte predominance Hodgkin's disease. N Engl J Med 1988;318:214–9.

57. Ohno T, Stribley JA, Wu G, et al. Clonality in nodular lymphocyte-predominant Hodgkin's disease. N Engl J Med 1997;337:459–66.

58. Marafioti T, Hummel M, Anagnostopoulos I, et al. Origin of nodular lymphocyte-predominant Hodgkin's disease from a clonal expansion of highly mutated germinal-center B cells. N Engl J Med 1997; 337:453–8.

59. Diehl V, Sextro M, Franklin J, et al. Clinical presentation, course, and prognostic factors in lymphocyte-predominant Hodgkin's disease and lymphocyte-rich classical Hodgkin's disease: report from the European task force on lymphoma project on lymphocyte-predominant Hodgkin's disease. J Clin Oncol 1999;17:776–83.

60. Hutchings M, Loft A, Hanson M, et al. Different histopathological subtypes of Hodgkin lymphoma show significantly different levels of FDG uptake. Hematol Oncol 2006;24:146–50.

61. Orlandi E, Lazzarino M, Brusamolino E, et al. Nodular lymphocyte predominance Hodgkin's disease:

long-term observation reveals a continuous pattern of recurrence. Leuk Lymphoma 1997;26:359–68.

62. Schulz H, Rehwald U, Morschhauser F, et al. Rituximab in relapsed lymphocyte-predominant Hodgkin lymphoma: long-term results of a phase 2 trial by the German Hodgkin Lymphoma Study Group (GHSG). Blood 2008;111:109–11.

63. Ekstrand BC, Lucas JB, Horwitz SM, et al. Rituximab in lymphocyte-predominant Hodgkin disease: results of a phase 2 trial. Blood 2003;101:4285–9.

64. Wright G, Tan B, Rosenwald A, et al. A gene expression-based method to diagnose clinically distinct subgroups of diffuse large B cell lymphoma. Proc Natl Acad Sci U S A 2003;100:9991–6.

65. Rosenwald A, Wright G, Chan WC, et al. The use of molecular profiling to predict survival after chemotherapy for diffuse large-B-cell lymphoma. N Engl J Med 2002;346:1937–47.

66. Shipp MA, Ross KN, Tamayo P, et al. Diffuse large B-cell lymphoma outcome prediction by gene-expression profiling and supervised machine learning. Nat Med 2002;8:68–74.

67. Hans CP, Weisenburger DD, Greiner TC, et al. Confirmation of the molecular classification of diffuse large B-cell lymphoma by immunohistochemistry using a tissue microarray. Blood 2004;103:275–82.

68. Lossos IS, Czerwinski DK, Alizadeh AA, et al. Prediction of survival in diffuse large-B-cell lymphoma based on the expression of six genes. N Engl J Med 2004;350:1828–37.

69. Lenz G, Wright G, Dave S, et al. Gene expression signatures predict overall survival in diffuse large B Cell lymphoma treated with rituximab and chop-like chemotherapy. Blood 2007;110:203A.

70. Rigacci L, Nassi L, di Lollo S, et al. Dose-Dense CHOP Plus Rituximab (R-CHOP14) Seems To Overcome, in Large B Cell Lymphoma, the Negative Prognostic Significance of B Cell Origin. Blood 2004;110(11):4577.

71. Nyman H, Adde M, Karjalainen-Lindsberg ML, et al. Prognostic impact of immunohistochemically defined germinal center phenotype in diffuse large B-cell lymphoma patients treated with immunochemotherapy. Blood 2007;109:4930–5.

72. Moskowitz C, Hamlin PA, Horwitz SM, et al. Phase II Trial of Dose-Dense R-CHOP Followed by Risk-Adapted Consolidation with Either ICE or ICE and ASCT, Based upon the Results of Biopsy Confirmed Abnormal Interim Restaging PET Scan, Improves Outcome in Patients with Advanced Stage DLBCL. Blood 2006;108(11):532A.

73. Winter JN, Weller EA, Horning SJ, et al. Prognostic significance of Bcl-6 protein expression in DLBCL treated with CHOP or R-CHOP: a prospective correlative study. Blood 2006;107:4207–13.

74. Moller MB, Pedersen NT, Christensen BE. Diffuse large B-cell lymphoma: clinical implications of extranodal versus nodal presentation—a population-based study of 1575 cases. Br J Haematol 2004;124:151–9.

75. Lopez-Guillermo A, Colomo L, Jimenez M, et al. Diffuse large B-cell lymphoma: clinical and biological characterization and outcome according to the nodal or extranodal primary origin. J Clin Oncol 2005;23:2797–804.

76. Zelenetz AD, Chen TT, Levy R. Histologic transformation of follicular lymphoma to diffuse lymphoma represents tumor progression by a single malignant B cell. J Exp Med 1991;173:197–207.

77. Montoto S, Davies AJ, Matthews J, et al. Risk and clinical implications of transformation of follicular lymphoma to diffuse large B-cell lymphoma. J Clin Oncol 2007;25:2426–33.

78. Yuen AR, Kamel OW, Halpern J, et al. Long-term survival after histologic transformation of low-grade follicular lymphoma. J Clin Oncol 1995;13:1726–33.

79. Bastion Y, Sebban C, Berger F, et al. Incidence, predictive factors, and outcome of lymphoma transformation in follicular lymphoma patients. J Clin Oncol 1997;15:1587–94.

80. Hollender A, Kvaloy S, Nome O, et al. Central nervous system involvement following diagnosis of non-Hodgkin's lymphoma: a risk model. Ann Oncol 2002;13:1099–107.

81. Haioun C, Besson C, Lepage E, et al. Incidence and risk factors of central nervous system relapse in histologically aggressive non-Hodgkin's lymphoma uniformly treated and receiving intrathecal central nervous system prophylaxis: a GELA study on 974 patients. Ann Oncol 2000;11:685–90.

82. Ryan GF, Roos DR, Seymour JF. Primary non-Hodgkin's lymphoma of the breast: retrospective analysis of prognosis and patterns of failure in two Australian centers. Clin Lymphoma Myeloma 2006;6:337–41.

83. Gholam D, Bibeau F, El Weshi A, et al. Primary breast lymphoma. Leuk Lymphoma 2003;44:1173–8.

84. Ganjoo K, Advani R, Mariappan MR, et al. Non-Hodgkin lymphoma of the breast. Cancer 2007;110:25–30.

85. Fisher RI, Gaynor ER, Dahlberg S, et al. Comparison of a standard regimen (CHOP) with three intensive chemotherapy regimens for advanced non-Hodgkin's lymphoma. N Engl J Med 1993;328:1002–6.

86. Pfreundschuh M, Schubert J, Ziepert M, et al. Six versus eight cycles of bi-weekly CHOP-14 with or without rituximab in elderly patients with aggressive CD20+ B-cell lymphomas: a randomised controlled trial (RICOVER-60). Lancet Oncol 2008;9:105–16.

87. Pfreundschuh M, Trumper L, Osterborg A, et al. CHOP-like chemotherapy plus rituximab versus CHOP-like chemotherapy alone in young patients with good-prognosis diffuse large-B-cell lymphoma: a randomised controlled trial by the Mab-Thera International Trial (MInT) Group. Lancet Oncol 2006;7:379–91.

88. Habermann TM, Weller EA, Morrison VA, et al. Rituximab-CHOP versus CHOP alone or with maintenance rituximab in older patients with diffuse large B-cell lymphoma. J Clin Oncol 2006;24:3121–7.

89. Coiffier B, Lepage E, Briere J, et al. CHOP chemotherapy plus rituximab compared with CHOP alone in elderly patients with diffuse large-B-cell lymphoma. N Engl J Med 2002;346:235–42.

90. Miller TP. Effect of adding rituximab to three cycles of CHOP plus invoved-field radiotherapy for limited-stage aggressive diffuse B-cell lymphoma (SWOG-0014). Blood 2004;104:158.

91. Reyes F, Lepage E, Ganem G, et al. ACVBP versus CHOP plus radiotherapy for localized aggressive lymphoma. N Engl J Med 2005;352:1197–205.

92. Wilson WH, Gutierrez M, O'Connor P, et al. The role of rituximab and chemotherapy in aggressive B-cell lymphoma: a preliminary report of dose-adjusted EPOCH-R. Semin Oncol 2002;29:41–7.

93. Gianni AM, Bregni M, Siena S, et al. High-dose chemotherapy and autologous bone marrow transplantation compared with MACOP-B in aggressive B-cell lymphoma. N Engl J Med 1997; 336:1290–7.

94. Savage KJ, Monti S, Kutok JL, et al. The molecular signature of mediastinal large B-cell lymphoma differs from that of other diffuse large B-cell lymphomas and shares features with classical Hodgkin lymphoma. Blood 2003;102:3871–9.

95. Staudt LM, Dave S. The biology of human lymphoid malignancies revealed by gene expression profiling. Adv Immunol 2005;87:163–208.

96. Jacobson JO, Aisenberg AC, Lamarre L, et al. Mediastinal large cell lymphoma. An uncommon subset of adult lymphoma curable with combined modality therapy. Cancer 1988;62:1893–8.

97. Hamlin PA, Portlock CS, Straus DJ, et al. Primary mediastinal large B-cell lymphoma: optimal therapy and prognostic factor analysis in 141 consecutive patients treated at Memorial Sloan Kettering from 1980 to 1999. Br J Haematol 2005;130:691–9.

98. Todeschini G, Secchi S, Morra E, et al. Primary mediastinal large B-cell lymphoma (PMLBCL): long-term results from a retrospective multicentre Italian experience in 138 patients treated with CHOP or MACOP-B/VACOP-B. Br J Cancer 2004;90:372–6.

99. van Besien K, Kelta M, Bahaguna P. Primary mediastinal B-cell lymphoma: a review of pathology and management. J Clin Oncol 2001;19:1855–64.

100. Ponzoni M, Ferreri AJ, Campo E, et al. Definition, diagnosis, and management of intravascular large B-cell lymphoma: proposals and perspectives from an international consensus meeting. J Clin Oncol 2007;25:3168–73.

101. Murase T, Yamaguchi M, Suzuki R, et al. Intravascular large B-cell lymphoma (IVLBCL): a clinicopathologic study of 96 cases with special reference to the immunophenotypic heterogeneity of CD5. Blood 2007;109:478–85.

102. Lopez-Guillermo A, Cabanillas F, McLaughlin P, et al. The clinical significance of molecular response in indolent follicular lymphomas. Blood 1998;91:2955–60.

103. Wilder RB, Jones D, Tucker SL, et al. Long-term results with radiotherapy for Stage I-II follicular lymphomas. Int J Radiat Oncol Biol Phys 2001;51:1219–27.

104. Richards MA, Gregory WM, Hall PA, et al. Management of localized non-Hodgkin's lymphoma: the experience at St. Bartholomew's Hospital 1972–1985. Hematol Oncol 1989;7:1–18.

105. Mac Manus MP, Hoppe RT. Is radiotherapy curative for stage I and II low-grade follicular lymphoma? Results of a long-term follow-up study of patients treated at Stanford University. J Clin Oncol 1996; 14:1282–90.

106. Horning SJ, Rosenberg SA. The natural history of initially untreated low-grade non-Hodgkin's lymphomas. N Engl J Med 1984;311:1471–5.

107. Toze CL, Barnett MJ, Connors JM, et al. Long-term disease-free survival of patients with advanced follicular lymphoma after allogeneic bone marrow transplantation. Br J Haematol 2004;127:311–21.

108. van Besien K, Loberiza FR Jr, Bajorunaite R, et al. Comparison of autologous and allogeneic hematopoietic stem cell transplantation for follicular lymphoma. Blood 2003;102:3521–9.

109. Dierlamm J, Pittaluga S, Wlodarska I, et al. Marginal zone B-cell lymphomas of different sites share similar cytogenetic and morphologic features. Blood 1996;87:299–307.

110. Thieblemont C, Berger F, Dumontet C, et al. Mucosa-associated lymphoid tissue lymphoma is a disseminated disease in one third of 158 patients analyzed. Blood 2000;95:802–6.

111. Pich A, Fraire F, Fornari A, et al. Intrasinusoidal bone marrow infiltration and splenic marginal zone lymphoma: a quantitative study. Eur J Haematol 2006;76:392–8.

112. Chacon JI, Mollejo M, Munoz E, et al. Splenic marginal zone lymphoma: clinical characteristics and prognostic factors in a series of 60 patients. Blood 2002;100:1648–54.

113. Saadoun D, Sellam J, Ghillani-Dalbin P, et al. Increased risks of lymphoma and death among patients with non-hepatitis C virus-related mixed

cryoglobulinemia. Arch Intern Med 2006;166: 2101–8.

114. Saadoun D, Suarez F, Lefrere F, et al. Splenic lymphoma with villous lymphocytes, associated with type II cryoglobulinemia and HCV infection: a new entity? Blood 2005;105:74–6.

115. Hermine O, Lefrere F, Bronowicki JP, et al. Regression of splenic lymphoma with villous lymphocytes after treatment of hepatitis C virus infection. N Engl J Med 2002;347:89–94.

116. Ohsawa M, Shingu N, Miwa H, et al. Risk of non-Hodgkin's lymphoma in patients with hepatitis C virus infection. Int J Cancer 1999;80:237–9.

117. Alinari L, Castellucci P, Elstrom R, et al. 18F-FDG PET in mucosa-associated lymphoid tissue (MALT) lymphoma. Leuk Lymphoma 2006;47: 2096–101.

118. Beal KP, Yeung HW, Yahalom J. FDG-PET scanning for detection and staging of extranodal marginal zone lymphomas of the MALT type: a report of 42 cases. Ann Oncol 2005;16:473–80.

119. Elstrom R, Guan L, Baker G, et al. Utility of FDG-PET scanning in lymphoma by WHO classification. Blood 2003;101:3875–6.

120. Wündisch T, Thiede C, Morgner A, et al. Long-term follow-up of gastric MALT lymphoma after *Helicobacter pylori* eradication. J Clin Oncol 2005;23: 8018–24.

121. Tsang RW, Gospodarowicz MK, Pintilie M, et al. Stage I and II MALT lymphoma: results of treatment with radiotherapy. Int J Radiat Oncol Biol Phys 2001;50:1258–64.

122. Fung CY, Grossbard ML, Linggood RM, et al. Mucosa-associated lymphoid tissue lymphoma of the stomach: long term outcome after local treatment. Cancer 1999;85:9–17.

123. Matasar MJ, Ritchie EK, Consedine N, et al. Incidence rates of the major leukemia subtypes among US Hispanics, Blacks, and non-Hispanic Whites. Leuk Lymphoma 2006;47:2365–70.

124. Tsimberidou AM, Keating MJ. Richter syndrome: biology, incidence, and therapeutic strategies. Cancer 2005;103:216–28.

125. Dohner H, Stilgenbauer S, Benner A, et al. Genomic aberrations and survival in chronic lymphocytic leukemia. N Engl J Med 2000;343:1910–6.

126. Hamblin TJ, Davis Z, Gardiner A, et al. Unmutated Ig V(H) genes are associated with a more aggressive form of chronic lymphocytic leukemia. Blood 1999;94:1848–54.

127. Oscier DG, Gardiner AC, Mould SJ, et al. Multivariate analysis of prognostic factors in CLL: clinical stage, IGVH gene mutational status, and loss or mutation of the p53 gene are independent prognostic factors. Blood 2002;100: 1177–84.

128. Cohen PL, Kurtin PJ, Donovan KA, et al. Bone marrow and peripheral blood involvement in mantle cell lymphoma. Br J Haematol 1998;101:302–10.

129. Pott C, Schrader C, Bruggemann M, et al. Blastoid variant of mantle cell lymphoma: late progression from classical mantle cell lymphoma and quantitation of minimal residual disease. Eur J Haematol 2005;74:353–8.

130. Raty R, Franssila K, Jansson SE, et al. Predictive factors for blastoid transformation in the common variant of mantle cell lymphoma. Eur J Cancer 2003;39:321–9.

131. Lenz G, Dreyling M, Hoster E, et al. Immunochemotherapy with rituximab and cyclophosphamide, doxorubicin, vincristine, and prednisone significantly improves response and time to treatment failure, but not long-term outcome in patients with previously untreated mantle cell lymphoma: results of a prospective randomized trial of the German Low Grade Lymphoma Study Group (GLSG). J Clin Oncol 2005;23:1984–92.

132. Evens AM, Winter JN, Hou N, et al. A phase II clinical trial of intensive chemotherapy followed by consolidative stem cell transplant: long-term follow-up in newly diagnosed mantle cell lymphoma. Br J Haematol 2008;140:385–93.

133. Khouri IF, Romaguera J, Kantarjian H, et al. Hyper-CVAD and high-dose methotrexate/cytarabine followed by stem-cell transplantation: an active regimen for aggressive mantle-cell lymphoma. J Clin Oncol 1998;16:3803–9.

134. Lim ST, Karim R, Nathwani BN, et al. AIDS-related Burkitt's lymphoma versus diffuse large-cell lymphoma in the pre-highly active antiretroviral therapy (HAART) and HAART eras: significant differences in survival with standard chemotherapy. J Clin Oncol 2005;23:4430–8.

135. Mead GM, Sydes MR, Walewski J, et al. An international evaluation of CODOX-M and CODOX-M alternating with IVAC in adult Burkitt's lymphoma: results of United Kingdom Lymphoma Group LY06 study. Ann Oncol 2002;13:1264–74.

136. Rizzieri DA, Johnson JL, Niedzwiecki D, et al. Intensive chemotherapy with and without cranial radiation for Burkitt leukemia and lymphoma: final results of Cancer and Leukemia Group B Study 9251. Cancer 2004;100:1438–48.

137. Sweetenham JW, Pearce R, Taghipour G, et al. Adult Burkitt's and Burkitt-like non-Hodgkin's lymphoma—outcome for patients treated with high-dose therapy and autologous stem-cell transplantation in first remission or at relapse: results from the European Group for Blood and Marrow Transplantation. J Clin Oncol 1996;14:2465–72.

138. Bunn PA Jr, Schechter GP, Jaffe E, et al. Clinical course of retrovirus-associated adult T-cell

lymphoma in the United States. N Engl J Med 1983; 309:257–64.

139. Kim YH, Liu HL, Mraz-Gernhard S, et al. Long-term outcome of 525 patients with mycosis fungoides and Sezary syndrome: clinical prognostic factors and risk for disease progression. Arch Dermatol 2003;139:857–66.

140. van Doorn R, Van Haselen CW, van Voorst Vader PC, et al. Mycosis fungoides: disease evolution and prognosis of 309 Dutch patients. Arch Dermatol 2000;136:504–10.

141. Jones GW, Wilson LD. The changing survival of patients with mycosis fungoides: a population-based assessment of trends in the United States. Cancer 1999;86:191–3.

142. Kim YH, Chow S, Varghese A, et al. Clinical characteristics and long-term outcome of patients with generalized patch and/or plaque (T2) mycosis fungoides. Arch Dermatol 1999;135:26–32.

143. Kim YH, Jensen RA, Watanabe GL, et al. Clinical stage IA (limited patch and plaque) mycosis fungoides. A long-term outcome analysis. Arch Dermatol 1996;132:1309–13.

144. Bekkenk MW, Geelen FA, van Voorst Vader PC, et al. Primary and secondary cutaneous CD30(+) lymphoproliferative disorders: a report from the Dutch Cutaneous Lymphoma Group on the long-term follow-up data of 219 patients and guidelines for diagnosis and treatment. Blood 2000;95: 3653–61.

145. Klemke CD, Mansmann U, Poenitz N, et al. Prognostic factors and prediction of prognosis by the CTCL Severity Index in mycosis fungoides and Sezary syndrome. Br J Dermatol 2005;153: 118–24.

146. Isobe K, Uno T, Tamaru J, et al. Extranodal natural killer/T-cell lymphoma, nasal type: the significance of radiotherapeutic parameters. Cancer 2006;106: 609–15.

147. Rodriguez J, Conde E, Gutierrez A, et al. Frontline autologous stem cell transplantation in high-risk peripheral T-cell lymphoma: a prospective study from The Gel-Tamo Study Group. Eur J Haematol 2007;79:32–8.

148. Strehl J, Mey U, Glasmacher A, et al. High-dose chemotherapy followed by autologous stem cell transplantation as first-line therapy in aggressive non-Hodgkin's lymphoma: a meta-analysis. Haematologica 2003;88:1304–15.

149. Schmitz N, Kloess M, Reiser M, et al. Four versus six courses of a dose-escalated cyclophosphamide, doxorubicin, vincristine, and prednisone (CHOP) regimen plus etoposide (megaCHOEP) and autologous stem cell transplantation: early dose intensity is crucial in treating younger patients with poor prognosis aggressive lymphoma. Cancer 2006;106:136–45.

150. Gallamini A, Zaja F, Patti C, et al. Alemtuzumab (Campath-1H) and CHOP chemotherapy as first-line treatment of peripheral T-cell lymphoma: results of a GITIL (Gruppo Italiano Terapie Innovative nei Linfomi) prospective multicenter trial. Blood 2007;110:2316–23.

151. Paolo C, Lucia F, Anna D. Hematopoietic stem cell transplantation in peripheral T-cell lymphomas. Leuk Lymphoma 2007;48:1496–501.

152. Kewalramani T, Zelenetz AD, Teruya-Feldstein J, et al. Autologous transplantation for relapsed or primary refractory peripheral T-cell lymphoma. Br J Haematol 2006;134:202–7.

# The Impact of Fluorodeoxyglucose–Positron Emission Tomography in Primary Staging and Patient Management in Lymphoma Patients

Martin Allen-Auerbach, MD[a], Sven de Vos, MD, PhD[b], Johannes Czernin, MD[a],*

**KEYWORDS**
- PET/CT • FDG • Lymphoma • Staging

Positron emission tomography (PET) imaging became a clinical force in the mid-to-late 1990s when the US Health Care Administration approved whole-body PET imaging for several oncological indications. Following the initial approval for fluorodeoxyglucose (FDG)-PET characterization of solitary lung nodules, several other indications were approved, among them diagnosing, staging, and restaging of lymphoma. FDG-PET has taken the place of gallium-67 (Ga-67) scintigraphy as the modality of choice for functional and metabolic imaging of patients who have lymphoma.

With the advance of combined PET/CT devices,[1] anatomic masses can be dissected simultaneously based on size criteria and molecular characteristics such as their glucose metabolism.[2] This is important, because clinical practice and clinical trials still rely on anatomic response criteria,[3] and the value of molecular and anatomic tumor characterizations for response predictions can be compared directly.[4] The ability to accurately characterize masses and PET's/CT's high sensitivity and specificity for staging, restaging, and treatment monitoring have led to wide-spread acceptance of PET/CT imaging in the imaging of lymphoma.[5–7]

The important role of FDG-PET imaging in lymphoma is emphasized by the recent report of the International Harmonization Project.[8,9] The harmonization project recommendations are among the first to formally acknowledge the importance of glucose metabolic imaging for managing patients who have cancer.

Taking into account variability among readers and equipment, the working group arrived at the following recommendations:

1. FDG-PET is recommended strongly before treatment in patients with routinely FDG avid lymphoma such as diffuse large B cell lymphoma (DLBCL) or Hodgkin lymphoma (HL).
2. Treatment effects should be assessed 6 to 8 weeks after completion of chemotherapy.
3. Quantification of FDG uptake with standardized uptake values (SUV) and measurement of changes are not necessary, because visual

a Department of Molecular and Medical Pharmacology, Ahmanson Biological Imaging Center/Nuclear Medicine, David Geffen School of Medicine at UCLA, 10833 Le Conte Avenue, Los Angeles, CA 90095-6948, USA
b Department of Medicine, Division of Hematology/Oncology, David Geffen School of Medicine at UCLA, 10833 Le Conte Avenue, Los Angeles, CA 90095-6948, USA
* Corresponding author.
*E-mail address:* jczernin@mednet.ucla.edu (J. Czernin).

Radiol Clin N Am 46 (2008) 199–211
doi:10.1016/j.rcl.2008.03.004
0033-8389/08/$ – see front matter © 2008 Elsevier Inc. All rights reserved.

assessments of treatment effects after completion of therapy are sufficient.[9]

## IMAGING WITH FLUORODEOXYGLUCOSE-6-PHOSPHATE

Increased glucose metabolic activity as a hallmark of malignant degeneration initially was described in 1924 by Warburg.[10] This increase in glycolytic activity takes place even in the presence of oxygen. The increased glycolytic activity of tumors has been exploited for imaging cancer with PET and the glucose analog FDG.[11,12]

Competing with serum glucose FDG targets membrane-bound glucose transporters (Glut-1 and Glut-3) that shuttle FDG into tumor cells and hexokinases (HK-1 and HK-2), which phosphorylate FDG to FDG-6-phosphate. Both of these enzymes are overexpressed in many cancers.[13] Unlike glucose-6-phosphate, FDG-6-phosphate is no longer a substrate for the subsequent steps in the glycolytic pathway. Furthermore, glucose-6-phosphatase that would reverse the actions of hexokinase is available only in very limited amounts in tumor cells. Thus, FDG-6-phosphate essentially is trapped in tumor cells in proportion to their glycolytic activity (**Fig. 1**).

In vivo detection of fluorine-18 (F-18) positron emission can be achieved by the PET scanner that was invented in the early 1970s.[14] Positrons, however, are not detected directly as they travel a few millimeters from the site of decay before undergoing an annihilation reaction with electrons in tissue.[15] This annihilation reaction results in the simultaneous emission of two photons with 511 keV (the mass energy of an electron/positron) that leave the annihilation site at and angle of approximately 180° and are detected by the PET scanner (**Fig. 2**).

## STANDARDIZED UPTAKE VALUES

PET images can be analyzed visually, semiquantitatively by means of SUV,[16] or quantitatively using

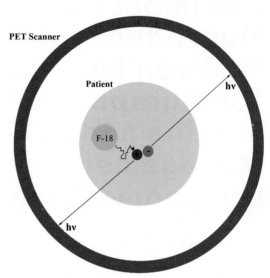

**Fig. 2.** Detection of photons (hν) originating from the annihilation reaction of a positron (resulting from the decay of the F-18 isotope) and a tissue electron.

appropriate tracer kinetic models.[17] Because of their simplicity, PET scans most frequently are analyzed visually or by means of SUV that is defined as:

$$\frac{\text{decay-corrected activity [kBq]}/\text{tissue volume[mL]}}{\text{injected-FDG activity [kBq]}/\text{body weight [g]}}$$

The reproducibility of SUVs and that of more sophisticated model-based quantitative approaches that for instance measure tumor glucose use in units of μmol/g/min was established by measuring tumor FDG uptake twice within 1 to 2 weeks in patients who had lung cancer.[17] This study demonstrated that simple SUV measurements are reproducible and suffice for estimating tumor glucose metabolic activity. The more computationally demanding modeling approach usually is reserved for research protocols.[18] Importantly, in lymphoma, visual assessments of treatment responses are sufficient in clinical practice.[8,9]

The following discussion will focus on the role of FDG PET and PET/CT for staging of lymphoma. In particular, the authors will discuss whether FDG PET adds to the staging information provided by CT and other conventional imaging modalities. Finally, they will examine whether and how PET/CT imaging findings translate into changes in patient management.

## FLUORODEOXYGLUCOSE–POSITRON EMISSION TOMOGRAPHY/CT COST AND AVAILABILITY

More than 1800 PET/CT and PET scanners are distributed throughout the United States.[19] With the emergence of commercial radio-pharmacies that produce FDG in small self-shielded

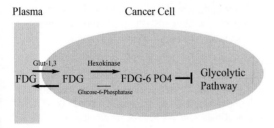

**Fig. 1.** Fluorodeoxyglucose (FDG) uptake by means of glucose transporters Glut 1 and 3, with subsequent phosphorylation and trapping of the phosphorylated FDG (FDG-PO4) in a cancer cell.

cyclotrons, more than 95% of all cancer patients now have access to PET/CT imaging. Thus, there are essentially no limitations to the use of PET and the old argument, that PET imaging is only available in selected centers, can be put to rest. Another outdated argument is that whole-body FDG PET imaging is expensive while CT imaging is considered inexpensive. Current technical and professional reimbursement rates for both whole-body contrast CT and PET/CT average around $1000. Moreover, combined FDG PET/CT does not increase health care costs. Providing the combined anatomic (CT) and glucose metabolic (PET) information is reimbursed at the same level as PET or CT alone.

## TECHNICAL CONSIDERATIONS

Most PET examinations in lymphoma and other cancers are performed as part of PET/CT studies that can be performed in less than 10 minutes in some patients.[20,21] PET/CT also increases patient comfort by reducing the need for multiple visits in clinics. PET image interpretation is facilitated by complementary anatomic information from CT, resulting in fewer equivocal findings, increased reader confidence[22,23], and more accurate assessments of the extent of disease.[24,25] PET/CT interpretations yield a higher diagnostic accuracy than side-by-side PET and CT interpretations in some[23,26] but not in other cancers (**Fig. 3**).[27]

Before treatment, most non-HL (NHL) and HL can be staged accurately with both CT and PET.

Arguments for the preferential use of CT include its high sensitivity (because of its superior spatial resolution) and accuracy, its wide availability, and its alleged relatively low cost. Disadvantages include its limited specificity, its inability to determine bone marrow involvement, and the high radiation dose to patients, which is estimated to average as much as 25 mSv.[28]

A recent study suggested that separate CT studies (in addition to PET/CT) are unnecessary in patients who have lymphoma.[29] The addition of PET/CT to CT changed the management decisions in 25% of NHL and 33% of HL patients, mostly in early disease stages.

Initial studies using PET/CT imaging demonstrated its diagnostic advantage over PET and CT alone.[24,30] This diagnostic advantage was achieved by using low-dose noncontrast-enhanced CT rather than fully diagnostic contrast CT studies. It remains unclear from the available literature whether the CT portion of PET/CT should be diagnostic (ie, performed after the administration of intravenous contrast) or whether a low-dose CT would suffice for this indication as suggested in one study. In this report of 47 patients, contrast-enhanced PET/CT resulted in a smaller number of indeterminate nodes and detected a larger number of extranodal sites but did not have a significant impact on patient management. PET and PET/CT arrived at a different disease stage in only one of the 47 patients.

Another study in 64 patients compared the diagnostic performance of unenhanced PET/CT with

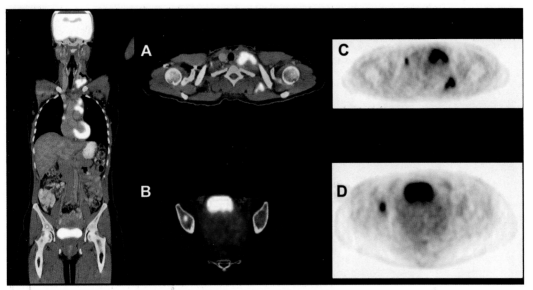

**Fig. 3.** 46-year-old woman with a history of nodular sclerosing HD. Selected fused positron emission tomography and axial slices demonstrate supraclavicular adenopathy (*A, C*) and bone involvement of the right acetabulum (*C, D*). Bone involvement would not have been identified on CT alone.

that of contrast-enhanced CT for lymphoma staging.[31] Nonenhanced PET/CT alone was superior to contrast CT, especially for staging of extranodal involvement. Sensitivity of nonenhanced PET/CT and enhanced CT was 88% and 50%, while specificities were 100% and 90%. Unfortunately, no direct comparison between contrast-enhanced and nonenhanced PET/CT was performed.

The ability of enhanced and nonenhanced PET/CT for staging pelvic and retroperitoneal nodes was evaluated by Morimoto and colleagues.[32] Standard clinical assessment and clinical follow up served as reference standards, and thus no true gold standard was available. The nodal stage was correct in 79% of the patients with contrast CT and in 71% on noncontrasted PET/CT ($P<.05$). Specifically, noncontrast CT was less accurate for assessing external and internal iliac node involvement.

More recently, Pfannenberg and colleagues[33] compared contrast-enhanced to nonenhanced PET/CT in a large group of cancer patients that also included some who had lymphoma. The CT protocol included standard multiphase acquisitions: an arterial phase thorax and liver scan, a portal–venous abdomen and pelvis scan, and if necessary, a postcontrast liver scan. The authors reported a considerable impact of intravenous contrast CT, specifically in patients who had metabolically faint lesions; in addition, and as expected, lesion localization and staging were improved. Finally, patient management was affected in 21 of 52 patients (42.7%). These findings

suggest that contrast-enhanced PET/CT might be the preferred protocol in patients who have low-grade lymphoma in whom lesions frequently exhibit low or faint FDG uptake.

The number of lymphoma patients in whom potential benefits of intravenous contrast administration have been evaluated systematically is still too low to permit firm conclusions. Several arguments, however, can be made for the use of oral and intravenous contrast with PET/CT. First, contrast enhancement is the current standard of care in CT imaging. Moreover, most lymphoma patients who receive a non-contrast-enhanced PET/CT will be referred for a separate additional contrast CT study, which adds to the radiation burden, the time spent in imaging clinics, and the complexity of image interpretation. For these reasons, the authors suggest performing PET/CT after oral and during intravenous contrast enhancement unless there are medical contraindications (**Fig. 4**).

Intravenous and oral contrast material (and metallic material) is dense, resulting in overcorrection for photon attenuation[34–36] in tissues, which in turn results in artificially increased FDG uptake, referred to as pseudo-FDG uptake. Clinically, however, this does not represent a significant problem. First, the origins of contrast-induced artifacts frequently are identified by blending PET and CT images. Secondly, in cases of ambiguity, nonattenuation-corrected images, which in case of artifact do not demonstrate increased uptake, are readily available for inspection.

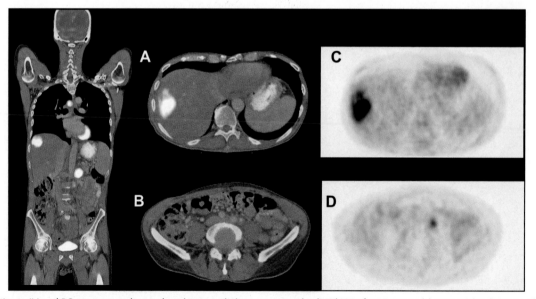

**Fig. 4.** IV and PO contrast-enhanced positron emission tomography (PET)/CT of a 55-year-old man with a history of anaplastic non-Hodgkin lymphoma. Selected fused PET and axial slices demonstrate liver involvement (*A, C*) and retroperitoneal adenopathy difficult to distinguish from ureteral activity without intravenous contrast (*C, D*).

## ARTIFACTS, PITFALLS, AND POTENTIALLY FALSE-POSITIVE STUDIES

Nonmalignant conditions such as inflammation, infection, and granulomatous eg, sarcoidosis[37,38] and physiologic FDG uptake such as in brown adipose tissue,[39] activated muscle (**Fig. 5**), or hyperplasia of the thymus[40] can cause focally increased FDG uptake, and potentially lead to false-positive studies. Similarly, abnormal FDG uptake has been associated with hyperplasia in the bone marrow and spleen after chemotherapy or in patients receiving granulocyte colony-stimulating factor after chemotherapy.[41] Conversely false-negative PET scans usually result from lesions below the resolution of the scanner, generally 5 to 10 mm.

## GLUCOSE METABOLIC ACTIVITY VARIES AMONG DIFFERENT TYPES OF NON-HODGKIN LYMPHOMA

Lymphomas differ with regard to their glucose metabolic activity. Systematic studies have shown that indolent lymphomas exhibit lower glucose metabolic activity and hence FDG uptake than the more aggressive ones.[42] For instance, diffuse large B-cell, and high-grade follicular lymphoma had, on average, threefold higher FDG SUVs than indolent lymphomas such as low grade follicular, lymphocytic–plasmocytic, mantle cell, marginal zone, or small cell lymphoma.[43]

These differences in glucose metabolic activity are explained among other factors by differing proliferative activities among lymphoma types and likely account for their variable detection rates as reported in the literature.[43,44]

The variability in glycolytic activity and FDG uptake has implications for both staging of disease and treatment monitoring. For instance, when baseline FDG uptake is low, treatment-induced changes in FDG uptake are difficult to quantify. Nevertheless, there might be a role of FDG PET

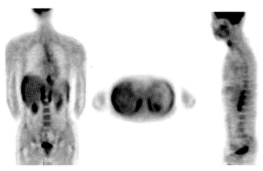

Fig. 5. Patient with chronic hiccups. Intense fluoro-deoxyglucose uptake throughout the muscle tissue of the diaphragm can be seen.

or PET/CT for staging and monitoring even in the few low-grade lymphomas with very low FDG uptake, since their transformation into high-grade lymphomas is associated with marked increases in glucose metabolic activity, which are detectable with PET.[45]

The staging accuracy of FDG PET is determined by the degree of FDG uptake in individual lesions. Because low-grade, indolent lymphomas grow more slowly than high-grade lymphomas, their energy requirements are lower, and consequently, their FDG uptake also would be expected to be lower. Nevertheless, not only high-grade, but also most low-grade lymphomas can be staged accurately with FDG PET (**Fig. 6**).

Limitations, however, do exist. For instance, Jerusalem and colleagues[46] demonstrated that in contrast to low-grade follicular lymphoma, small lymphocytic lymphomas were staged more successfully with CT than with FDG PET. No semi-quantitative analysis by means of SUV was performed in their study. Lower detection rates (sensitivity of 67%) of FDG PET in marginal zone lymphoma (MALT) and peripheral T cell lymphoma (sensitivity of 40%) have been reported by others.[43] No semiquantitative analysis, however, was available in this report.

T cell lymphomas are frequently primarily extra-nodal or involve extranodal sites. Limited experience suggests that FDG PET may be useful in primary extranodal T cell lymphomas such as enteropathy-associated T cell lymphoma (EATCL) and cutaneous T cell lymphomas such as mycosis fungoides.[47,48] Newer studies[49] suggest a higher rate of FDG-positive T cell lymphoma (**Table 1**), and standardized uptake values in T cell lymphoma show a wide range. Some T cell lymphomas are weakly FDG PET avid.

In another retrospective study,[50] the follicular, nontransformed type had a significantly higher SUV (7.7+-4.6) than marginal zone tumors (3.8, +- 1.3), or small lymphocytic lymphoma/chronic lymphocytic lymphoma type (2.5+- 0.7). Perry and colleagues[51] evaluated FDG uptake in 33 patients with extra-nodal MALT lymphoma. While overall disease detection was low at around 55% detectability was site and grade dependent. For instance, gastric MALT was detected in less than 40% of the patients while lung involvement was correctly identified in 5/5 patients. FDG PET correctly detected disease in all seven patients who had stage 3 or 4 disease, while sensitivity dropped to 42% in patients who had stage 1 or 2 MALT. Similar observations of site and grade dependency were made by others.[52]

The notion that follicular lymphoma of any grade can be staged reliably with FDG PET was

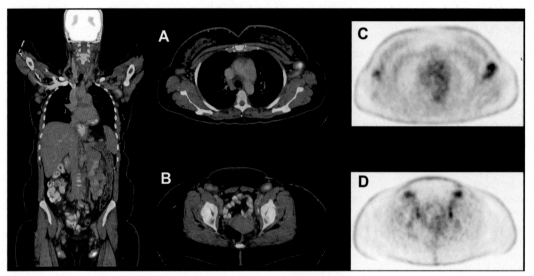

**Fig. 6.** 48-year-old woman with a history of cutaneous T cell lymphoma. Despite this being a low-grade lymphoma, selected fused and PET and axial slices demonstrate significant FDG uptake in axillary (*A, C*) and inguinal (*B, C*) adenopathy. Increased FDG uptake in the skin, best seen on the PET images (*C, D*), reflects cutaneous lymphomatous involvement.

confirmed by Wohrer and colleagues[53] in a study of 64 patients with grade 1 through 3 disease. There was only a trend toward higher maximum SUV (SUVmax) in aggressive versus indolent lymphoma (median SUVmax: 11.4 versus 5.7; *P* = .085).

In a more recent study, the SUVmax varied substantially among different lymphoma types and ranged from 3.2 in diffuse small-cleaved lymphoma to 43.0 in recurrent diffuse large B cell lymphoma.[42] Aggressive lymphomas (n = 63) had on average a three times higher SUVmax than indolent lymphoma (n = 28; *P*<.01). Using an SUV of 10 as a cutoff, FDG PET separated aggressive from indolent lymphoma with a sensitivity of 71% and a specificity of 81%.

Another study in low-grade follicular lymphoma[54] reported SUVmax that ranged from 5.2 to 8.1. Grades 1 and 2 follicular lymphomas appeared to have a comparable SUVmax, again suggesting that low-grade follicular lymphoma can be imaged with FDG PET.

| Table 1 | |
|---|---|
| **Fluorodeoxyglucose uptake of selected lymphoma** | |
| Diffuse large B-cell lymphoma | Moderate to high |
| Follicular lymphoma | Low to moderate |
| Mantle cell lymphoma | Low to high |
| T cell lymphoma | Low to high[a] |
| Marginal zone lymphoma (including MALT lymphoma) | None to high[b] |
| Small lymphocytic lymphoma of chronic lymphocytic lymphoma type | Low to moderate |
| Hodgkin lymphoma (classic form) | High |
| Hodgkin lymphoma (nodular lymphocyte predominant) | Moderate |

Please note that there is a significant range for the reported standardized uptake values (SUV)max in patients with similar lymphoma.
[a] Despite high positive rates of peripheral T cell lymphoma, fluorodeoxyglucose (FDG)–positron emission tomography results in a change of stage in a small number of patients (many patients are stage 4 by conventional modalities). Includes: peripheral T-cell lymphoma, NOS, mycosis fungoides, angioimmunoblastic T cell lymphoma, adult T-cell/human T-lymphotropic virus-1 associated lymphoma, NK/T-cell nasal-type lymphoma, anaplastic large-cell lymphoma, and others.
[b] Approximately 35% of marginal zone lymphomas have no FDG uptake. One publication[52] showed SUV as low as 1.4 but also high as 26.

## FLUORODEOXYGLUCOSE UPTAKE IN HODGKIN LYMPHOMA

Since the cytologic and immunochemical atypical cells (Reed-Sternberg cells and variants) may represent 1% to 3% of the tumor bulk, PET activity in classical HL almost exclusively reflects the reactive microenvironment (lymphoid hyperplasia) within which the malignant cells are found, rather than the neoplastic population itself. This is in contrast to NHLs, where, with few exceptions, most of the tumor bulk consists of neoplastic cells.

Few studies have examined differences among glucose metabolism of the different histopathologic subtypes of HL. These include classical HL (nodular sclerosing, mixed cellularity, lymphocyte rich, and lymphocyte depleted) as well as the non-classical nodular lymphocyte-predominant HL, an entity that behaves and is being treated more like a low-grade NHL.

Döbert and colleagues[55] reported SUVmax values of 5.2 for the nodular sclerosing, 3 for the mixed cellularity, and 2.6 for the nodular lymphocyte-predominant subgroup (a nonclassical HL). In this group of 44 patients who had HL, tumor FDG uptake did not seem to be affected significantly by the histopathological subtype. The number of patients, however, was too small for a reliable statistical analysis. A more recent prospective study by Hutchings and colleagues[56] studied FDG uptake in 60 patients who had newly diagnosed HL. Contrary to Dobert and colleagues, SUVmax of the different subtypes differed significantly and ranged from 8.3 in nodular lymphocyte-predominant HL up to 14.6 in the mixed cellularity subtype.

Differences in SUVs among studies likely are explained by differences in image acquisition protocols, region of interest (ROI) approaches, and differences in imaging equipment. This emphasizes the need for standardization of image acquisition and interpretation approaches across institutions.

## THE ROLE OF POSITRON EMISSION TOMOGRAPHY AND POSITRON EMISSION TOMOGRAPHY/CT IMAGING IN STAGING OF LYMPHOMA

Lymphoma is a tissue biopsy-based diagnosis. Once established, the assumption that most (if not all) enlarged lymph nodes and most (if not all) extranodal lesions are lymphoma involved is reasonable. Therefore, CT-based initial staging has remained the mainstay of the noninvasive diagnostic workup. On the other hand, because all lymphoma patients who have potentially curable disease undergo chemotherapy or chemo/radiation treatment, and FDG PET is far superior to CT for treatment monitoring and response assessment, a baseline PET/CT scan represents a more rational initial staging approach.

The Ann Arbor Staging[57] accounts for number of tumor sites (nodal and extra-nodal), location, and the presence or absence of systemic ("B") symptoms. The disease stage has considerable impact on treatment. For example stage I follicular lymphoma is treated with local radiation only, and systemic therapy is reserved for higher stages of disease[58] The majority of patients with aggressive lymphomas have advanced stage disease (ie, stage 4) at presentation. There appear to be limited therapeutic consequences from distinguishing stage 3 from stage 4 disease in NHL, because treatment options are nearly identical. In HL the stage also dictates the appropriate treatment.[59]

Several studies have suggested a superior staging accuracy of PET when compared with CT[60] as also listed in **Table 2**.[30,61–65] The consequence is a significant upward stage migration of patients who have HL and NHL.[66] This stage migration effect has the potential to improve reported patient outcomes in both the lower stage and the higher stage patient populations, independent of treatment program.

In addition, given that lymphoma is treatable and curable, and several lines of treatment are available, the imaging modality that allows not only for staging but also for treatment monitoring should be selected. Other arguments for using FDG-PET/CT as the primary staging modality include: its ability to assess bone marrow involvement, andits relatively low radiation dose when compared with diagnostic CT or with PET and CT interpreted side by side. As discussed previously, limitations include its inability to stage some of the less FDG-avid lymphomas[42,43] and its limited spatial resolution.

Functional imaging in lymphoma was provided for a long time by whole-body Ga-67 imaging. An early study in aggressive NHL and HL[67] reported significantly higher site and patient sensitivity for FDG PET than Ga-67 scintigraphy (100% versus 71.5% and 100% versus 80.3%, respectively). In a more recent and apparently prospective study, Tsukamoto and colleagues[64] compared in 191 of 222 lymphoma patients the staging accuracy of FDG PET to that of Ga-67 imaging (see **Table 2**). FDG PET was superior to Ga imaging for follicular lymphoma, for mantle cell lymphoma, and for the nasal type of natural killer/T cell lymphoma. Although this study had limitations (ie, lack of true gold standard and reference standard of limited value) it still strongly underscores the usefulness

Table 2
Staging accuracy of PET versus CT and gallium

| Author | Year | Type | Indication | N | PET | | | CT[a] or Gallium[b] | | | | p value |
|---|---|---|---|---|---|---|---|---|---|---|---|---|
| | | | | | Sens | Spec | Acc | Sens | Spec | Acc | | |
| Wirth[63] | 2002 | NHL/HD | ST/RST | 50 | 82 | — | — | 69[b] | — | — | | 0.01 |
| Kostakoglu[61] | 2002 | NHL/HD | ST/RST | 51 | 100 | — | — | 81[b] | — | — | | Not reported |
| Freudenberg[30] | 2004 | NHL/HD | RST | 27 | 96 (PET/CT) | 99 | 98 | 61[a] | 89 | 84 | | 0.005 (Sens) 0.003 (Spec) |
| La Fougre[62] | 2006 | NHL/HD | ST/RST | 50 | 98 | 99 | — | 87[a] | 80 | — | | Not reported |
| Tsukamoto[64] | 2007 | NHL/HD | ST/RST | 191 | 90.5 | — | — | 56.7[b] | — | — | | Not reported |
| Nogami[65] | 2007 | NHL | RST | 50 | 86.1 | 99.4 | 91 | 59.4[a] | 96.1 | 91 | | <.001 |

Abbreviations: Acc, Accuracy; HD, Hodgkin disease; N, number of patients; NHL, non-Hodgkin lymphoma; PET, positron emission tomography; RST, restaging; Sens, sensitivity; Spec, specificity; ST, staging.
[a] Versus CT
[b] Versus Gallium

of PET imaging for staging of a range of lymphoma types and its superiority over Ga imaging.

## EVALUATION OF BONE MARROW INVOLVEMENT

One important aspect of staging is the evaluation of bone marrow involvement.[68] In a prospective study the accuracy of PET/CT, bone marrow biopsy and MRI for detecting marrow involvement was compared in 47 patients with aggressive, most frequently diffuse large B-cell lymphoma. Both MRI and PET/CT identified 9 patients with bone marrow involvement while bone marrow aspiration identified only two patients. It seems likely that the noninvasively identified lesions truly represented areas of marrow involvement since all disappeared or had markedly reduced FDG uptake halfway through or at the end of treatment. No image-guided biopsies were performed to confirm this finding, however.

Using stringent inclusion criteria for a meta-analysis, Pakos and colleagues[69] identified 13 appropriate studies that enrolled a total of 587 patients. The sensitivity rates of 18F-FDG PET for identifying lymphomatous bone marrow involvement ranged from 0% to 100% across the studies with specificities ranging from 72% to 100%. When all patients were lumped, the sensitivity and specificity of FDG PET for identifying bone marrow involvement were 51% and 91%.

These results clearly indicate that PET alone is not sufficient to replace biopsy for bone marrow staging. FDG PET, however, could provide valuable information in patients with heterogeneous bone marrow involvement, in whom biopsy sampling errors can occur. For instance, in six patients, all of whom had negative bone marrow biopsies, FDG PET revealed focal bone marrow infiltrates.[70]

## IMPACT OF FLUORODEOXYGLUCOSE POSITRON EMISSION TOMOGRAPHY ON DISEASE MANAGEMENT

Patient prognosis depends upon histopathology and clinical parameters that are used to calculate disease-specific prognostic indices (international prognostic index, Follicular Lymphoma International Prognostic Index[71]). Because stage usually depends upon the location and number of disease sites, it is not a true measure of tumor burden. Staging is an important prognostic determinant in NHL, and it affects the overall therapeutic strategy. It is performed to identify the small number of patients with early stage disease who can be treated with local therapy or combined modality treatment; it is also useful to stratify within histologic subtypes to determine prognosis and identify the best treatment approach.

**Table 3**
**Impact of fluorodeoxyglucose –positron emission tomography on patient management**

| Author/# | Year | Type | Indication | N | R/P | Δ Stage (%) | Δ Management (%) |
|----------|------|------|-----------|---|-----|-------------|------------------|
| Montravers[72] | 2002 | Pediatric HD/NHL | ST/RST | 12 | R | 50 | 23 |
| Depas[73] | 2004 | Pediatric HD/NHL | ST | 19 | R | 10.5 | 10.5 |
| Hermann[74] | 2005 | Pediatric HD/NHL | ST | 25 | R | 24 | NA |
| Shah[75] | 2000 | HD/NHL | ST | 29 | R | — | 31 |
| Schöder[76] | 2002 | HD/NHL | ST/RST Monitoring | 52 | P | 44 | 42 |
| Sasaki[77] | 2002 | NHL | ST | 42 | R | NA | 17 |
| Talbot[78] | 2002 | HD/NHL | ST/RST | 43 | P | 43 | 39 |
| Naumann[79] | 2004 | HD | ST | 88 | P | 20 | 18[a] |
| Raannani[29] | 2005 | HD/NHL | ST | 103 | R | 36 | 45 |
| Hutchings[56] | 2006 | HD | Radiation Planning | 30 | P | — | 33 8 |
| Rigacci[80] | 2007 | HD | ST | 186 | P | 16 | NA |
| Hernandez[81] | 2006 | HD/NHL | ST | 47 | P | 23 | 15 |

*Abbreviations:* HD, Hodgkin disease; N, number of patients; NHL, non-Hodgkin lymphoma; RST, restaging; ST, staging.
[a] Potential management change; R/P, Retrospective/Prospective.

The impact of FDG PET imaging on patient management has been investigated by several groups (**Table 3**).[29,56,72–81] In a simple questionnaire study[76] comparable in design to the current National Outpatient PET Registry (NOPR) study,[82] referring physicians were asked among others to indicate: patient stage and intended management before PET, and changes in stage and management following PET. The response rate was only around 50% in this study. The completed questionnaires, however, revealed a substantial impact of FDG PET on stage and patient management that was affected in 39% of patients who had HL and 44% of those who had NHL.

The impact of FDG PET staging on patient management ranged from 8 to 45% in other prospective and retrospective studies (see **Table 3**). It tended to be lower in three studies that were conducted in pediatric patients (ranging from 10%–23%)[72–74] when compared with the adults in which FDG-PET affected treatment decisions in 8%–45% of the patients.[29,56,75–81]

A recent prospective multicentric study by Rigacci and colleagues[80] investigated the contribution of PET scanning to the staging of HL by CT and attempted to determine whether it has any impact on the therapeutic approach. Out of 186 patients, six consecutive patients who had HL from six Italian centers, PET stage in comparison with CT stage was higher in 27 patients (14%) and lower in 3 patients (1%). PET scanning upstaged 10 patients (8%) from localized to advanced disease and resulted in a change of treatment plan. FDG PET was shown to be a relevant, noninvasive method that supplements conventional procedures and therefore should be used routinely to stage HL, particularly in early stage patients, where a change in stage may modify disease management.

The impact of FDG PET staging on patient management ranged from 8% to 45% in other prospective and retrospective studies (see **Table 3**). It tended to be lower in three studies that were conducted in pediatric patients[72–74] (ranging from 10% to 23%) when compared with the adults in whom FDG-PET affected treatment decisions in 8% to 45% of the patients.

## TREATMENT RESPONSE ASSESSMENT

Many studies have reported the prognostic significance of changes in glucose metabolic activity in response to treatment.[83–88] The value of PET for monitoring of treatment is reflected in the recently published guidelines of the International Harmonization Project.[9,89] Please refer to the articles by Schoeder and Cheson in this issue, which discuss this topic in detail.

## SUMMARY

Fully diagnostic PET/CT scans acquired during oral and intravenous contrast can be provided to patients and referring physicians in a single imaging session. Although FDG uptake varies, most low-grade lymphomas exhibit sufficient FDG avidity to also be staged reliably with FDG PET/CT.

PET/CT imaging is more accurate for lymphoma staging than PET or CT alone and has substantial impact on patient management. This accurate whole-body glucose metabolic survey should serve as the baseline for subsequent treatment response evaluations. PET/CT has evolved to become the modality of choice for staging of nodal and extranodal lymphoma, for assessing therapeutic response, and for establishing patient prognosis.

## REFERENCES

1. Beyer T, Townsend DW, Brun T, et al. A combined PET/CT scanner for clinical oncology. J Nucl Med 2000;41(8):1369–79.
2. Czernin J, Allen-Auerbach M, Schelbert HR. Improvements in cancer staging with PET/CT: literature-based evidence as of September 2006. J Nucl Med 2007;48(Suppl 1):78S–88S.
3. Moertel C, Hanley J. The effect of measuring error on the results of therapeutic trials in advanced cancer. Cancer 1976;38:388–94.
4. Evilevitch V, Weber WA, Tap WD, et al. Reduction of glucose metabolic activity is more accurate than change in size at predicting histopathologic response to neoadjuvant therapy in high-grade soft-tissue sarcomas. Clin Cancer Res 2008;14(3):715–20.
5. Seam P, Juweid ME, Cheson BD. The role of FDG-PET scans in patients with lymphoma. Blood 2007;110(10):3507–16.
6. Jerusalem G, Hustinx R, Beguin Y, et al. Evaluation of therapy for lymphoma. Semin Nucl Med 2005;35(3):186–96.
7. Kasamon YL, Jones RJ, Wahl RL. Integrating PET and PET/CT into the risk-adapted therapy of lymphoma. J Nucl Med 2007;58(Suppl 1):19S–27S.
8. Cheson BD, Pfistner B, Juweid ME, et al. Revised response criteria for malignant lymphoma. J Clin Oncol 2007;25(5):579–86.
9. Juweid ME, Stroobants S, Hoekstra OS, et al. Use of positron emission tomography for response assessment of lymphoma: consensus of the Imaging Subcommittee of International Harmonization Project in Lymphoma. J Clin Oncol 2007;25(5):571–8.

10. Warburg O, Posener K, Negelein E. VIII. The metabolism of cancer cells. Biochem Z 1924;152:129–69.

11. Phelps M. Positron emission tomography provides molecular imaging of biological processes. Proc Natl Acad Sci U S A 2000;97(16):9226–33.

12. Czernin J, Phelps ME. Positron emission tomography scanning: current and future applications. Annu Rev Med 2002;53:89–112.

13. Flier J, Mueckler M, McCall A, et al. Distribution of glucose transporter messenger RNA transcripts in tissues of rat and man. J Clin Invest 1987;79: 657–61.

14. Phelps M, Hoffmann E, Mullani N, et al. Application of annihilation coincidence detection to transaxial reconstruction tomography. J Nucl Med 1975;16: 210–24.

15. Czernin J. PET/CT: imaging function and structure. J Nucl Med 2004;45(Suppl):1S–103S.

16. Huang S-C. Anatomy of SUV. Nucl Med Biol 2000; 27(7):643–6.

17. Weber W, Ziegler S, Thodtmann R, et al. Reproducibility of metabolic measurements in malignant tumors using FDG PET. J Nucl Med 1999;40:1771–7.

18. Czernin J, Phelps ME. Positron emission tomography scanning: current and future applications. Molecular Genetics and Metabolism 2002;53:89–112.

19. Czernin J, Schelbert HR. Introduction. J Nucl Med 2007;48:2S–3S.

20. Halpern B, Dahlbom M, Quon A, et al. Impact of patient weight and emission scan duration on PET/CT image quality and lesion detectability. J Nucl Med 2004;45:797–801.

21. Halpern BS, Dahlbom M, Auerbach MA, et al. Optimizing imaging protocols for overweight and obese patients: a lutetium orthosilicate PET/CT study. J Nucl Med 2005;46(4):603–7.

22. Tatsumi M, Cohade C, Nakamoto Y, et al. Direct comparison of FDG PET and CT findings in patients with lymphoma: initial experience. Radiology 2005; 237(3):1038–45.

23. Lardinois D, Weder W, Hany T, et al. Staging of non-small cell lung cancer with integrated positron emission tomography and computed tomography. N Engl J Med 2003;348:2500–7.

24. Allen-Auerbach M, Quon A, Weber WA, et al. Comparison between 2-deoxy-2-[18F]fluoro-D-glucose positron emission tomography and positron emission tomography/computed tomography hardware fusion for staging of patients with lymphoma. Mol Imaging Biol 2004;6(6):411–6.

25. Freudenberg L, Antoch G, Mueller S, et al. Whole-body FDG-PET/CT in restaging of lymphoma. J Nucl Med 2003;44(Suppl 5):83P.

26. Veit-Haibach P, Luczak C, Wanke I, et al. TNM staging with FDG-PET/CT in patients with primary head and neck cancer. Eur J Nucl Med Mol Imaging 2007;34(12):1953–62.

27. Veit-Haibach P, Antoch G, Beyer T, et al. FDG-PET/CT in restaging of patients with recurrent breast cancer: possible impact on staging and therapy. Br J Radiol 2007;80(955):508–15.

28. Barentsz J, Takahashi S, Oyen W, et al. Commonly used imaging techniques for diagnosis and staging. J Clin Oncol 2006;24(20):3234–44.

29. Raanani P, Shasha Y, Perry C, et al. Is CT scan still necessary for staging in Hodgkin and non-Hodgkin lymphoma patients in the PET/CT era? Ann Oncol 2006;17(1):117–22.

30. Freudenberg LS, Antoch G, Schutt P, et al. FDG-PET/CT in restaging of patients with lymphoma. Eur J Nucl Med Mol Imaging 2004;31(3):325–9.

31. Schaefer NG, Hany TF, Taverna C, et al. Non-Hodgkin lymphoma and Hodgkin disease: coregistered FDG PET and CT at staging and restaging—do we need contrast-enhanced CT? Radiology 2004;232(3): 823–9.

32. Morimoto T, Tateishi U, Maeda T, et al. Nodal status of malignant lymphoma in pelvic and retroperitoneal lymphatic pathways: comparison of integrated PET/CT with or without contrast enhancement. Eur J Radiol 2007; [epub ahead of print].

33. Pfannenberg AC, Aschoff P, Brechtel K, et al. Value of contrast-enhanced multiphase CT in combined PET/CT protocols for oncological imaging. Br J Radiol 2007;80(954):437–45.

34. Kinahan P, Townsend D, Beyer T, et al. Attenuation correction for a combined 3D PET/CT scanner. Med Phys 1998;25:2046–53.

35. Cohade C, Osman M, Nakamoto Y, et al. Initial experience with oral contrast in PET/CT: phantom and clinical studies. J Nucl Med 2003;44(3):412–6.

36. Halpern BS, Dahlbom M, Waldherr C, et al. Cardiac pacemakers and central venous lines can induce focal artifacts on CT-corrected PET images. J Nucl Med 2004;45(2):290–3.

37. de Hemricourt E, De Boeck K, Hilte F, et al. Sarcoidosis and sarcoid-like reaction following Hodgkin's disease. Report of two cases. Mol Imaging Biol 2003;5(1):15–9.

38. Hollister D Jr, Lee MS, Eisen RN, et al. Variable problems in lymphomas: CASE 2. Sarcoidosis mimicking progressive lymphoma. J Clin Oncol 2005;23(31): 8113–6.

39. Yeung HW, Grewal RK, Gonen M, et al. Patterns of (18)F-FDG uptake in adipose tissue and muscle: a potential source of false-positives for PET. J Nucl Med 2003;44(11):1789–96.

40. Sugawara Y, Fisher SJ, Zasadny KR, et al. Preclinical and clinical studies of bone marrow uptake of fluorine-1-fluorodeoxyglucose with or without granulocyte colony-stimulating factor during chemotherapy. J Clin Oncol 1998;16(1):173–80.

41. Sugawara Y, Zasadny KR, Kison PV, et al. Splenic fluorodeoxyglucose uptake increased by granulocyte

colony-stimulating factor therapy: PET imaging results. J Nucl Med 1999;40(9):1456–62.

42. Schoder H, Noy A, Gonen M, et al. Intensity of 18fluorodeoxyglucose uptake in positron emission tomography distinguishes between indolent and aggressive non-Hodgkin's lymphoma. J Clin Oncol 2005;23(21):4643–51.

43. Elstrom R, Guan L, Baker G, et al. Utility of FDG-PET scanning in lymphoma by WHO classification. Blood 2003;101(10):3875–6.

44. Jerusalem G, Beguin Y, Najjar F, et al. Positron emission tomography (PET) with 18F-fluorodeoxyglucose (18F-FDG) for the staging of low-grade non-Hodgkin's lymphoma (NHL). Ann Oncol 2001; 12(6):825–30.

45. Rodriguez M, Rehn S, Ahlstrom H, et al. Predicting malignancy grade with PET in non-Hodgkin's lymphoma. J Nucl Med 1995;36:1790–6.

46. Jerusalem G, Beguin Y, Najjar F, et al. Positron emission tomography (PET) with 18F-fluorodeoxyglucose (18F-FDG) for the staging of low-grade non-Hodgkin's lymphoma (NHL). Ann Oncol 2001;12:825–30.

47. Tsai EY, Taur A, Espinosa L, et al. Staging accuracy in mycosis fungoides and sezary syndrome using integrated positron emission tomography and computed tomography. Arch Dermatol 2006;142(5): 577–84.

48. Hadithi M, Mallant M, Oudejans J, et al. 18F-FDG PET versus CT for the detection of enteropathy-associated T cell lymphoma in refractory celiac disease. J Nucl Med 2006;47(10):1622–7.

49. Horwitz S, Foss F, Goldfarb S, et al. FDG-PET scans as a staging study for T cell lymphomas: high rates of positivity do not result in frequent changes in stage. Blood 2006;108(11):2399.

50. Karam M, Novak L, Cyriac J, et al. Role of fluorine-18 fluoro-deoxyglucose positron emission tomography scan in the evaluation and follow-up of patients with low-grade lymphomas. Cancer 2006;107:175–83.

51. Perry C, Herishanu Y, Metzer U, et al. Diagnostic accuracy of PET/CT in patients with extranodal marginal zone MALT lymphoma. Eur J Haematol 2007; 79(3):205–9.

52. Beal KP, Yeung HW, Yahalom J. FDG-PET scanning for detection and staging of extranodal marginal zone lymphomas of the MALT type: a report of 42 cases. Ann Oncol 2005;16(3):473–80.

53. Wohrer S, Jaeger U, Kletter K, et al. 18F-fluoro-deoxy-glucose positron emission tomography (18F-FDG-PET) visualizes follicular lymphoma irrespective of grading. Ann Oncol 2006;17(5):780–4.

54. Bishu S, Quigley J, Bishu S, et al. Predictive value and diagnostic accuracy of F-18-fluoro-deoxy-glucose positron emission tomography treated grade 1 and 2 follicular lymphoma. Leuk Lymphoma 2007;48:1548–55.

55. Döbert N, Menzel C, Berner U, et al. Positron emission tomography in patients with Hodgkin's disease: correlation to histopathologic subtypes. Cancer Biother Radiopharm 2003;18:565–71.

56. Hutchings M, Loft A, Hansen M, et al. Position emission tomography with or without computed tomography in the primary staging of Hodgkin's lymphoma. Haematologica 2006;91(4):482–9.

57. Carbone PP, Kaplan HS, Musshoff K, et al. Report of the Committee on Hodgkin's Disease Staging Classification. Cancer Res 1971;31(11):1860–1.

58. Ansell S, Armitage J. Non-Hodgkin lymphoma: diagnosis and treatment. Mayo Clin Proc 2005;80: 1087–97.

59. Diehl V, Fuchs M. Early, intermediate, and advanced Hodgkin's lymphoma: modern treatment strategies. Ann Oncol 2007;18(Suppl 9):ix71–9.

60. Hernandez-Maraver D, Hernandez-Navarro F, Gomez-Leon N, et al. Positron emission tomography/computed tomography: diagnostic accuracy in lymphoma. Br J Haematol 2006;135(3):293–302.

61. Kostakoglu L, Leonard J, Kuji I, et al. Comparison of fluorine-18 fluorodeoxyglucose positron emission tomography and Ga-67 scintigraphy in evaluation of lymphoma. Cancer 2002;94:879–88.

62. la Fougere C, Hundt W, Brockel N, et al. Value of PET/CT versus PET and CT performed as separate investigations in patients with Hodgkin's disease and non-Hodgkin's lymphoma. Eur J Nucl Med Mol Imaging 2006;33(12):1417–25.

63. Wirth A, Seymour JF, Hicks RJ, et al. Fluorine-18 fluorodeoxyglucose positron emission tomography, gallium-67 scintigraphy, and conventional staging for Hodgkin's disease and non-Hodgkin's lymphoma. Am J Med 2002;112(4):262–8.

64. Tsukamoto N, Kojima M, Hasegawa M, et al. The usefulness of (18)F-fluorodeoxyglucose positron emission tomography ([18]F-FDG-PET) and a comparison of (18)F-FDG-pet with (67)gallium scintigraphy in the evaluation of lymphoma: relation to histologic subtypes based on the World Health Organization classification. Cancer 2007;110(3): 652–9.

65. Nogami M, Nakamoto Y, Sakamoto S, et al. Diagnostic performance of CT, PET, side-by-side, and fused image interpretations for restaging of non-Hodgkin lymphoma. Ann Nucl Med 2007;21(4):189–96.

66. Hutchings M, Specht L. PET/CT in the management of haematological malignancies. Eur J Haematol 2008;80(5):369–80.

67. Kostakoglu L, Coleman M, Leonard JP, et al. PET predicts prognosis after 1 cycle of chemotherapy in aggressive lymphoma and Hodgkin's disease. J Nucl Med 2002;43(8):1018–27.

68. Ribrag V, Vanel D, Leboulleux S, et al. Prospective study of bone marrow infiltration in aggressive lymphoma by three independent methods: whole-body MRI,

PET/CT, and bone marrow biopsy. Eur J Radiol 2008; 66(2):325–31.

69. Pakos EE, Fotopoulos AD, Ioannidis JP. 18F-FDG PET for evaluation of bone marrow infiltration in staging of lymphoma: a meta-analysis. J Nucl Med 2005;46(6):958–63.

70. Kabickova E, Sumerauer D, Cumlivska E, et al. Comparison of 18F-FDG-PET and standard procedures for the pretreatment staging of children and adolescents with Hodgkin's disease. Eur J Nucl Med Mol Imaging 2006;33(9):1025–31.

71. Hasenclever D, Diehl V. A prognostic score for advanced Hodgkin's disease. International prognostic factors project on advanced Hodgkin's disease. N Engl J Med 1998;339(21):1506–14.

72. Montravers F, McNamara D, Landman-Parker J, et al. [18F]FDG in childhood lymphoma: clinical utility and impact on management. Eur J Nucl Med Mol Imaging 2002;29(9):1155–65.

73. Depas G, De Barsy C, Jerusalem G, et al. 18F-FDG PET in children with lymphomas. Eur J Nucl Med Mol Imaging 2005;32(1):31–8.

74. Hermann S, Wormanns D, Pixberg M, et al. Staging in childhood lymphoma: differences between FDG-PET and CT. Nuklearmedizin 2005;44:1–7.

75. Shah N, Hoskin P, McMillan A, et al. The impact of FDG positron emission tomography imaging on the management of lymphomas. Br J Radiol 2000; 73(869):482–7.

76. Schöder H, Meta J, Yap C, et al. Effect of whole-body 18 F-FDG PET imaging on clinical staging and management of patients with malignant lymphoma. J Nucl Med 2001;42:1139–43.

77. Sasaki M, Kuwabara Y, Koga H, et al. Clinical impact of whole body FDG-PET on the staging and therapeutic decision making for malignant lymphoma. Ann Nucl Med 2002;16:337–45.

78. Talbot J, Rain J, Meignan M, et al. Impact de la TEP au [18F]-FDG sur la décision médicale en cancérologie: évaluation par les prescripteurs durant la première année de fonctionnement. Bulletin du Cancer Radiotherapie 2002;89:313–21 [in French].

79. Naumann R, Beuthien-Baumann B, Rei A, et al. Substantial impact of FDG PET imaging on the therapy decision in patients with early-stage Hodgkin's lymphoma. Br J Cancer 2004;90:620–5.

80. Rigacci L, Vitolo U, Nassi L, et al. Positron emission tomography in the staging of patients with Hodgkin's lymphoma. A prospective multicentric study by the Intergruppo Italiano Linfomi. Ann Hematol 2007; 86(12):897–903.

81. Hernandez-Maraver D, Hernandez-Navarro F, Gomez-Leon N, et al. Positron emission tomography/computed tomography: diagnostic accuracy in lymphoma. 2006;135:293–302.

82. Hillner BE, Liu D, Coleman RE, et al. The National Oncologic PET Registry (NOPR): design and analysis plan. J Nucl Med 2007;48(11):1901–8.

83. Jerusalem G, Beguin Y, Fassotte MF, et al. Whole-body positron emission tomography using 18F-fluorodeoxyglucose for post-treatment evaluation in Hodgkin's disease and non-Hodgkin's lymphoma has higher diagnostic and prognostic value than classical computed tomography scan imaging. Blood 1999;94(2):429–33.

84. Spaepen K, Stroobants S, Dupont P, et al. Prognostic value of positron emission tomography (PET) with fluorine-18 fluorodeoxyglucose ([18F]FDG) after first-line chemotherapy in non-Hodgkin's lymphoma: is [18F]FDG-PET a valid alternative to conventional diagnostic methods? J Clin Oncol 2001;19(2):414–9.

85. Haioun C, Itti E, Rahmouni A, et al. [18F]fluoro-2-deoxy-D-glucose positron emission tomography (FDG-PET) in aggressive lymphoma: an early prognostic tool for predicting patient outcome. Blood 2005;106(4):1376–81.

86. Mikhaeel NG, Hutchings M, Fields PA, et al. FDG-PET after two to three cycles of chemotherapy predicts progression-free and overall survival in high-grade non-Hodgkin lymphoma. Ann Oncol 2005;16(9):1514–23.

87. Kostakoglu L, Goldsmith SJ, Leonard JP, et al. FDG-PET after 1 cycle of therapy predicts outcome in diffuse large cell lymphoma and classic Hodgkin disease. Cancer 2006;107(11):2678–87.

88. Gallamini A, Hutchings M, Rigacci L, et al. Early interim 2-[18F] fluoro-2-deoxy-D-glucose positron emission tomography is prognostically superior to international prognostic score in advanced-stage Hodgkin's lymphoma: a report from a joint Italian–Danish study. J Clin Oncol 2007;25(24): 3746–52.

89. Cheson BD. The international harmonization project for response criteria in lymphoma clinical trials. Hematol Oncol Clin North Am 2007;21(5): 841–54.

# New Staging and Response Criteria for Non-Hodgkin Lymphoma and Hodgkin Lymphoma

Bruce D. Cheson, MD

**KEYWORDS**
- Response criteria • Non-Hodgkin lymphoma
- Hodgkin lymphoma
- Positron emission tomography scan

Standardized methods for staging and response assessment are an integral component of clinical trials. In turn, clinical trials are essential to the development of new and more effective therapy for patients with lymphomas. In the absence of effective agents, response criteria are almost irrelevant. With the increasing number of effective therapies, however, standardized criteria are critical to reliably assess and compare them, and to provide a framework upon which regulatory agencies can assess the efficacy of such treatments.

Before 1999, considerable variability among clinical trials groups in how patients were evaluated impeded comparisons of study results. Response sometimes was assessed prospectively, other times retrospectively, with disparity as to the size of a normal lymph node. The importance of standardization was emphasized by an analysis of data from the rituximab pivotal trial in which minor differences in the definition of a normal-sized lymph node resulted in major differences in the percentage of patients considered to have attained a complete remission.[1] To address these issues, an international working group (IWG) composed of clinicians, radiologists, and pathologists with expertise in the evaluation and management of patients with lymphoma developed guidelines that standardized the size of a normal lymph node, when and how responses were assessed, and response category and endpoint definitions.[2]

These recommendations were adopted widely by clinical trials groups and regulatory agencies.

With their application over time, however, it became clear that revisions were indicated. For example, the IWG criteria relied on physical examination, with its marked inter- and intraobserver variability, CT scans, and single photon emission computed tomography (SPECT) gallium scans, the latter no longer being used widely.

A major problem with the original IWG criteria was the misinterpretation of the term complete remission/unconfirmed (CRu). CRu originally was proposed to designate two types of responses. The first responses were in those patients who had curable histologies, such as Hodgkin lymphoma or diffuse large B-cell lymphoma, who had lymphadenopathy that included a large mass before therapy and for whom treatment resulted in a disappearance of all detectable tumor except for persistence of that mass, which had decreased by at least 75% on CT scan. In as many as 90% of cases, these lesions are scar tissue or fibrosis rather than active tumor.[3,4] Instead, CRu often was applied to situations in which the sum of the product of the diameters (SPD) of multiple nodes decreased by at least 75%, even in patients who had incurable histologies, which more appropriately would be considered partial responses. One consequence has been an artificial inflation of complete remission (CR) rates. The second type of CRu included patients with bone marrow involvement before treatment who fulfilled all of the conditions for a CR following therapy except that the bone marrow was considered by the

Georgetown University Hospital, Lombardi Comprehensive Cancer Center, 3800 Reservoir Road Northwest, Washington, DC 20007, USA
*E-mail address:* bdc4@georgetown.edu

Radiol Clin N Am 46 (2008) 213–223
doi:10.1016/j.rcl.2008.03.003
0033-8389/08/$ – see front matter © 2008 Elsevier Inc. All rights reserved.

pathologist to be morphologically indeterminate. Instead, the term also was assigned to patients who did not undergo a repeat biopsy to confirm response.

The increasing availability of fluorodeoxyglucose (FDG) positron emission tomography (PET) resulted in a major shift in lymphoma patient management. PET has been proposed for diagnosis, where it is not useful because of a lack of specificity, staging, prognosis, directing therapy, restaging, and post-treatment surveillance.[5-28]

Pretreatment staging determines the extent of disease and helps direct therapy. The Ann Arbor system that is used most commonly initially was designed to distinguish patients who might be candidates for radiation therapy from those who would benefit from systemic treatment.[29] Traditionally, the Ann Arbor staging system was based on physical examination and bone marrow evaluation, but CT scans subsequently have been incorporated. Whether PET should be incorporated into the Ann Arbor staging system is controversial. PET is highly sensitive in detecting nodal and extranodal involvement by most histologic subtypes of lymphoma and may provide complementary information to conventional staging methods, such as CT and bone marrow biopsy.[5,9,11,12,17,22,30-40]

Most common types of lymphoma (eg, diffuse large B-cell non-Hodgkin lymphoma [NHL], follicular NHL, mantle cell NHL, Hodgkin lymphoma [HL]) are routinely FDG-avid with a sensitivity that exceeds 80% and a specificity of about 90%, which is superior to CT.[30,31,34] PET and CT are 80% to 90% concordant in staging of patients who have diffuse large B-cell lymphoma, follicular lymphoma, and mantle cell lymphoma.[11,34] In those patients who have discordant results, PET typically results in upstaging because of the additional presumed sites of nodal, hepatic, or splenic disease. In contrast, concordance of PET and CT in determining clinical stage occurs in only about 60% to 80% of patients who have Hodgkin lymphoma. Discordant findings occur with a comparable frequency in both directions.[5,9,17,22,36-38] Although PET identifies more lesions than CT, PET alone cannot replace CT for pretreatment staging.[5,9,17,37]

In a meta-analysis of FDG PET in staging of patients who had lymphoma,[40] the pooled sensitivity for 14 studies with patient-based data was 90.9% (95% CI, 88.0 to 93.4) with a false-positive rate of 10.3% (95% CI, 7.4 to 13.8). The maximum joint sensitivity and specificity were 87.8% (95% CI, 85.0 to 90.7) with an apparently higher sensitivity and false-positive rate in patients who had HL compared with NHL. The pooled sensitivity for seven studies with lesion-based data was 95.6% (95% CI, 93.9 to 97.0), with a false-positive rate of only 1.0% (95% CI, 0.6 to 1.3). The maximum sensitivity and specificity were 95.6% (95% CI, 93.1 to 98.1). Thus, PET detects more occult lymphomatous sites than contrast-enhanced CT and bone marrow biopsy.[11,17,22,33,34,39,41]

PET can detect bone or bone marrow involvement in lymphoma patients with a negative iliac crest bone marrow biopsy, confirmed by histopathology or MRI.[41-43] PET alone is unreliable in detecting limited bone marrow involvement.[43] In patients with extensive bone/bone marrow involvement by PET, the bone marrow biopsy is typically positive. Diffusely increased bone marrow uptake on PET may also be due to reactive myeloid hyperplasia, such as with the use of myeloid growth factors.[42] PET-positive bone/bone marrow findings should be confirmed by biopsy or MR imaging if a change in treatment will be based on these findings. Thus, PET cannot substitute for bone marrow biopsy in lymphoma staging.

Despite its superior sensitivity and specificity compared with CT, PET is currently not part of standard lymphoma staging, primarily because of its expense and the generally small percentage of patients (approximately 15% to 20%) in whom PET detects additional disease sites that modify clinical stage, and even fewer patients (approximately 10% to 15%) for whom this modification alters management or outcome.[12,34,44]

PET/CT offers important advantages compared with contrast-enhanced, full-dose diagnostic CT or PET alone. PET/CT performed even without intravenous contrast (unenhanced PET/CT) with the CT portion typically acquired as low-dose CT (40 to 80 mAs) is more sensitive and specific than contrast-enhanced full-dose CT for evaluation of nodal and extranodal lymphomatous involvement.[39,45,46] Schaefer and colleagues[39] reported that the sensitivity of PET/CT and contrast-enhanced CT for lymph node involvement in patients who had HL or high-grade NHL was 94% and 88%, while the specificity was 100% and 86%, respectively. For organ involvement, the sensitivity of PET/CT and contrast-enhanced CT was 88% and 50%, while the specificity was 100% and 90%, respectively. Tatsumi and colleagues[46] evaluated 1537 anatomic sites in 20 patients who had HL and 33 patients who had NHL on an unenhanced low-dose PET/CT scanner. There were 1489 sites concordant between PET and CT, and among the 48 discordant sites, PET correctly identified 40 sites as true positives or true negatives by biopsy or clinical follow-up.

The CT portion of the PET/CT examination for initial staging using intravenous contrast may permit a more accurate assessment of the liver and spleen compared with unenhanced CT.[26] A recently published study showed no significant difference between the typically acquired unenhanced low-dose PET/CT (80 mAs) and a contrast-enhanced full-dose PET/CT acquired with up to 300 mAs in the assessment of nodal and extranodal lymphoma at initial staging.[44] The enhanced full-dose PET/CT, however, resulted in fewer indeterminate findings and identified a larger number of extranodal sites compared with the unenhanced, low-dose PET/CT. The authors attributed this slight advantage to the use of intravenous contrast rather than the use of high-dose radiograph. In aggregate, the published data suggest that enhanced low-dose PET/CT may represent a reasonable choice as a single imaging modality for staging routinely FDG-avid lymphomas. The increased radiation associated with PET would be offset, in part, by the reduced radiation dose associated with the low- compared with full-dose CT.

PET/CT may be of particular value before therapy for patients who appear to have stage 1 or 2 disease and for whom radiation therapy is being considered (**Fig. 1**). Additional sites of involvement would result in altering the treatment to systemic therapy. Thus, although PET may identify additional lesions during staging, prospective trials are needed to document an impact on patient outcome.

In a recent systematic review, Kwee and colleagues[47] evaluated the role of CT and FDG PET in staging of lymphomas. Of the 19 studies that were eligible for their analysis, three investigated CT and 17 PET. Nine of the latter included patients who had Hodgkin lymphoma, but only one of these was as part of initial staging, with sensitivity and specificity of 87.5% and 100%, respectively. In the single staging study including patients with non-Hodgkin lymphoma, the sensitivity was 83.3% with 100% lesion-based specificity. Four studies evaluated PET/CT fusion scans, but only one for initial staging.[48] The authors concluded that CT remains the standard for staging, with FDG PET being superior for restaging. Although PET/CT was found to be superior to either modality alone, the authors felt that further study was needed to determine the most accurate and cost-effective method for lymphoma staging.

## THE USE OF POSITRON EMISSION TOMOGRAPHY IN CLINICAL TRIALS

Juweid and colleagues[20] were the first to integrate PET into the IWG criteria in NHL. PET not only resulted in an increased number of patients with diffuse large B-cell NHL classified as a CR, but also eliminated CRus and provided a better separation of the progression-free survival curves between CR and partial recovery (PR) patients. This information, along with the increasing availability of FDG PET, stimulated interest in revising the IWG response criteria.

The German Competence Network Malignant Lymphoma facilitated this process by convening the International Harmonization Project, including an international committee of lymphoma clinical investigators, pathologists, and nuclear medicine physicians to review the IWG and other proposed response criteria (eg, response evaluation criteria in solid tumors [RECIST]), and to determine how best to clarify and improve on them to ensure transparency among clinical trials groups.[49]

The two major outcomes of the International Harmonization Project were a standardization of performance and interpretation of PET in lymphoma clinical trials[26] and new response criteria incorporating PET and bone marrow immunohistochemistry.[27] A positive scan was defined as focal or diffuse FDG uptake above background in a location incompatible with normal anatomy or physiology. Exceptions include mild and diffusely increased FDG uptake at the site of moderate- or large-sized masses with an intensity that is lower than or equal to the mediastinal blood pool, hepatic or splenic nodules 1.5 cm with FDG uptake lower than the surrounding liver/spleen uptake, and diffusely increased bone marrow uptake within weeks following treatment.[26] Areas of necrosis may be FDG-avid within an otherwise negative residual mass, and a follow-up scan in a few months often is indicated to confirm this clinical impression. Residual masses of at least 2 cm in greatest transverse diameter (GTD) with FDG activity visually exceeding that of mediastinal blood pool structures are considered PET-positive, whereas residual masses 1.1 to 1.9 cm are considered PET-positive only if their activity exceeds surrounding background activity. Visual assessment is considered adequate for determining whether a PET scan is positive, and using the standardized uptake value (SUV) is not necessary.[26] What proportion of a reduction in SUV correlates with response is being evaluated. The numerous causes of false-positive scans, however, must be ruled out including sarcoidosis, infection, or inflammation.[50]

Using the new IHP definitions, Olsen and colleagues[51] evaluated 50 consecutive patients with HL (n = 26) or aggressive NHL (n = 24) who underwent PET/CT within 3 to 12 weeks after therapy with at least a year of follow-up after treatment. Fifty-one residual masses were found in 28 patients (56%); 31 were at least 2 cm in GTD and 20 1.1 to 1.9 cm in GTD but with a short axis diameter greater than 1 cm. The proposed IHP

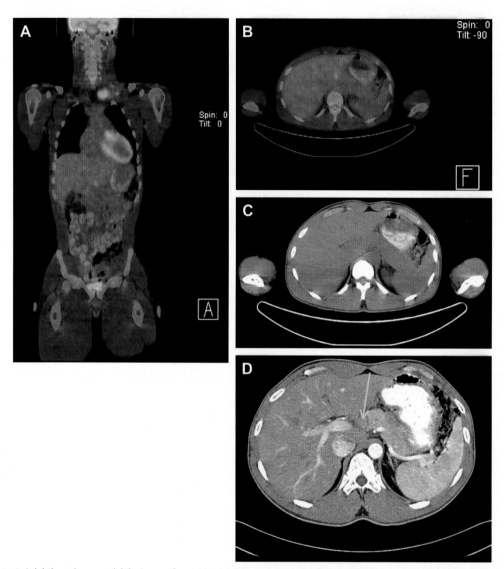

Fig. 1. Axial (A) and coronal (B) views of a patient with nodular sclerosing Hodgkin lymphoma who underwent CT/PET, which demonstrated supradiaphragmatic disease, with a suggestion of an intra-abdominal lymph node. Unenhanced PET/CT failed to confirm abdominal disease (C). Contrast- enhanced CT (D) was required to confirm that the patient had stage 3 disease (arrow).

interpretation resulted in high predictive value in post-treatment evaluation of residual masses both in both histologies. The 2-year event-free survival in patients who had PET-positive residual masses by the IHP definitions[26] was 0% compared with 95% in patients who had PET-negative residual masses and 85% in patients without residual masses.

## IHP RECOMMENDATIONS FOR THE USE OF FLUORODEOXYGLUCOSE POSITRON EMISSION TOMOGRAPHY IN CLINICAL TRIALS

The new recommendations for PET scans in clinical trials took into consideration the variability in

FDG-avidity among the various lymphoma histologic subtypes and the relevant endpoints of clinical trials (Table 1). For example, PET was recommended as standard for the initial evaluation of patients who had routinely FDG-avid, potentially curable lymphomas (eg, diffuse large B-cell lymphoma, Hodgkin lymphoma) to define the extent of disease and to provide a baseline against which to compare post-treatment studies. It is also useful in confirming whether a patient has limited stage disease and, thus, who might be a candidate for local radiation only. For the FDG-avid but incurable histologies (eg, follicular lymphoma and low-grade, and mantle cell lymphoma), PET is warranted only if complete response is a primary

**Table 1**
**Recommended timing of positron emission tomography (positron emission tomography/CT) scans in lymphoma clinical trials**

| Histology | Pretreatment | Midtreatment | Response Assessment | Posttreatment Surveillance |
|---|---|---|---|---|
| Routinely fluorodeoxyglucose (FDG)-avid | | | | |
| DLBCL | Yes[a] | Clinical trial | Yes | No |
| Hodgkin lymphoma (HL) | Yes[a] | Clinical trial | Yes | No |
| Follicular non –HL (NHL) | No[b] | Clinical trial | No[b] | No |
| Mantle cell lymphoma | No[b] | Clinical trial | No[b] | No |
| Variably FDG-avid | | | | |
| Other aggressive NHLs | No[b] | Clinical trial | No[b,c] | No |
| Other indolent NHLs | No[b] | Clinical trial | No[b,c] | No |

[a] Strongly recommended but not mandated pretreatment.
[b] Recommended only if overall response rate/complete remission is a primary study endpoint.
[c] Recommended only if PET is positive pretreatment and ORR/CR is a primary study endpoint.

endpoint of the trial, because time-dependent endpoints (eg, progression-free survival) are generally of greater importance.

Numerous studies have demonstrated that PET scans performed after one or more cycles of chemotherapy predict progression-free and overall survival.[6–8,21,22,24,25,52–54] Gallamini and colleagues[54] demonstrated that PET after two cycles of chemotherapy was a more potent predictor of outcome in Hodgkin lymphoma than the standard international prognostic score. Several investigators have demonstrated that PET after one or two cycles has stronger predictive value than a scan performed later during or after therapy.[22,25,53,54] Unfortunately, no available data demonstrate that altering treatment on the basis of PET results improves patient outcome. This critically important issue is being addressed in several clinical trials.

When indicated, PET scans should not be performed until at least 6 to 8 weeks following completion of therapy to reduce the likelihood of a false-positive result.[26] PET is essential for restaging the potentially curable lymphoma histologies following completion of therapy. In these patients, a complete remission is required for cure, and therapeutic intervention generally is indicated if residual disease is present. PET, however, is not recommended in the post-treatment assessment of the remaining histologies unless the PET scan was positive before treatment and if complete response rate is a primary endpoint of a clinical study.

The second major outcome of the IHP was a revision of the IWG response criteria.[27]

## REVISED RESPONSE CRITERIA

Complete remission requires (**Table 2**):

1. Complete disappearance of all clinical evidence of disease and disease-related symptoms.
2. a. Typically FDG-avid lymphoma exists in patients who have no pretreatment PET scan or when the FDG PET scan was positive before therapy: a post-treatment residual mass of any size is permitted as long as it is PET-negative. Variably FDG-avid lymphomas or FDG with unknown avidity exist in patients without pretreatment PET scan, or if pretreatment PET scans were negative. All lymph nodes and nodal masses must have regressed on CT to normal size (no more than 1.5 cm in their greatest transverse diameter for nodes greater than 1.5 cm before therapy). Previously involved nodes that were 1.1 to 1.5 cm in their long axis and greater than 1.0 cm in their short axis before treatment must have decreased to no more than 1.0 cm in their short axis after treatment.
3. The spleen and/or liver, if considered enlarged before therapy on the basis of a physical examination or CT scan, should not be palpable on physical examination and should be considered normal size by imaging studies, and nodules related to lymphoma should disappear. Determination of splenic involvement, however, is not always reliable, as a spleen considered normal in size still may contain lymphoma, whereas an enlarged spleen may reflect variations in anatomy, blood volume, the use of

**Table 2**
**Response definitions for clinical trials**

| Response | Definition | Nodal Masses | Spleen, Liver | Bone Marrow |
|---|---|---|---|---|
| Complete remission (CR) | Disappearance of all evidence of disease | a. Fluorodeoxyglucose (FDG)-avid or positron emission tomography (PET) + before therapy: mass of any size permitted if PET-<br>b. Variably FDG-avid or PET-: regression to normal size on CT | Not palpable, nodules disappeared | Infiltrate cleared on repeat biopsy, if indeterminate by morphology immunohistochemistry should be negative |
| Partial remission (PR) | Regression of measurable disease and no new sites | ≥ 50% decrease in sum of the product of the diameters (SPD) of up to six largest dominant masses. No increase in size of other nodes<br>a. FDG-avid or PET + before therapy: one or more PET + at previously involved site<br>b. Variably FDG-avid or PET-: regression on CT | ≥ 50% decrease in SPD of nodules (for single nodule in greatest transverse diameter), no increase in size of liver or spleen | Irrelevant if positive before therapy; cell type should be specified. |
| Stable disease (SD) | Failure to attain CR/PR or PD | a. FDG-avid or PET + before therapy: PET + at prior sites of disease and no new sites on CT or PET<br>b. Variably FDG-avid or PET-: no change in size of previous lesions on CT | | |
| Relapsed or progressive disease | Any new lesion or increase from nadir by ≥ 50% of previously involved sites | Appearance of a new lesion >1.5 in any axis<br>≥ 50% increase in the longest diameter of a previously identified node >1 cm in short axis or in the SPD of more than one node<br>Lesions PET + if FDG-avid lymphoma or PET + before therapy | ≥ 50% increase from nadir in the SPD of any previous lesions | New or recurrent involvement |

*From* Cheson BD, Pfistner B, Juweid ME, et al. Revised response criteria for malignant lymphoma. J Clin Oncol 2007;25:579–86. Reprinted with permission of the American Society of Clinical Oncology.

hematopoietic growth factors, or other causes rather than lymphoma.

4. If the bone marrow was involved by lymphoma before treatment, the infiltrate must have cleared on repeat bone marrow biopsy. The biopsy sample on which this determination is made must be adequate (with a goal of at least 20 mm unilateral core). If the sample is indeterminate by morphology, it should be negative by immunohistochemistry. A sample that is negative by immunohistochemistry but demonstrating a small population of clonal lymphocytes by flow cytometry will be considered a CR until data become available demonstrating a clear difference in patient outcome.

Using the definition for CR and that which follows for PR eliminates the category of Cru (complete remission/unconfirmed).

Partial remission requires all of the following:

1. At least a 50% decrease in SPD of up to six of the largest dominant nodes or nodal masses. These nodes or masses should be selected if: they are clearly measurable in at least two perpendicular dimensions; they are from disparate regions of the body, and they include mediastinal and retroperitoneal areas of disease whenever these sites are involved.
2. No increase in the size of other nodes, liver or spleen
3. Splenic and hepatic nodules must regress by at least 50% in their SPD or, for single nodules, in the greatest transverse diameter.
4. With the exception of splenic and hepatic nodules, involvement of other organs is usually evaluable and not measurable disease.
5. Bone marrow assessment is irrelevant for determination of a PR if the sample was positive before treatment. If positive, however, the cell type should be specified (eg, large-cell lymphoma or small neoplastic B cells). Patients who achieve a complete remission by the previously mentioned criteria, but who have persistent morphologic bone marrow involvement, will be considered partial responders.
   In cases where the bone marrow was involved before therapy that resulted in a clinical CR, but with no bone marrow assessment following treatment, patients should be considered partial responders.
6. No new sites of disease
7. Typically FDG-avid lymphoma. For patients who have no pretreatment PET scan or if the PET scan was positive before therapy, the post-treatment PET scan should be positive in at least one previously involved site.

8. Variably FDG-avid lymphomas/FDG-avidity unknown. For patients without a pretreatment PET scan, or if a pretreatment PET scan was negative, CT criteria should be used.

Stable disease is described by the following:

1. Failing to attain the criteria needed for a CR or PR, but not fulfilling those for progressive disease
2. Typically FGD-avid lymphomas. The FDG-PET should be positive at prior sites of disease with no new areas of involvement on the post-treatment CT or PET.
3. Variably FDG-avid lymphomas/FDG-avidity unknown. For patients without a pretreatment PET scan or if the pretreatment PET was negative, there must be no change in the size of the previous lesions on the post-treatment CT scan.

### Relapsed Disease (After Complete Remission)/ Progressive Disease (After Partial Remission, Stable Disease)

Lymph nodes should be considered abnormal if the long axis is greater than 1.5 cm regardless of the short axis. If a lymph node has a long axis of 1.1 to 1.5 cm, it should be considered abnormal only if its short axis is greater than 1.0. Lymph nodes less than or equal to 1.0 cm by less than or equal to 1.0 cm will not be considered as abnormal for relapse or progressive disease.

Relapse is defined as:

1. Appearance of any new lesion greater than 1.5 cm in any axis during or at the end of therapy, even if others are decreasing in size. Increased FDG uptake in a previously unaffected site only should be considered relapsed or progressive disease after confirmation with other modalities. In patients who have no prior history of pulmonary lymphoma, new lung nodules identified by CT are mostly benign. Thus, a therapeutic decision should not be made solely on the basis of the PET scan without histologic confirmation.
2. At least a 50% increase from nadir in the SPD of any previously involved nodes, or in a single involved node, or the size of other lesions (eg, splenic or hepatic nodules). To be considered progressive disease, a lymph node with a diameter of the short axis of less than 1.0 cm must increase by at least 50% and to a size of $1.5 \times 1.5$ cm or greater than 1.5 cm in the long axis.
3. At least a 50% increase in the longest diameter of any single previously identified node greater than 1 cm in its short axis.

4. Lesions should be PET-positive if a typical FDG-avid lymphoma or one that was PET-positive before therapy unless the lesion is too small to be detected with current PET systems (less than 1.5 cm in its long axis by CT)

Measurable extranodal disease should be assessed in a manner similar to nodal disease. Disease that is only evaluable (eg, pleural effusions, bone lesions) are recorded as present or absent only, unless, while an abnormality remains noted by imaging studies or physical examination, it is found to be histologically negative.

In clinical trials where PET is unavailable to most participants, or where PET is not deemed necessary or appropriate, response should be assessed as previously described, but only using CT scans. In this setting, residual masses should not be considered a CRu, but should be designated as partial responses.

## FOLLOW-UP EVALUATION

There are limited data on the role of imaging studies in routine surveillance following response to therapy. The most important components of monitoring patients following treatment are a careful history and physical examination along with complete blood cell count (CBC) and serum chemistries, including lactate dehydrogenase (LDH) and other relevant blood tests. Recently, the National Comprehensive Cancer Network published recommendations for follow-up of patients who have HL and NHL[55,56]: for patients who have NHL in an initial complete remission, follow-up should include an interim history and physical examination every 2 to 4 months for 1 to 2 years, then every 3 to 6 months for the next 3 to 5 years, with annual monitoring for late effects after 5 years. For follicular or other indolent histology lymphoma patients in a complete remission, the recommendation for follow-up was every 3 months for a year then every 3-6 months. For diffuse large B-cell NHL, the guidelines proposed every 3 months for 24 months then every 6 months for 36 months. Imaging studies should be performed when clinically indicated.

Although widely used in clinical practice, there is no evidence to support regular surveillance CT or PET scans. Several studies in the pre-PET era demonstrated that it is the patient or physician who identifies the relapse more than 80% of the time.[57–60]

Jerusalem and colleagues[61] reported a series of 36 patients who underwent PET following therapy and every 4 to 6 months thereafter. There were five events detected by PET, one in a patient with known residual disease. Two of the four patients whose relapse 5 to 24 months following treatment was identified by PET already had developed disease-related symptoms, In addition, there were six false-positive studies. Zinzani and colleagues[62] conducted a prospective evaluation of 160 patients who had HL and 261 patients with indolent or aggressive NHL who underwent PET at 6, 12, 18, and 24 months after therapy. For the patients who had HL, the likelihood of relapse was negligible after 12 months and after 18 months for the aggressive NHL. There was a continuous risk of relapse for the indolent NHLs. Patients who had suspected relapse were biopsied, and more than 40% of those who had a positive PET but negative CT had a negative biopsy. The authors concluded that there was no benefit from continued surveillance studies after 18 months.

## ISSUES WITH POSITRON EMISSION TOMOGRAPHY/CT

Several important limitations of PET remained to be resolved. Differences in equipment, technique, and variability in interpretation among readers impair comparisons among studies. Newer technology, such as PET/CT, makes comparisons with older data difficult. Histologic subtypes also differ in FDG-avidity.[11,63–66] Moreover, there are many common causes of false-positive and false-negative PET scans.[20,26,50,67] In addition, the usefulness of PET in clinical trials requires additional prospective validation as is being conducted by the Cancer and Leukemia Group B (CALGB) Lymphoma Committee in multicenter studies.

## SUMMARY

The International Harmonization Project developed recommendations for the use of PET for managing patients who have lymphoma. It provided guidance as to the interpretation of FDG PET and generated response definitions incorporating metabolic imaging with the goal of improving interpretation of response comparability among studies, leading to accelerated new agent development, more rapid availability of more effective therapies, and enhanced outcome for patients who have lymphoma.

## REFERENCES

1. Grillo-López AJ, Cheson BD, Horning SJ, et al. Response criteria for NHL: importance of normal lymph node size and correlations with response rates. Ann Oncol 2000;11:399–408.

2. Cheson BD, Horning SJ, Coiffier B, et al. Report of an International Workshop to standardize response criteria for non-Hodgkin lymphomas. J Clin Oncol 1999;17:1244–53.

3. Surbone A, Longo DL, DeVita VT Jr, et al. Residual abdominal masses in aggressive non-Hodgkin lymphoma after combination chemotherapy: significance and management. J Clin Oncol 1988;6: 1832–7.

4. Radford JA, Cowan RA, Flanagan M, et al. The significance of residual mediastinal abnormality on the chest radiograph following treatment for Hodgkin disease. J Clin Oncol 1988;6:940–6.

5. Bangerter M, Moog F, Buchmann I, et al. Whole-body 2-[18F]-fluoro-2-deoxy-D-glucose positron emission tomography (FDG-PET) for accurate staging of Hodgkin disease. Ann Oncol 1998;9: 1117–22.

6. Spaepen K, Stroobants S, Dupont P, et al. Prognostic value of positron emission tomography (PET) with fluorine-18 fluorodeoxyglucose ([18F]FDG) after first-line chemotherapy in non-Hodgkin lymphoma: is [18F]FDG-PET a valid alternative to conventional diagnostic methods? J Clin Oncol 2001;19:414–9.

7. Spaepen K, Stroobants S, Dupont P, et al. Prognostic value of pretransplantation positron emission tomography using fluorine 18-fluorodeoxyglucose in patients with aggressive lymphoma treated with high-dose chemotherapy and stem cell transplantation. Blood 2003;102:53–9.

8. Spaepen K, Stroobants S, Dupont P, et al. Early restaging positron emission tomography with 18F-fluorodeoxyglucose predicts outcome in patients with aggressive non-Hodgkin lymphoma. Ann Oncol 2002;13:1356–63.

9. Jerusalem G, Beguin Y, Fassotte MF, et al. Whole-body positron emission tomography using 18F-fluorodeoxyglucose compared to standard procedures for staging patients with Hodgkin disease. Haematologica 2001;86:266–73.

10. Jerusalem G, Beguin Y, Fassotte MF, et al. Whole-body positron emission tomography using 18F-fluorodeoxyglucose for posttreatment evaluation in Hodgkin disease and non-Hodgkin lymphoma has higher diagnostic and prognostic value than classical computed tomography scan imaging. Blood 1999;94:429–33.

11. Jerusalem G, Beguin Y, Najjar F, et al. Positron emission tomography (PET) with 18F-fluorodeoxyglucose (18F-FDG) for the staging of low-grade non-Hodgkin lymphoma (NHL). Ann Oncol 2001;12:825–30.

12. Jerusalem G, Warland V, Najjar F, et al. Whole-body 18F-FDG PET for the evaluation of patients with Hodgkin disease and non-Hodgkin lymphoma. Nucl Med Commun 1999;20:13–20.

13. Zinzani PL, Magagnoli M, Chierichetti F, et al. The role of positron emission tomography (PET) in the management of lymphoma patients. Ann Oncol 1999;10:1141–3.

14. Weihrauch MR, Re D, Scheidhauer K, et al. Thoracic positron emission tomography using 18F-fluorodeoxyglucose for the evaluation of residual mediastinal Hodgkin disease. Blood 2001;98: 2930–4.

15. Naumann R, Vaic A, Beuthien-Baumann B, et al. Prognostic value of positron emission tomography in the evaluation of post-treatment residual mass in patients with Hodgkin disease and non-Hodgkin lymphoma. Br J Haematol 2001;115: 793–800.

16. Kostakoglu L, Leonard JP, Kuji I, et al. Comparison of fluorine-18 fluorodeoxyglucose positron emission tomography and Ga-67 scintigraphy in evaluation of lymphoma. Cancer 2002;94:879–88.

17. Naumann R, Beuthien-Baumann B, Reiss A, et al. Substantial impact of FDG PET imaging on the therapy decision in patients with early-stage Hodgkin lymphoma. Br J Cancer 2004;90:620–5.

18. Munker R, Glass J, Griffeth LK, et al. Contribution of PET imaging to the initial staging and prognosis of patients with Hodgkin disease. Ann Oncol 2004;15: 1699–704.

19. Mikhaeel NG, Hutchings M, Fields PA, et al. FDG-PET after two to three cycles of chemotherapy predicts progression-free and overall survival in high-grade non-Hodgkin lymphoma. Ann Oncol 2005;16:1514–23.

20. Juweid M, Wiseman GA, Vose JM, et al. Response assessment of aggressive non-Hodgkin lymphoma by integrated International Workshop criteria (IWC) and 18F-fluorodeoxyglucose positron emission tomography (PET). J Clin Oncol 2005;23:4652–61.

21. Haioun C, Itti E, Rahmouni A, et al. [18F]fluoro-2-deoxy-D-glucose positron emission tomography (FDG-PET) in aggressive lymphoma: an early prognostic tool for predicting patient outcome. Blood 2005;106:1376–81.

22. Hutchings M, Loft A, Hansen M, et al. Positron emission tomography with or without computed tomography in the primary staging of Hodgkin lymphoma. Haematologica 2006;91:482–9.

23. Querellou S, Valette F, Bodet-Milin C, et al. FDG-PET/CT predicts outcome in patients with aggressive non-Hodgkin lymphoma and Hodgkin disease. Ann Hematol 2006;85:759–67.

24. Gallamini A, Rigacci L, Merli F, et al. Predictive value of positron emission tomography performed after two courses of standard therapy on treatment outcome in advanced stage Hodgkin disease. Haematologica 2006;91:475–81.

25. Hutchings M, Loft A, Hansen M, et al. FDG-PET after two cycles of chemotherapy predicts treatment failure and progression-free survival in Hodgkin lymphoma. Blood 2006;107:52–9.

26. Juweid ME, Stroobants S, Hoekstra OS, et al. Use of positron emission tomography for response assessment of lymphoma: consensus recommendations of the Imaging Subcommittee of the International Harmonization Project in Lymphoma. J Clin Oncol 2007;25:571–8.

27. Cheson BD, Pfistner B, Juweid ME, et al. Revised response criteria for malignant lymphoma. J Clin Oncol 2007;25:579–86.

28. Seam P, Juweid ME, Cheson BD. The role of FDG-PET scans in patients with lymphoma. Blood 2007; 110:3507–16.

29. Carbone PP, Kaplan HS, Musshoff K, et al. Report of the committee on Hodgkin disease staging classification. Cancer Res 1971;31:1860–1.

30. Newman JS, Francis JR, Kaminski MS, et al. Imaging of lymphoma with PET with 2-[F-18]-fluoro-2-deoxy-D-glucose: correlation with CT. Radiology 1994;190:111–6.

31. Thill R, Neuerburg J, Fabry U, et al. [Comparison of findings with 18-FDG PET and CT in pretherapeutic staging of malignant lymphoma]. Nuklearmedizin 1997;36:234–9 [in German].

32. Moog F, Bangerter M, Diederichs CG, et al. Lymphoma: role of whole-body 2-deoxy-2-[F-18]-D-glucpse)FDG) PET in nodal staging. Radiology 1997;203:795–800.

33. Moog F, Bangerter M, Diederichs CG, et al. Extranodal malignant lymphoma: detection with FDG PET versus CT. Radiology 1998;206:475–81.

34. Buchmann I, Reinhardt M, Elsner K, et al. 2-(fluorine-18)fluoro-2-deoxy-D-glucose positron emission tomography in the detection and staging of malignant lymphoma. A bicenter trial. Cancer 2001;91:889–99.

35. Blum RH, Seymour JF, Wirth A, et al. Frequent impact of [18F] Fluorodeoxyglucose positron emission tomography on the staging and management of patients with indolent non-Hodgkin lymphoma. Clin Lymphoma 2004;4:43–9.

36. Partridge S, Timothy A, O'Doherty MJ, et al. 2-Fluorine-18-fluoro-2-deoxy-D glucose positron emission tomography in the pretreatment staging of Hodgkin disease: influence on patient management in a single institution. Ann Oncol 2000;11:1273–9.

37. Weihrauch MR, Re D, Bischoff S, et al. Whole-body positron emission tomography using 18F-fluorodeoxyglucose for initial stsaging of patients with Hodgkin disease. Ann Hematol 2002;81:20–5.

38. Menzel C, Dobert N, Mitrou P, et al. Positron emission tomography for the staging of Hodgkin lymphoma - increasing the body of evidence in favor of the method. Ann Oncol 2002;41:430–6.

39. Schaefer NG, Hany TF, Taverna C, et al. Non-Hodgkin lymphoma and Hodgkin disease: coregistered FDG PET and CT at staging and restaging - do we need contrast-enhanced CT? Radiology 2004;232:823–9.

40. Isasi CR, Lu P, Blaufox MD. A metaanalysis of $^{18}$F-2-deoxy-2-fluoro-D-glucose positron emission tomography in the stasging and restaging of patients with lymphoma. Cancer 2005;104:1066–74.

41. Moog F, Bangerter M, Kotzerke J, et al. 18-F-fluorodeoxyglucose-positron emission tomography as a new approach to detect lymphomatous bone marrow. Blood 1998;16:603–9.

42. Carr R, Barrington SF, Madan B, et al. Detection of lymphoma in bone marrow by whole-body positron emission tomography. Blood 1998;91:3340–6.

43. Pakos EE, Fotopoulos AD, Ioannidis JP. 18F-FDG PET for evaluation of bone marrow infiltration in staging of lymphoma: a meta-analysis. J Nucl Med 2005; 46:958–63.

44. Rodriguez-Vigil B, Gomez-Leon N, Pinilla I, et al. PET/CT in lymphoma: prospective study of enhanced full-dose PET/CT versus unenhanced low-dose PET/CT. J Nucl Med 2006;47:1643–8.

45. Freudenberg LS, Antoch G, Schütt P, et al. FDG-PET/CT in restaging of patients with lymphoma. Eur J Nucl Med Mol Imaging, in press.

46. Tatsumi M, Cohade C, Nakamoto Y, et al. Direct comparison of FDG PET and CT findings in patients with lymphoma: initial experience. Radiology 2005; 237:1038–45.

47. Kwee TC, Kwee RM, Nievelstein RA. Imaging in stagin of malignant lymphoma: a systematic review. Blood 2008;111:504–16.

48. La Fougere C, Hundt W, Brockel N, et al. Value of PET/CT versus PET and CT performed as separate investigations in patients with Hodgkin disease and non-Hodgkin lymphoma. Eur J Nucl Med Mol Imaging 2006;33:1417–25.

49. Pfistner B, Diehl V, Cheson B. International harmonization of trial parameters in malignant lymphoma. Eur J Haematol Suppl 2005;75(66):53–4.

50. Castellucci P, Nanni C, Farsad M, et al. Potential pitfalls of $^{18}$F-FDG PET in a large series of patients treated for malignant lymphoma: prevalence and scan interpretation. Nucl Med Commun 2005;26: 689–94.

51. Olsen K, Sohi J, Abraham T, et al. Initial validation of standardized quantitative (visual) criteria for FDG PET assessment of residual masses following lymphoma therapy. Proc Radiol Soc North Amer 2006;323 [abstract 355:E323–302].

52. Zinzani PL, Tani M, Fanti S, et al. Early positron emission tomography (PET) restaging: a predictive final response in Hodgkin disease patients. Ann Oncol 2006;17:1296–300.

53. Kostakoglu L, Goldsmith SJ, Leonard JP, et al. FDG-PET after 1 cycle of therapy predicts outcome in diffuse large cell lymphoma and classic Hodgkin disease. Cancer 2006;107:2678–87.

54. Gallamini A, Hutchings M, Rigacci L, et al. Early interim 2-[18F]fluoro-2-D-glucose positron emission

tomography is prognostically superior to international prognostic score in advanced stage Hodgkin lymphoma: a report from a joint Italian–Danish study. J Clin Oncol 2007;25:3746–52.

55. Hoppe RT, Advani RH, Bierman PJ, et al. Hodgkin disease/lymphoma. Clinical practice guidelines in oncology. J Natl Compr Canc Netw 2006;4(3): 210–30.

56. Zelenetz AD, Advani RH, Buadi F, et al. Non-Hodgkin lymphoma: clinical practice guidelines in oncology. J Natl Compr Canc Netw 2006;4(3): 258–310.

57. Weeks JC, Yeap BY, Canellos GP, et al. Value of follow-up procedures in patients with large-cell lymphoma who achieve a complete remission. J Clin Oncol 1991;9:1196–203.

58. Oh YK, Ha CS, Samuels BI, et al. Stages I-III follicular lymphoma: role of CT of the abdomen and pelvis in follow-up studies. Radiology 1999;210:483–6.

59. Foltz LM, Song KW, Connors JM. Who actually detects relapse in Hodgkin lymphoma: patient or physician. Blood 2004;104(part 1):853–4 [abstract 3124].

60. Liedtke M, Hamlin PA, Moskowitz CH, et al. Surveillance imaging during remission identifies a group of patients with more favorable aggressive NHL at time of relapse: a retrospective analysis of a uniformly treated patient population. Ann Oncol 2006;17: 909–13.

61. Jerusalem G, Beguin Y, Fassotte MF, et al. Early detection of relapse by whole-body positron emission tomography in the follow-up of patients with Hodgkin disease. Ann Oncol 2003;14:123–30.

62. Zinzani PL, Stefoni V, Ambrosini V, et al. FDG-PET in the serial assessment of patients with lymphoma in complete remission. Blood 2007;110(part 1):71 [abstract 216].

63. Hoffmann M, Kletter K, Diemling M, et al. Positron emission tomography with fluorine-18-2-fluoro-2-deoxy-D-glucose (F18-FDG) does not visualize extranodal B-cell lymphoma of the mucosa-associated lymphoid tissue (MALT)-type. Ann Oncol 1999;10:1185–9.

64. Elstrom R, Guan L, Baker G, et al. Utility of FDG-PET scanning in lymphoma by WHO classification. Blood 2003;101:3875–6.

65. Karam M, Novak L, Cyriac J, et al. Role of fluorine-18 fluoro-deoxyglucose positron emission tomography scan in the evaluation and follow-up of patients with low-grade lymphomas. Cancer 2006;107:175–83.

66. Hoffmann M, Wöhrer S, Becherer A, et al. 18F-fluoro-deoxy-glucose positron emission tomography in lymphoma of mucosa-associated lymphoid tissue: histology makes the difference. Ann Oncol 2006; 17:1761–5.

67. Lewis PJ, Salama A. Uptake of fluorine-18-flouorodeoxyglucose in sarcoidosis. J Nucl Med 1994;35:1647–9.

# PET Imaging for Response Assessment in Lymphoma: Potential and Limitations

Heiko Schöder, MD[a,b,*], Craig Moskowitz, MD[b,c]

**KEYWORDS**
• Lymphoma • FDG • PET • PET-CT • Response

*As long as we know little, we know; as our knowledge expands, so grows our doubt.*
*Johann Wolfgang von Goethe*

Much has been said and written about treatment monitoring and response assessment in lymphoma with fluorodeoxyglucose (FDG) positron emission tomography (PET). This article clarifies the potential and limitations of FDG for determining the presence of residual disease during chemotherapy (interim PET), or at the end of chemotherapy. Briefly discussed are treatment strategies for lymphoma. Some clinical scenarios of how and when interim PET or end-of-treatment PET may be helpful in guiding the management of patients with lymphoma are outlined. Although recognizing the limitations of many published studies, response assessment with FDG-PET can provide clinically meaningful information and will be an essential tool in most future trials in Hodgkin lymphoma (HL) and aggressive non-Hodgkin lymphoma (NHL).

## CLINICAL BACKGROUND

HL and NHL are the most common hematologic malignancies in the United States; they account for 4% to 5% of all new cancer cases and are the fifth leading cause of cancer death in the United States.

Among HL, nodular sclerosis is the most common subtype in the United States and Western Europe, followed by mixed cellularity phenotype, lymphocyte-predominant subtype, and lymphocyte-depleted subtype. The international prognostic score is used for risk stratification.[1] Treatment decisions for classical HL are based on stage and symptoms. All patients receive combination chemotherapy, whereas radiotherapy tends to be reserved for patients with bulky disease. The response rates and prognosis (best in the lymphocyte-predominant subtype, worst in the lymphocyte-depleted subtype) vary with tumor histology and clinical stage. A 5-year progression-free survival (PFS) for nonbulky stage I to IIIA disease can be achieved in as many as 85% of patients[2] and in stage IV in about 65% of patients.[3]

NHL can be subdivided into indolent, aggressive, and highly aggressive histologic entities.[4] The international prognostic index (IPI) is used for risk stratification.[5] Patient classification by IPI into groups with low, low-intermediate, high-intermediate, and high risk can be applied in aggressive lymphoma and other histologies[6–9]; it has proved valuable in interpreting trial results and

a Department of Radiology, Memorial Sloan-Kettering Cancer Center, 1275 York Avenue, Box 77, New York, NY 10065, USA
b Weill Cornell Medical College, 1305 York Avenue, New York, NY 10021, USA
c Department of Medicine, Memorial Sloan-Kettering Cancer Center, 1275 York Avenue, Box 77, New York, NY 10065, USA
* Corresponding author. Department of Radiology/Nuclear Medicine, Memorial Sloan-Kettering Cancer Center, 1275 York Avenue, Box 77, New York, NY 10065.
*E-mail address:* schoderh@mskcc.org (H. Schöder).

Radiol Clin N Am 46 (2008) 225–241
doi:10.1016/j.rcl.2008.04.002
0033-8389/08/$ – see front matter © 2008 Elsevier Inc. All rights reserved.

for designing prospective trials in patients with similar risk.

Response assessment with PET is mainly of interest in aggressive NHL; of these, diffuse large B-cell lymphoma (DLBCL) is the most common form, accounting for 31% of all NHL cases.[10] In localized DLBCL, the 5-year PFS ranges from 65% to 75%.[11–13] The prognosis is worse in disseminated DLBCL, with a 3-year failure-free survival in the 40% range and an overall survival in the 50% range.[14]

The treatment for aggressive NHL has evolved over the past decades. For more than 25 years, the CHOP regimen (eight cycles of cyclophosphamide, doxorubicin, vincristine, and prednisone with a 3-week break) has been the standard of care for aggressive lymphomas.[15,16] Recent modifications include the addition of the monoclonal anti-CD20 antibody rituximab (R-CHOP-21),[17] leading to improved response rates and outcome in large B-cell lymphoma.[17–21] Other groups have focused on reducing the number of chemotherapy cycles from eight to six, and on shortening the intervals between treatment cycles from 3 weeks to 2 weeks (CHOP-14).[22] The latter regimen is also known as "dose-dense" therapy.

Most patients with HL and a significant fraction of patients with aggressive NHL can be cured with current treatment regimens. There is increasing emphasis on achieving long-term survival with the least amount of treatment-related toxicities. Such potential toxicities include myelosuppression, neuropathy, pulmonary fibrosis, and cardiomyopathy from chemotherapy, and mucositis and an increased risk for second malignancy from radiation therapy. It is hoped that these toxicities can be avoided, or at least reduced, with abbreviated therapies (fewer cycles of chemotherapy) or the elimination of radiation therapy in certain subgroups of patients. At the same time it is important to identify patients with resistant disease who have failed conventional therapy regimens, so that they may undergo salvage treatment, including high-dose chemotherapy and stem cell transplantation.

## POSITRON EMISSION TOMOGRAPHY IMAGING

FDG-PET is now widely used for the staging, restaging, and detection of recurrence in many patients with HL and NHL. It is also increasingly used for monitoring the response to chemotherapy in these patients. For meaningful clinical use, the specific lymphoma entity has to be FDG-avid. Although this information may be inferred from past studies,[23,24] it is clearly desirable to obtain a baseline scan to assess the extent of disease

and to establish the degree and intensity of FDG uptake in lymphoma sites in a given patient; this should always be done when PET is to be used in the follow-up and response assessment.

The intensity of FDG uptake in lymphoma is determined by many factors, including histology (HL versus NHL); grade (indolent versus aggressive NHL[23]); viable tumor cell fraction; tumor cell proliferation; up-regulation of glucose metabolism; salvage pathways and tumor-specific pathways; local perfusion (which determines substrate delivery to the cancer cell); and the presence of hypoxia. Of note, in HL, more than 90% of cells in a given lesion may be inflammatory, and less than 10% tumor cells. Because FDG uptake is a multifactorial process, it should come as no surprise that there is (sometimes large) heterogeneity between lesions of the same histologic entity and some overlap between tumor grades.[23] In contrast to some soft tissue malignancies, there is no convincing evidence that the intensity of FDG uptake in lymphoma in a baseline scan is an independent prognostic factor. It is now clearly established that changes in FDG uptake do reflect the response to chemotherapy, and that residual abnormal FDG uptake after completion of chemotherapy identifies patients with poor prognosis.[25,26] It is less clear what degree of change in FDG uptake should be expected during chemotherapy. In addition to the number of treatment cycles after which the scan is obtained, that parameter (qualitatively or quantitatively) is likely to vary with tumor histology (generally more rapid response in HL than in aggressive NHL); tumor subentity (large B-cell lymphoma versus other aggressive NHL); and treatment regimen. The following technical aspects are also important:

- Patient-related: blood glucose level; duration of uptake phase; positioning during the uptake phase (may affect FDG uptake in brown adipose tissue or skeletal muscles)
- Equipment and data acquisition: time per bed position and acquisition matrix; coincidence versus time of flight acquisition; two-dimensional versus three-dimensional acquisition; material, size, and shape of the PET crystal; PET scanner electronics (recent technical developments emphasize speed of data processing and handling of image noise [ie, scatter and random counts])
- Image processing: reconstruction and smoothing filter settings

Although blood glucose and uptake time should be standardized (eg, <200 mg/dL and 60–90 minutes), some of the technical parameters cannot be standardized easily or decreed, because most commercially available PET and PET-CT scanners vary with regard to their crystal material; electronics; suggested acquisition modes (some only permit acquisition in three-dimensional mode, others promote time of flight acquisition); and suggested filtering techniques. Rather than demanding uniform acquisition settings, images must be processed in a manner that is considered optimal by the physicians interpreting the scan. For multicenter trials, the accuracy and reproducibility of quantitative measurements should be established in phantom studies. Ideally, patients enrolled in response assessment protocols should be imaged under the same conditions and on the same scanner at baseline and during follow-up. As a minimum requirement, all images should be acquired on a full-ring dedicated PET scanner (or PET-CT scanner). Attenuation-corrected images should be reviewed in all three orthogonal planes; non–attenuation-corrected images should be available for review in all cases.

In HL and aggressive NHL, the advantage of FDG-PET, when compared with conventional imaging modalities, lies in the high tumor-to-background contrast, resulting in high sensitivity. Because of the relatively poor visualization of normal organs and tissues on PET images, however, lesion localization is suboptimal. This is particularly problematic for NHL, in which disease is frequently extranodal and can occur in almost any site and organ in the body. Combined PET-CT has clearly improved diagnostic abilities in lymphoma.[27–32]

## Goals and Prerequisites for Positron Emission Tomography Response Assessment in Lymphoma

Once the diagnosis of lymphoma has been established, physicians and patients like to know if a given treatment regimen is likely to succeed (ie, if the patient can be cured or if at least durable remission can be achieved). This desire has led to efforts to predict the likely treatment outcome and prognosis of patient subgroups based on prognostic indices,[1,5,33] and use imaging studies to monitor the response to chemotherapy and determine the probability for complete response versus presence of residual disease.

With recent advances in the imaging sciences, and with the development of new chemotherapy regimens, the widespread clinical introduction of immunotherapy with rituximab, and increasing availability of experimental drugs,[34,35] response assessment has become an area of growing interest for imaging physicians and hemato-

oncologists alike. The goals of response assessment are defined in **Box 1**.

It is apparent that these goals are demanding an imaging test that combines high sensitivity (not to miss any patient with residual disease who might benefit from alternate or additional therapies) with a reasonable specificity (to avoid a high number of false-positives). Because it is virtually impossible to design an imaging test that combines very high sensitivity and very high specificity, a trade-off must always be made. Test results are either interpreted with emphasis on high sensitivity (so as not to miss residual disease when it is likely to be present, a more likely scenario in aggressive NHL than in most rapidly responding HL) or with emphasis on high specificity (to avoid false-positives in a setting when disease is likely to be absent or cured, which applies to most HL cases at the end of therapy). The decision whether to emphasize sensitivity or specificity depends on the disease under study, the time point of imaging, and the goals of the study protocol.

In contrast to sensitivity and specificity, which are characteristics of a given test, positive and negative predictive values (PPV and NPV) depend on the disease prevalence in the study cohort.[36] In lymphoma, the prevalence of (residual) disease at the end of planned therapy can be estimated from large studies. Up to 80% to 90% of patients with HL and approximately half as many patients with aggressive NHL can be cured with current chemotherapy or combined chemotherapy and radiation therapy regimens. Based on average historical relapse rates of 10% to 20% for HL and approximately 30% to 50% for DLBCL (and assuming

---

**Box 1**
**The goals of response assessment**

*At the end of standard chemotherapy*

- To identify accurately patients with residual disease (nonresponders) who may benefit from additional treatment, such as autologous stem cell transplant; this is of particular interest in patients with residual structural abnormalities (residual mass) after end of therapy
- To help in designing the radiation field in patients undergoing "involved field irradiation"

*During the course of planned chemotherapy*

- To assess the initial response after a few cycles of chemotherapy and predict the ultimate patient outcome with that therapy (likelihood the patient will achieve a complete response at the end of planned therapy)

that relapses originate from surviving cancer cell clones at the time of the original disease), residual viable cancer must have been present in 10% to 20% and 30% to 50% of cases, respectively. Further, in HL up to 50% of patients may present with residual mediastinal masses, but viable tumor is eventually found in only 20% to 30% of these.[37]

From these statistics it is apparent that the NPV of any imaging test in HL is bound to be high: residual disease after completion of therapy is rare and a negative imaging test is most likely true-negative. Conversely, because few patients have residual disease, a positive test has a relatively higher likelihood of being false-positive. Assuming a similar test performance of FDG-PET in aggressive NHL, the higher prevalence of residual disease with standard CHOP chemotherapy should translate into a somewhat lower NPV but higher PPV. This is shown in the following example: Assume a sensitivity and specificity of 80% for FDG-PET in HL and aggressive NHL. With an expected 10% prevalence of residual disease in HL, the test has a PPV of 31% and an NPV of 97%. Assuming a similar sensitivity and specificity in aggressive NHL, but a 35% prevalence for residual disease, the PPV is 68% and the NPV 88%.

## Indications for Positron Emission Tomography Response Assessment in Lymphoma

The recently revised response criteria for lymphoma[38] suggested the following indications for PET imaging in lymphoma:

- PET is strongly recommended before treatment for patients with routinely FDG-avid, potentially curable lymphomas (eg, DLBCL and HL) to delineate better the extent of disease.
- For incurable, routinely FDG-avid, indolent, and aggressive histologies (eg, follicular lymphoma and mantle-cell lymphoma), and for most variably FDG-avid lymphomas, the primary end points for clinical trials generally include PFS, event-free survival, and overall survival. Routine PET was not recommended before treatment unless the response rate (presumably response to alternate chemotherapy regimens or newer experimental drugs) is a major end point in a clinical trial.
- Interim PET should only be obtained as part of clinical trials.

## Positron Emission Tomography Methods of Response Assessment

Most published studies have used qualitative assessment of FDG uptake in lymphoma to determine whether or not residual disease is present,

and to grade treatment response on interim PET scans. These methods of visual assessment used varying criteria to define abnormal FDG uptake:

- Any FDG uptake greater than surrounding local background activity and outside normal anatomic structures.
- Same as before and standardized uptake value greater than 2.5 if visual analysis is inconclusive.[39]
- PET-, PET+, and minimal residual uptake.[40,41] Minimal residual uptake is defined as any activity slightly above background. This criterion has been criticized as "rather vague" and observer-dependent. It does, however, reflect daily clinical practice in that sometimes findings cannot be categorized clearly as abnormal or normal. Instead, such findings require further evaluation with other methods or particular attention on follow-up.
- Compare all lesions with activity in mediastinal blood pool.
- Compare chest lesions with mediastinal blood pool and abdominal lesions with background activity in the liver.
- Compare lesions in the abdomen with activity in gluteal muscle.[42]

In the recently revised lymphoma response criteria,[43] lesion size has been introduced as a new parameter for treatment evaluation with PET. Depending on lesion size, residual FDG uptake should be compared with local background activity or mediastinal blood pool. Specific criteria apply for lesions in liver, spleen, and bone (**Table 1**). For the first time, response assessment in lymphoma is based on the combination of structural imaging and FDG-PET.[38] It remains to be seen if the new criteria are practical in the clinical setting, if they reduce interobserver and interstudy variability, and if they are more accurate in evaluating treatment response and predicting patient outcome. Given the interobserver variability among radiologists, one might wonder how accurately a lesion of 1.5 cm or 2 cm (see **Table 1**) could be measured, and why different reference standards should be used for a 1.9-cm lesion as compared with a 2.1-cm lesion.

Standardized uptake value (SUV) numbers may be helpful in characterizing lymphoma subentities.[23,24,44] They are not necessary in evaluating treatment response,[43] but can be used to measure the intensity of FDG uptake in suspected residual lesions and uptake in reference regions. SUV numbers should be used judiciously, sparingly, in light of their known limitations,[45,46] and never in isolation. No absolute SUV number can tell whether or not residual viable tumor is present. Most patients show some degree of decline in FDG uptake

**Table 1**
**Revised response criteria for malignant lymphoma**

| Criteria | Interpretation |
| --- | --- |
| Residual mass ≥2 cm | Uptake greater than mediastinal blood pool is abnormal, regardless of location |
| Residual lesions <2 cm | Any uptake greater than surrounding background is abnormal |
| New lung nodules and complete response elsewhere | Consider infection or inflammation |
| Residual liver/spleen nodules | >1.5 cm: abnormal if SUV greater than or equal to surrounding liver/spleen<br><1.5 cm: abnormal if SUV greater than liver/spleen<br>Diffuse spleen greater than liver: abnormal unless recent cytokine therapy |
| Bone | Focal uptake is abnormal |

Lesion size should be measured on the CT component of a PET-CT or separate contrast CT.
*Data from* Juweid ME, Stroobants S, Hoekstra OS, et al. Use of positron emission tomography for response assessment of lymphoma: consensus of the Imaging Subcommittee of International Harmonization Project in Lymphoma. J Clin Oncol 2007;25:571–8.

during treatment, whereas few patients have a completely negative scan in particular after only one or two cycles of chemotherapy. Recent studies demonstrated considerable overlap in SUV of disease sites considered negative or positive by visual analysis on interim PET. After two cycles of chemotherapy PET-negative sites in HL had an SUV of 1.8 to 5 compared with PET-positive sites with 3 to 11.[47] In aggressive NHL, these numbers were 0.9 to 4.5 and 1.9 to 20.8, respectively.[42] Such statements as "all metabolic responders had an SUV of less than 3" are probably meaningless; these exact numbers are not reproducible in other institutions with varying equipment, patient population, and study conditions. In contrast to absolute SUV, changes in SUV (ΔSUV) from baseline to interim scan may potentially provide meaningful clinical information. ΔSUV indicates the slope of treatment-induced decline in FDG uptake from baseline to interim scan, and should predict the likelihood of achieving a complete response at the end of planned therapy. As long as repeat studies are acquired under the same conditions (blood glucose in the acceptable range, same uptake time and equipment) this parameter may also reduce some of the variability in visual PET interpretation. In a recent study in patients with DLBCL, a ΔSUV of 66% after cycle 2 of therapy distinguished well between patients with poor and good prognosis, with a 2-year event-free survival of 21% versus 79% in PET-positive and PET-negative patients.[42] In contrast, visual analysis of PET scans was less predictive (2-year event-free survival 51% versus 79%).

Note, however, that the exact 66% decline in SUV was obtained in a homogenous patient group with DLBCL after two cycles of chemotherapy; it may not be applicable in other patient populations and at other time points.

### Reasons for False-positive and False-negative Positron Emission Tomography Scans

There are numerous reasons for false-positive findings at the end of therapy or on an interim PET scan. In addition to physiologic variants, such as intense uptake in brown adipose tissue[48] or skeletal muscle, the intensity of normal FDG uptake in the stomach, gastroesophageal junction, and small and large bowel varies considerably. Nonspecific uptake in normal-sized or mildly enlarged inguinal nodes is a common finding. Dose infiltration in the forearm can cause FDG uptake in normal axillary lymph nodes. New foci of uptake in the lungs in a patient showing otherwise good response to therapy are more likely inflammatory or infectious, rather than sites or new disease. Because of the many reasons for false-positive findings, it is mandatory to confirm suspicious FDG uptake with biopsy if scan findings are to be used to alter therapy at interim, or to continue with additional therapy in cases with suspected residual disease after completion of standard chemotherapy.

In some studies of HL patients with residual mass after the end of first-line therapy, the PPV was as low as 50%.[49] Similarly, in a mixed group of patients with HL and NHL showing residual

FDG uptake in the mediastinum after first-line chemotherapy, the rate of false-positive PET scans was 43% (PPV 56%).[50] PET was performed 1 month after chemotherapy or 3 months after radiation therapy, and any FDG uptake greater than background was defined as abnormal. This study is noteworthy because all positive PET findings were pursued with core biopsy, mediastinoscopy, or open surgical biopsy. This also included three cases with essentially normal CT scan, where persistent disease was proved in small nodes or mediastinal soft tissue.

A high number of false-positive cases were also reported for interim PET imaging. Preliminary analysis of the CALGB trial 50203 in patients with early stage HL treated with an AVG (doxorubicin, vinblastine, gemcitabine) regimen showed a PPV of 58% after two cycles of chemotherapy.[51] In the authors' own experience, interim PET had a PPV of only 32% in patients with DLBCL treated with an R-CHOP-14 regimen.[52]

Small volume and microscopic foci of residual disease cannot be detected by PET. Mildly elevated uptake is detected more easily against low background (lungs, axilla) than against high background activity (abdomen, pelvis). Diffuse bone marrow uptake is common after the end of therapy, indicating marrow rebound, and in patients treated with granulocyte colony–stimulating factor. Against this high background activity, sites of successfully treated lymphoma (but also some sites with residual disease) may appear photopenic.

## END OF THERAPY ASSESSMENT
### Background

Historically, imaging studies were obtained at baseline and after completion of therapy, for the purpose of staging and restaging. Investigators realized increasingly that a lack of complete normalization on structural imaging, either conventional radiograms[53,54] or CT,[55] did not necessarily indicate the presence of residual viable tumor tissue. This led to the introduction of a category "complete response, unconfirmed" in the 1999 lymphoma response criteria.[55] That is, clinicians presumed that treatment had been successful, but uncertainty remained. Among the functional imaging techniques, [67]gallium scintigraphy was first used to predict the presence of residual disease after completion of therapy in lymphoma.[56] In subsequent studies of patients with HL and NHL, the NPV of CT and [67]gallium were very similar at about 85%, but the PPV was 73% to 80% for [67]gallium compared with 30% to 35% for CT.[57] In lymphoma (and most other indications), [67]gallium

scintigraphy has now been replaced completely by FDG-PET, because of the better image contrast and overwhelming clinical benefits.[58,59] It is a testament to the clinical success of FDG-PET that this imaging study has now been adopted as part of the newly revised lymphoma response criteria.[38]

### Positron Emission Tomography Findings

The results of FDG-PET after completion of chemotherapy in HL and NHL have been summarized in two recent meta-analyses.[25,26] In their meta-analysis in 2006, Zijlstra and colleagues[25] included a total of 15 studies with 705 patients. The pooled sensitivity and specificity for the detection of residual disease in HL were 84% and 90%, and in NHL 72% and 100%, respectfully. This meta-analysis pointed out significant methodologic problems with many studies; only six had been prospective, and in only two studies patients were enrolled consecutively. The time interval between end of therapy and PET varied widely. In 2008, Terasawa and colleagues[26] published another meta-analysis for end-of-treatment PET in lymphoma. Some studies considered in the Zijlstra article were excluded by Terasawa because of poor methodologic quality. In total, these authors evaluated 19 studies in 474 patients with HL and 274 patients with aggressive NHL. Six studies included mixed patient populations with HL and NHL, whereas 10 included only patients with HL and 3 studies only patients with NHL. The time interval between end of therapy and PET ranged widely from 1 month to 55 months, and most studies were retrospective.

Among patients with HL, most had nodular sclerosis subtype. Some studies did not report clinical stage, and most other studies included patients with all stages (I–IV) of HL. Most, but not all, patients had been treated with either ABVD (doxorubicin, bleomycin, vinblastine, dacarbazine) or MOPP (nitrogen mustard, vincristine, procarbazine, prednisone) regimens with or without additional radiation therapy. Relapse rates were similar for patients in whom PET was ordered for posttherapy evaluation (4%–55%) and patients with residual mass after therapy (35%–70% of all patients, relapse rate 0%–50%). Studies in aggressive NHL often included patients with various histologies, although DLBCL was the most common subtype. Most patients were treated with CHOP regimens, some received additional radiation therapy. The relapse rates were similar for patients with residual mass posttherapy (26%–55% of patients, relapse in 33%–67% of them) and those without (relapse rate 33%–60%).

In this meta-analysis, the sensitivity and specificity of FDG-PET after first-line chemotherapy in HL ranged from 50% to 100% and 67% to 100%, respectively (residual mass: 43%–100% and 67%–100%). In patients with aggressive NHL, the sensitivity and specificity were 33% to 77% and 82% to 100% (residual mass: 33%–87% and 75%–100%). Unfortunately, many studies suffered from poor-quality design and reporting. When the authors separately evaluated the studies that included at least 30 adult patients (imaged on a full-ring PET scanner with attenuation correction of PET emission data, and fully accessible in English language) the fraction of PET-positive patients was 25% to 60% in HL studies and 20% to 35% in aggressive NHL studies. Of note, the fraction of PET-positive scans was considerably lower in some studies done without attenuation correction[60,61] or on a PET scanner that would not meet today's requirements.[62] At the same time, the PPV in these studies was uniformly 100%,[60–62] suggesting that areas of mild residual FDG uptake were probably not detected with these techniques. It also emphasizes that mild FDG uptake in residual HL masses may often be false-positive. When obtained with state of the art technique, the PPV of PET was 50% to 92% in HL studies,[49,63–65] and 74% to 100% in NHL.[66,67] In contrast, the NPV of an end-of-treatment scan was greater than 90% in these HL studies, and 83% in the NHL studies. Patients with negative end-of-treatment PET scan can generally be followed clinically, with surveillance intervals adjusted to clinical risk for relapse. In contrast, positive PET findings need to be confirmed with biopsy before embarking on additional therapy. Alternatively, depending on the level of clinical suspicion one might opt to repeat the PET scan in 6 to 8 weeks. Finally, in many patients with DLBCL, immunotherapy with rituximab is now part of the standard regimen; although this is expected to increase response rates, it may potentially also increase the number of false-positive PET findings.

## Potential Problems and Pitfalls with End-of-Therapy Positron Emission Tomography

There are some conceptual problems inherent to response assessment at the end of treatment. Early response assessment may be more accurate than assessment after completion of chemotherapy.[68] For instance, some tumor shrinkage is often observed even in patients who still harbor residual disease at the end of therapy. Because smaller tumor masses are more prone to partial volume effects, the degree of FDG uptake in these masses is underestimated, potentially leading to misinterpretation as "nonspecific post-treatment change." If only a small amount of residual viable tumor remains, it becomes increasingly difficult to distinguish residual disease from physiologic background activity. Conversely, tumor masses may not regress completely because of some degree of treatment-induced fibrosis and remaining necrotic debris. Nonspecific inflammation (caused by accumulation of white cells and macrophages removing the debris of dead tumor cells) may then cause false-positive study interpretations. This has led to the recommendation that PET not be performed before 3 weeks after the end of chemotherapy (8–12 weeks after chemoradiotherapy),[43] because with increasing time the surviving viable tumor cells may recover their ability to grow and proliferate, whereas inflammatory changes subside. This waiting period represents a trade-off between the clinical demand for a reliable answer and the desire to avoid false-positive and false-negative imaging findings.

## Can One Eliminate Radiotherapy if the End-of-treatment Positron Emission Tomography Scan is Negative?

One recent study addressed the role of PET in determining the need for consolidative radiotherapy in HL patients with initial soft tissue masses greater than 5 cm.[69] Following standard chemotherapy, a total of 160 patients had an FDG-negative residual soft tissue mass. They were randomized to observation or radiotherapy with 32 Gy. Among the 80 patients receiving radiotherapy the relapse rate was 2.5% (N = 2), and among the 80 patients who were followed clinically without further intervention, it was 14% (N = 11); of note 10 of these 11 relapses in the observation-only group occurred at the site of the residual mass. Although the difference in relapse rates was significant and may seem striking, the NPV of PET in this study was 86%, which is consistent with reports in most other studies. Assuming similar propensity for relapse in the observation group and intervention group, radiotherapy could potentially have prevented 18 relapses in 160 patients, but at the expense of irradiating the other 142 patients without clear benefit. A clearer picture may emerge from ongoing trials. In the current EORTC trial 20051 (http://www.cancer.gov/clinicaltrials/EORTC-20051), patients with stage I or II supra-diaphragmatic HL are randomized into three treatment arms. The standard treatment consists of three to four cycles of ABVD chemotherapy followed by involved nodal irradiation. In the experimental arms, patients are randomized based on PET findings after two cycles of chemotherapy: group A receives an additional two to four cycles of ABVD only (depending on risk profile), whereas group B is treated with escalated BEACOPP chemotherapy (cyclophosphamide, doxorubicin, vincristine, bleomycin, etoposide, procarbazine, prednisone) followed by involved nodal irradiation. A major problem with these study designs is the definition of bulky disease. In United States intergroup clinical trials, bulk is defined as a mass greater than 10 cm in size, and this cohort receives radiotherapy. In German HL studies patients are irradiated if there is a single nodal mass of greater than 7 cm pretreatment or a residual mass post-chemotherapy of greater than 2 cm. Other countries and cooperative groups use greater than 5 cm as the cut-off. Before one can answer the question "Can planned radiotherapy be eliminated when the end of treatment PET is negative," there needs to be a consensus on the definition of bulky disease. It is prudent, however, first to study this question in patients with nonbulky disease once this definition is universally accepted.

A recent study in HL clearly indicated that a persistent positive PET scan after the end of first-line chemotherapy indicates a poor prognosis, which apparently cannot be remedied by involved field radiation therapy. In that study of 81 patients, four of six patients with persistent PET positivity relapsed within 4 years, but only 3 of 75 patients whose PET had become negative with chemotherapy.[70]

## EARLY RESPONSE ASSESSMENT
### Background

Early response assessment, although much en vogue nowadays, is not new. As early as 1986, Armitage and colleagues[71] reported that "rapidly responding patients with DLBCL have more durable remissions." They used conventional response criteria and chest radiograph and abdominal CT. With the advent of functional imaging, Front and colleagues[72] used [67]gallium scintigraphy for similar purpose and in 1999 published that a "negative test after one cycle of chemotherapy is a good early predictor of outcome" in HL. Failure-free survival differed significantly between patients with positive and patients with negative [67]gallium scintigrams after one cycle of treatment. At about the same time, in 1993, Hoekstra and colleagues[73] used planar scintigraphy with a high energy collimator to image FDG distribution in lymphoma patients. In patients who eventually achieved complete remission, the FDG distribution had normalized after two cycles of chemotherapy; high uptake reflected treatment failure and faint uptake was associated with variable outcome. Römer and colleagues[74] then conducted the first pilot study on a dedicated full-ring PET scanner. Eleven patients with mixed histologies of NHL underwent PET at baseline, at 1 week, and at 6 weeks after initiation of chemotherapy. The authors reported a 60% decrease in SUVmax on day 7 and a 79% decrease from baseline on day 42. The study emphasized that early decline in FDG uptake in aggressive lymphoma is not uncommon and may be useful in predicting ultimate treatment outcome and survival. Changes in SUV at 6 weeks were more predictive of long-term outcome than the early scan after 1 week.

## Rationale for Interim Positron Emission Tomography

A growing number of studies now suggest that interim PET can provide an insight into patient prognosis. There are tumor biologic and technical reasons for this clinical observation. The resolution limit of modern PET scanners ranges from 5 to 10 mm,[75] which may correspond to a tumor size of approximately 0.1 to 1 g, or $10^8$ to $10^9$ cells.[29] That is, small amounts of residual viable cancer cannot be excluded based on a negative end-of-treatment PET. If the PET is already negative after a few cycles of chemotherapy and treatment is continued as planned, however, it becomes rather unlikely that viable cancer still persist at the end of therapy. Essentially, the change in FDG uptake between baseline and interim scan provides an insight into the kinetics of tumor cell kill. Accordingly, the earlier the PET scan becomes negative (eg, after 1 day or 1 week), the greater the chemotherapy responsiveness of the tumor cell clone, and the greater the chance for a complete response and cure. This model is based on several assumptions: all cancer cells are killed by first-order kinetics (same fraction of cells is killed with each treatment cycle; "logarithmic cell kill")[76]; there are no resistant cell clones; no tumor cell repair occurs between treatment sessions; and FDG uptake is directly proportional to the number of tumor cells.

The early detection of treatment failure (ie, after a few cycles of chemotherapy or at mid of scheduled treatment) could alter the treatment strategy in two ways. Immediately, if the predictive value of the imaging test is very high, all nonresponders may be diverted immediately to a different, non–cross resistant chemotherapy regimen with the potential still to achieve a complete response at the end of eight cycles of chemotherapy.

Conversely, patients showing a very rapid response to therapy may not need the entire amount of planned therapy. This does not mean that treatment should be stopped as soon as the PET scan becomes negative (small amounts of residual cancer cannot be excluded because of sensitivity and resolution limits), but it may open a chance for abbreviated therapy in particular in patients with early stage or low-risk disease. These two approaches are also known as "response-adapted therapy."

In the second way, after end of therapy, patients showing a slow response to chemotherapy but with negative PET after the end of therapy might harbor more aggressive (chemoresistant) tumor cell clones and may require closer surveillance during follow-up.

## Potential Problems with Interim Positron Emission Tomography

First, to be clinically meaningful, the interim PET scan should reliably identify patients who will fail standard chemotherapy, and there should be an effective alternative therapy for these individuals. Moreover, the outcome of patients receiving such alternative therapy early should be equal to, or superior to, the outcome of patients receiving the same therapy at the time of clinical treatment failure at a later point of time (ie, salvage therapy). At present there is no clearly established alternative therapy, however, and the effect of early intervention on patient outcome is unproved.

Second, tumor response to therapy is often associated with temporary inflammation related to migrating white cells and macrophages that remove necrotic material and cellular debris. The time course of these events was investigated in mouse lymphoma model.[77] With a single dose of cyclophosphamide on day 0, the fraction of viable tumor cells declined until day 10, after which repopulation occurred and tumor growth resumed. The fraction of necrotic material and host macrophages peaked around day 10. By comparison, FDG uptake in the tumor bed declined only until day 3 and then rose again, suggesting a significant radiotracer uptake in inflammatory white cells. The inflammatory change subsided around day 15 after treatment. Although the time course of these events may not be identical in humans, the data suggest that a higher fraction of false-positive findings is likely when the interim PET is performed too early after chemotherapy, which is more likely to happen when patients are treated with accelerated chemotherapy regimens (dose-dense treatment every 2 weeks instead of standard treatment every 3 weeks).

## Critical Review of Interim Positron Emission Tomography Studies

A plethora of original studies (and innumerable review articles) have been published addressing the role of FDG-PET in early response assessment for lymphoma. In some of these studies, PET was performed as early as 1 day[78] after initiation of chemotherapy. Imaging at this early time point may provide interesting insights into tumor biology, but is probably meaningless for the clinical management of lymphoma patients. Other studies have investigated the treatment response after one cycle of chemotherapy,[68] after two to three cycles,[40–42,47,79–82] or at mid treatment after four cycles.[52,79,83]

Some of the early studies raised considerable excitement, because the presence or absence of FDG uptake on an interim PET scan seemed to predict patient outcome with high certainty. In particular in patients with aggressive NHL, it has been somewhat difficult to reproduce these early promising data. For instance, Spaepen and colleagues[83] performed FDG-PET after three to four cycles of chemotherapy in 70 patients with aggressive NHL (including 47 with DLBCL and 10 with anaplastic large cell lymphoma). Patients with all stages of disease were included; 48 patients had a low or low-intermediate IPI score, and 22 a high or high-intermediate score. Two different treatment regimens were used. On nonattenuation corrected PET images, 33 patients showed residual FDG uptake and none of them achieved durable complete remission. In contrast, 37 patients already showed a complete metabolic response (PET-negative) on the interim scan, and 31 of them remained in complete remission with a median follow-up of about 3 years. The 3-year PFS was almost 90% in patients with negative interim PET compared with less than 10% in patients with positive interim PET. By comparison, Haioun and colleagues[79] performed interim PET after two cycles of chemotherapy in a cohort of 90 patients with aggressive NHL (94% with DLBCL, 37 low risk, and 57 high risk by IPI score). The event-free survival at 2 years was 82% in patients with negative interim PET and 43% in those with positive interim PET. Interim PET continued to show an excellent NPV, but the PPV was only moderate. PET was equally predictive of outcome in patients with low-risk and those with high-risk disease. A subset of patients was also imaged after four cycles of chemotherapy, with results similar to those obtained with the earlier interim scan.

Unfortunately, many studies investigating the use of interim PET in lymphoma suffer from limitations, which makes if difficult to interpret the findings and apply them in the clinical setting. These limitations include:

- Retrospective analysis with selection bias
- Suboptimal gold standard for extent of disease assessment
- Aggregate analysis of patients with HL and NHL
- Aggregate analysis of patients with various subtypes of NHL (this is important because NHL is a heterogenous disease with regard to tumor biology, histology, and prognosis)
- Aggregate analysis of patients with widely varying disease stages with no attention to IPI or international prognostic score
- Nonuniform treatment regimens
- Use of a gamma camera or outdated PET equipment (rather than dedicated full-ring PET scanner) for FDG imaging
- Lack of attenuation correction in some studies

To some degree the comparability of study results may also be handicapped by the increasing use of PET-CT. It is the authors' observation that residual abnormalities, which may have been ignored or not even been detected on PET only, can now easily be identified on combined PET-CT, thereby perhaps improving sensitivity but also risking a higher number of potentially false-positive findings.

To date, several hundreds of patients with HL and aggressive NHL have been imaged with PET after a few cycles of chemotherapy. Studies including at least 40 patients with advanced-stage HL show a sensitivity of 67% to 100% and a specificity of 90% to 97%.[40,47,80–82] The larger interim PET studies in aggressive NHL show a sensitivity of 80% to 90% and a specificity of 63% to 100%.[41,79,83] This analysis is confounded by the inclusion of patients with a variety of histologic subtypes and clinical stages in almost all studies. Overall, the data seem somewhat more consistent in HL, but should be interpreted with greater caution in aggressive NHL. Minimal residual uptake on interim PET scan is likely irrelevant in patients with HL,[40] but in NHL it may identify a subgroup of patients with dubious prognosis.[41] Taken with a grain of salt, patients with early complete response to chemotherapy probably have good long-term prognosis, whereas a lack of response or delayed response probably identifies a more aggressive tumor phenotype with higher likelihood for relapse. Of note, the interim PET results may predict patient outcome better than the international prognostic score in HL[80] or the IPI score in NHL.[83] **Table 2** summarizes data from some large recent studies with reasonably good quality. In these series, the event-free survival or

PFS was clearly better in patients with negative interim PET.

In the recently revised response criteria for malignant lymphoma,[38] PET imaging at interim is only recommended as part of clinical trials; it should not be used to alter patient management in daily routine practice. Most importantly, a positive PET scan needs to be confirmed by biopsy if it is used to change the treatment plan (**Figs. 1** and **2**).

## Response-adapted Therapy Modification After Interim Positron Emission Tomography

Interim PET not only provides prognostic information, but may be used to change patient management with the goal to improve survival rates in high-risk patients and reduce treatment-related side effects in low-risk patients. One example for applying this approach in HL is the ongoing EORTC trial 20051 (http://www.cancer.gov/clinicaltrials/EORTC-20051, discussed previously).

In patients with DLBCL, the authors recently completed a risk-adapted, phase II study (stages IIx, III, or IV and one to three risk factors by age-adjusted IPI score). Following induction therapy with four cycles of R-CHOP-14, all patients underwent FDG-PET. PET-negative patients then received non–cross-resistant chemotherapy with three cycles of ICE (ifosfamide, carboplatin, etoposide). All positive interim PET findings were confirmed by biopsy. If the PET was true-positive, therapy was continued with three cycles of ICE followed by HDT and autologous stem cell transplant. If the interim PET was false-positive, however, the treatment was the same as for patients with negative interim PET. In this study, the NPV of interim PET was more than 80%, but the PPV was only 32%. There was no difference in outcome for patients with true-negative and patients with a false-positive interim PET scan, with a 3-year PFS of about 83% in both groups. Only five patients had a true-positive interim PET; they underwent autologous stem cell transplant and three of them remain progression free.[52] Based on these data, a higher number of false-positive interim PET should be expected with dose-dense treatment regimens and in particular when rituximab is part of the therapy. Similar studies in HL and NHL are now ongoing in the United States and Europe.

## Is There an Optimal Time Point for Interim Positron Emission Tomography in Lymphoma?

The answer to this question may depend on the clinical scenario. If physicians would like to know whether the current treatment will ultimately lead to a complete response with a chance for cure,

**Table 2**
Summary of the results in selected interim positron emission tomography studies

| | Prosp. or Retrosp. | N | No. of Cycles | No. PET+ | PPV % | NPV % | PFS PET+%, (Years) | PFS PET-%, (Years) | Median f/u (Months) |
|---|---|---|---|---|---|---|---|---|---|
| *Hodgkin lymphoma* | | | | | | | | | |
| Gallamini et al[80] | P | 260 | 2 | 50 | 92 | 95 | 13 (2) | 95 (2) | 27 |
| Hutchings et al[40] | R | 85 | 2 or 3 | 13 (+ 9 w/ MRU) | 62 | 94 | 46[a] (2) 38[a] (5) | 97[a] (2) 91[a] (5) | 40 |
| Hutchings et al[47] | P | 77 | 2 | 16 | 69 | 95 | 0 (2) | 96 (2) | 23 |
| | | 64 | 4 | 13 | 85 | 96 | 19 (2) | 96 (2) | 23 |
| *Aggressive non-Hodgkin lymphoma* | | | | | | | | | |
| Mikhaeel et al[41] | R | 121 | 2 or 3 | 52 19 w/MRU | 71 MRU: 36 | 90 — | 30 (2) 16 (5) MRU: 59 (2) 59 (5) | 93 (2) 89 (2) | 24 |
| Haioun et al[79] | P | 90 | 2 | 36 | 42 | 83 | 43 (2) | 82 (2) | 24 |
| Lin et al[42,b] | P | 92 | 2 | 34 | V: 50 S: 81 | V: 74 S: 75 | V: 51 (2) S: 21 (2) | V: 79 (2) S: 79 (2) | 42 |

Only studies done on dedicated PET scanners with attenuation correction are included. Study selection was based on size, quality, and completeness of data reporting.
*Abbreviations:* MRU, minimal residual uptake; NPV, negative predictive value; PFS, progression-free survival; PPV, positive predictive value; S, SUV-based using ΔSUV of 66% that discriminated best between responders and nonresponders; V, visual.
[a] MRU considered negative; Mikhaeel 2005 and Haioun 2005 included mixed histologies of aggressive non-Hodgkin lymphoma.
[b] Included only patients with diffuse large B-cell lymphoma, but substantial overlap with patients included in Haioun 2005.

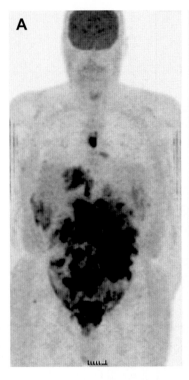

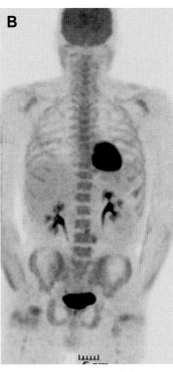

Fig. 1. Maximum intensity projection images of a patient with diffuse large B-cell lymphoma. (A) At baseline there is intense abnormal FDG uptake in numerous lymph node regions in the chest, abdomen, and pelvis. (B) At mid treatment all abnormal FDG uptake has resolved (complete metabolic response); the increased uptake in bone marrow indicates marrow rebound and is a normal response.

PET after cycle 2 of chemotherapy may predict outcome accurately. Whether PET after cycle 2 is truly more accurate than PET after cycle 4 could only be answered in a prospective study, which has never been done. If physicians would like to know whether the current treatment regimen should be changed when the interim PET remains positive, the answer may vary with local practice patterns. If one believes that therapy should generally not be changed until mid treatment (cycle 4 in DLBCL) so as not to deprive the patient of the best chance for cure with the primary (most powerful) therapy regimen, PET after cycle 4 is most appropriate. In contrast, if one believes that lack of complete metabolic response after cycle 2 predestines to ultimate treatment failure, it might be argued that change in therapy at this early time may be appropriate. Importantly, whenever the interim PET is to be used for management change, positive findings require confirmation by biopsy.

## PEDIATRIC PATIENTS

In children and adolescents, HL and Burkitt's lymphoma, lymphoblastic, and DLBCL are the most common histopathologic subtypes. These tumors are generally FDG-avid. These considerations should also apply to PET response assessment in pediatric patients, but this needs to be proved in prospective studies.

## IMAGING WITH [18]F FLUOROTHYMIDINE

This article is entirely focused on PET imaging with FDG. Among the many other PET radiotracers, the proliferation marker [18]F fluorothymidine (FLT) seems particularly promising for treatment monitoring.[84] FLT uptake depends on the activity of nucleoside transporters and the activity of the enzyme thymidine kinase 1.[85] Thymidine kinase 1 activity correlates well with other indicators of cellular proliferation, and tumor FLT uptake correlates with the tissue proliferation marker ki-67.[86] In experimental lymphoma studies in mice, treatment with a single dose of cyclophosphamide caused a clear and rapid decline in tumor FLT uptake within 48 hours, whereas no change was observed with rituximab or radioimmunotherapy with [90]yttrium anti-CD20 moAb.[87] In a small group of patients, a 77% decline in tumor SUV was observed as early as day 7 after treatment with R-CHOP, with some additional decline on day 40 with that treatment.[88] It is widely believed that FLT will become the next successful PET radiotracer for clinical use within the next 3 years.

## OPEN QUESTIONS

Among several open questions regarding the use of FDG-PET in lymphoma response assessment, **Box 2** offers some that may be of particular interest to oncologists and imaging physicians.

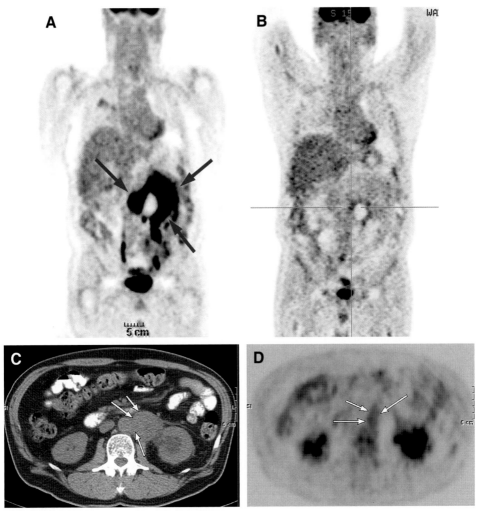

Fig. 2. Images of a patient with diffuse large B-cell lymphoma in a retroperitoneal mass. (*A*) Coronal PET at base-line; arrows indicate the mass. Note ametabolic center indicating necrosis. (*B*) Coronal PET at interim, with mild residual uptake (standardized uptake value 3.6). (*C, D*) Corresponding axial CT and PET images; arrows indicate the mass. This was biopsy-proved residual lymphoma.

## SUMMARY

FDG-PET is currently the most accurate tool for the assessment of treatment response and prognosis in lymphoma; it is certainly more accurate than structural imaging or clinical indices. Unfortunately, many published studies suffer from suboptimal methodology and incomplete data reporting. In general, the data seem more consistent in HL than in aggressive NHL. A negative PET excludes residual disease with reasonably high certainty. In contrast, positive PET findings should always be confirmed by biopsy before a treatment regimen is changed or additional (salvage) therapy is initiated.

End-of-treatment PET aims to establish the completeness of response or the presence of residual viable tumor tissue. In contrast, interim PET demonstrates the degree of response to standard chemotherapy; it provides an insight into the kinetics of tumor cell kill and is used to predict the likelihood for a complete response at the end of such therapy. In light of the detection limits of current PET and PET-CT scanners and based on tumorbiologic considerations, interim PET may be more accurate than an end-of-therapy scan for predicting PFS; however, this is not clearly established.

Interim PET is increasingly used for response-adapted therapy modifications. This might include the adoption of more aggressive therapy in patients with advanced-stage HL or aggressive NHL with a true-positive interim PET, or the abbreviation of therapy in subsets of patients with HL

Box 2
**Open questions regarding the use of FDG-PET in lymphoma response assessment**

*Clinical questions*

- What really is the earliest time point to predict treatment results with reasonable certainty?
- Which alternate treatment strategy exists for patients who are likely to fail standard chemotherapy based on a persistent positive interim PET? Is such alternate treatment going to affect ultimate patient outcome? (The answer to the latter question requires a randomized study because any comparison with historical control groups is limited by changes in treatment regimens, improvements in imaging techniques, and so forth)
- Can one avoid overtreatment of patients with apparently good prognosis, based on negative interim PET scan?

*Imaging questions*

- Is the accuracy of interim and end-of-therapy PET affected by recent changes in treatment regimens, in particular the increasing use of rituximab?
- Will the accuracy of PET interpretation improve when applying the new response criteria? Should one mechanically apply standardized response criteria in daily practice, or will PET interpretation continue to be part of the "art of medicine"?
- What is the role of FLT in lymphoma response assessment?

and a priori good prognosis. There is considerable hope that these response-adapted treatment strategies may improve patient outcome. Until the results of ongoing clinical trials emerge over the next 5 years, however, interim PET should be considered investigational and should not be used for patient management outside of study protocols.

# REFERENCES

1. Hasenclever D, Diehl V. A prognostic score for advanced Hodgkin's disease. International Prognostic Factors Project on Advanced Hodgkin's Disease. N Engl J Med 1998;339:1506–14.

2. Straus DJ, Portlock CS, Qin J, et al. Results of a prospective randomized clinical trial of doxorubicin, bleomycin, vinblastine, and dacarbazine (ABVD) followed by radiation therapy (RT) versus ABVD alone for stages I, II, and IIIA nonbulky Hodgkin disease. Blood 2004;104:3483–9.

3. Duggan DB, Petroni GR, Johnson JL, et al. Randomized comparison of ABVD and MOPP/ABV hybrid for the treatment of advanced Hodgkin's disease: report of an intergroup trial. J Clin Oncol 2003;21:607–14.

4. Harris NL, Jaffe ES, Diebold J, et al. World Health Organization classification of neoplastic diseases of the hematopoietic and lymphoid tissues: report of the Clinical Advisory Committee meeting-Airlie House, Virginia, November 1997. J Clin Oncol 1999;17:3835–49.

5. A predictive model for aggressive non-Hodgkin's lymphoma. The International Non-Hodgkin's Lymphoma Prognostic Factors Project. N Engl J Med 1993;329:987–94.

6. Hermans J, Krol AD, van Groningen K, et al. International Prognostic Index for aggressive non-Hodgkin's lymphoma is valid for all malignancy grades. Blood 1995;86:1460–3.

7. Wilder RB, Rodriguez MA, Medeiros LJ, et al. International prognostic index-based outcomes for diffuse large B-cell lymphomas. Cancer 2002;94:3083–8.

8. Moskowitz CH, Nimer SD, Glassman JR, et al. The International Prognostic Index predicts for outcome following autologous stem cell transplantation in patients with relapsed and primary refractory intermediate-grade lymphoma. Bone Marrow Transplant 1999;23:561–7.

9. Hamlin PA, Zelenetz AD, Kewalramani T, et al. Age-adjusted International Prognostic Index predicts autologous stem cell transplantation outcome for patients with relapsed or primary refractory diffuse large B-cell lymphoma. Blood 2003;102:1989–96.

10. Armitage JO, Weisenburger DD. New approach to classifying non-Hodgkin's lymphomas: clinical features of the major histologic subtypes. Non-Hodgkin's Lymphoma Classification Project. J Clin Oncol 1998;16:2780–95.

11. Miller TP, Dahlberg S, Cassady JR, et al. Chemotherapy alone compared with chemotherapy plus radiotherapy for localized intermediate- and high-grade non-Hodgkin's lymphoma. N Engl J Med 1998;339:21–6.

12. Horning SJ, Weller E, Kim K, et al. Chemotherapy with or without radiotherapy in limited-stage diffuse aggressive non-Hodgkin's lymphoma: Eastern Cooperative Oncology Group study 1484. J Clin Oncol 2004;22:3032–8.

13. Bonnet C, Fillet G, Mounier N, et al. CHOP alone compared with CHOP plus radiotherapy for localized aggressive lymphoma in elderly patients: a study by the Groupe d'Etude des Lymphomes de l'Adulte. J Clin Oncol 2007;25:787–92.

14. Friedberg JW, Mauch PM, Rimsza LM, et al. Non-Hodgkin lymphoma. In: DeVita VT, Lawrence TS, Rosenberg SA, editors. Cancer: principles & practice of oncology. Philadelphia: Lippincott Williams & Wilkins; 2008.

15. McKelvey EM, Gottlieb JA, Wilson HE, et al. Hydrox-yldaunomycin (adriamycin) combination chemotherapy in malignant lymphoma. Cancer 1976;38: 1484–93.

16. Fisher RI, Gaynor ER, Dahlberg S, et al. Comparison of a standard regimen (CHOP) with three intensive chemotherapy regimens for advanced non-Hodgkin's lymphoma. N Engl J Med 1993;328:1002–6.

17. Coiffier B, Lepage E, Briere J, et al. CHOP chemotherapy plus rituximab compared with CHOP alone in elderly patients with diffuse large-B-cell lymphoma. N Engl J Med 2002;346:235–42.

18. Mounier N, Briere J, Gisselbrecht C, et al. Rituximab plus CHOP (R-CHOP) overcomes bcl-2–associated resistance to chemotherapy in elderly patients with diffuse large B-cell lymphoma (DLBCL). Blood 2003;101:4279–84.

19. Feugier P, Van Hoof A, Sebban C, et al. Long-term results of the R-CHOP study in the treatment of elderly patients with diffuse large B-cell lymphoma: a study by the Groupe d'Etude des Lymphomes de l'Adulte. J Clin Oncol 2005;23:4117–26.

20. Pfreundschuh M, Schubert J, Ziepert M, et al. Six versus eight cycles of bi-weekly CHOP-14 with or without rituximab in elderly patients with aggressive CD20+ B-cell lymphomas: a randomised controlled trial (RICOVER-60). Lancet Oncol 2008;9:105–16.

21. Pfreundschuh M, Trumper L, Osterborg A, et al. CHOP-like chemotherapy plus rituximab versus CHOP-like chemotherapy alone in young patients with good-prognosis diffuse large-B-cell lymphoma: a randomised controlled trial by the MabThera International Trial (MInT) Group. Lancet Oncol 2006;7: 379–91.

22. Pfreundschuh M, Trumper L, Kloess M, et al. Two-weekly or 3-weekly CHOP chemotherapy with or without etoposide for the treatment of elderly patients with aggressive lymphomas: results of the NHL-B2 trial of the DSHNHL. Blood 2004;104: 634–41.

23. Schoder H, Noy A, Gonen M, et al. Intensity of 18fluorodeoxyglucose uptake in positron emission tomography distinguishes between indolent and aggressive non-Hodgkin's lymphoma. J Clin Oncol 2005;23:4643–51.

24. Elstrom R, Guan L, Baker G, et al. Utility of FDG-PET scanning in lymphoma by WHO classification. Blood 2003;101:3875–6.

25. Zijlstra JM, Lindauer-van der Werf G, Hoekstra OS, et al. 18F-fluoro-deoxyglucose positron emission tomography for post-treatment evaluation of malignant lymphoma: a systematic review. Haematologica 2006;91:522–9.

26. Terasawa T, Nihashi T, Hotta T, et al. 18F-FDG-PET for posttherapy assessment of Hodgkin's disease and aggressive non-Hodgkin's lymphoma: a systematic review. J Nucl Med 2008;49:13–21.

27. Allen-Auerbach M, Quon A, Weber WA, et al. Comparison between 2-deoxy-2-[18F]fluoro-D-glucose positron emission tomography and positron emission tomography/computed tomography hardware fusion for staging of patients with lymphoma. Mol Imaging Biol 2004;6:411–6.

28. Bar-Shalom R. Normal and abnormal patterns of 18F-fluorodeoxyglucose PET/CT in lymphoma. Radiol Clin North Am 2007;45:677–88.

29. Kasamon YL, Jones RJ, Wahl RL. Integrating PET and PET/CT into the risk-adapted therapy of lymphoma. J Nucl Med 2007;48(Suppl 1):19S–27S.

30. Hicks RJ, Mac Manus MP, Seymour JF. Initial staging of lymphoma with positron emission tomography and computed tomography. Semin Nucl Med 2005; 35:165–75.

31. Tatsumi M, Cohade C, Nakamoto Y, et al. Direct comparison of FDG-PET and CT findings in patients with lymphoma: initial experience. Radiology 2005; 237:1038–45.

32. Schaefer NG, Hany TF, Taverna C, et al. Non-Hodgkin lymphoma and Hodgkin disease: coregistered FDG-PET and CT at staging and restaging. Do we need contrast-enhanced CT? Radiology 2004;232:823–9.

33. Eghbali H, Raemaekers J, Carde P. The EORTC strategy in the treatment of Hodgkin's lymphoma. Eur J Haematol 2005;66(Suppl):135–40.

34. Fisher RI, Bernstein SH, Kahl BS, et al. Multicenter phase II study of bortezomib in patients with relapsed or refractory mantle cell lymphoma. J Clin Oncol 2006;24:4867–74.

35. Paoluzzi L, Gonen M, Gardner JR, et al. Targeting Bcl-2 family members with the BH3 mimetic AT-101 markedly enhances the therapeutic effects of chemotherapeutic agents in in vitro and in vivo models of B-cell lymphoma. Blood 2008; [epub ahead of print].

36. Schoder H, Gonen M. Screening for cancer with PET and PET/CT: potential and limitations. J Nucl Med 2007;48(Suppl 1):4S–18S.

37. Weihrauch MR, Re D, Scheidhauer K, et al. Thoracic positron emission tomography using 18F-fluoro-deoxyglucose for the evaluation of residual mediastinal Hodgkin disease. Blood 2001;98:2930–4.

38. Cheson BD, Pfistner B, Juweid ME, et al. Revised response criteria for malignant lymphoma. J Clin Oncol 2007;25:579–86.

39. Filmont JE, Gisselbrecht C, Cuenca X, et al. The impact of pre- and post-transplantation positron emission tomography using 18-fluorodeoxyglucose on poor-prognosis lymphoma patients undergoing autologous stem cell transplantation. Cancer 2007; 110:1361–9.

40. Hutchings M, Mikhaeel NG, Fields PA, et al. Prognostic value of interim FDG-PET after two or three cycles of chemotherapy in Hodgkin lymphoma. Ann Oncol 2005;16:1160–8.

41. Mikhaeel NG, Hutchings M, Fields PA, et al. FDG-PET after two to three cycles of chemotherapy predicts progression-free and overall survival in high-grade non-Hodgkin lymphoma. Ann Oncol 2005;16:1514–23.

42. Lin C, Itti E, Haioun C, et al. Early 18F-FDG-PET for prediction of prognosis in patients with diffuse large B-cell lymphoma: SUV-based assessment versus visual analysis. J Nucl Med 2007;48:1626–32.

43. Juweid ME, Stroobants S, Hoekstra OS, et al. Use of positron emission tomography for response assessment of lymphoma: consensus of the Imaging Subcommittee of International Harmonization Project in Lymphoma. J Clin Oncol 2007;25:571–8.

44. Bruzzi JF, Macapinlac H, Tsimberidou AM, et al. Detection of Richter's transformation of chronic lymphocytic leukemia by PET/CT. J Nucl Med 2006;47:1267–73.

45. Keyes JW Jr. SUV: standard uptake or silly useless value? J Nucl Med 1995;36:1836–9.

46. Huang SC. Anatomy of SUV. standardized uptake value. Nucl Med Biol 2000;27:643–6.

47. Hutchings M, Loft A, Hansen M, et al. FDG-PET after two cycles of chemotherapy predicts treatment failure and progression-free survival in Hodgkin lymphoma. Blood 2006;107:52–9.

48. Yeung HW, Grewal RK, Gonen M, et al. Patterns of (18)F-FDG uptake in adipose tissue and muscle: a potential source of false-positives for PET. J Nucl Med 2003;44:1789–96.

49. Friedberg JW, Fischman A, Neuberg D, et al. FDG-PET is superior to gallium scintigraphy in staging and more sensitive in the follow-up of patients with de novo Hodgkin lymphoma: a blinded comparison. Leuk Lymphoma 2004;45:85–92.

50. Zinzani PL, Tani M, Trisolini R, et al. Histological verification of positive positron emission tomography findings in the follow-up of patients with mediastinal lymphoma. Haematologica 2007;92:771–7.

51. Straus D, LaCase A, Juweid M. Doxorubicin, vinblastine and gemcitabine (AVG), a novel regimen excluding bleomycin for the treatment of early stage Hodgkin lymphoma (HL): results of CALGB 50203. Blood 2007;110:70A–1A.

52. Moskowitz C, Hamlin P, Horwitz S, et al. Phase II trial of dose-dense R-CHOP followed by risk-adapted consolidation with either ICE or ICE and ASCT, based upon the results of biopsy confirmed abnormal interim restaging PET scan, improves outcome in patients with advanced stage DLBCL (abstr 532). Blood 2006;108(11):532.

53. Jochelson M, Mauch P, Balikian J, et al. The significance of the residual mediastinal mass in treated Hodgkin's disease. J Clin Oncol 1985;3:637–40.

54. Radford JA, Cowan RA, Flanagan M, et al. The significance of residual mediastinal abnormality on the chest radiograph following treatment for Hodgkin's disease. J Clin Oncol 1988;6:940–6.

55. Cheson BD, Horning SJ, Coiffier B, et al. Report of an international workshop to standardize response criteria for non-Hodgkin's lymphomas. NCI Sponsored International Working Group. J Clin Oncol 1999;17:1244.

56. Front D, Israel O, Epelbaum R, et al. Ga-67 SPECT before and after treatment of lymphoma. Radiology 1990;175:515–9.

57. Front D, Ben-Haim S, Israel O, et al. Lymphoma: predictive value of Ga-67 scintigraphy after treatment. Radiology 1992;182:359–63.

58. Kostakoglu L, Leonard JP, Kuji I, et al. Comparison of fluorine-18 fluorodeoxyglucose positron emission tomography and Ga-67 scintigraphy in evaluation of lymphoma. Cancer 2002;94:879–88.

59. Wirth A, Seymour JF, Hicks RJ, et al. Fluorine-18 fluorodeoxyglucose positron emission tomography, gallium-67 scintigraphy, and conventional staging for Hodgkin's disease and non-Hodgkin's lymphoma. Am J Med 2002;112:262–8.

60. Spaepen K, Stroobants S, Dupont P, et al. Can positron emission tomography with [(18)F]-fluorodeoxyglucose after first-line treatment distinguish Hodgkin's disease patients who need additional therapy from others in whom additional therapy would mean avoidable toxicity? Br J Haematol 2001;115:272–8.

61. Spaepen K, Stroobants S, Dupont P, et al. Prognostic value of positron emission tomography (PET) with fluorine-18 fluorodeoxyglucose ([18F]FDG) after first-line chemotherapy in non-Hodgkin's lymphoma: is [18F]FDG-PET a valid alternative to conventional diagnostic methods? J Clin Oncol 2001;19:414–9.

62. Jerusalem G, Beguin Y, Fassotte MF, et al. Whole-body positron emission tomography using 18F-fluorodeoxyglucose for posttreatment evaluation in Hodgkin's disease and non-Hodgkin's lymphoma has higher diagnostic and prognostic value than classical computed tomography scan imaging. Blood 1999;94:429–33.

63. Filmont JE, Yap CS, Ko F, et al. Conventional imaging and 2-deoxy-2-[(18)F]fluoro-D-glucose positron emission tomography for predicting the clinical outcome of patients with previously treated Hodgkin's disease. Mol Imaging Biol 2004;6:47–54.

64. Guay C, Lepine M, Verreault J, et al. Prognostic value of PET using 18F-FDG in Hodgkin's disease for posttreatment evaluation. J Nucl Med 2003;44:1225–31.

65. Mikosch P, Gallowitsch HJ, Zinke-Cerwenka W, et al. Accuracy of whole-body 18F-FDP-PET for restaging malignant lymphoma. Acta Med Austriaca 2003;30:41–7.

66. Mikhaeel NG, Timothy AR, Hain SF, et al. 18-FDG-PET for the assessment of residual masses on CT

following treatment of lymphomas. Ann Oncol 2000; 11(Suppl 1):147–50.

67. Juweid ME, Wiseman GA, Vose JM, et al. Response assessment of aggressive non-Hodgkin's lymphoma by integrated International Workshop Criteria and fluorine-18-fluorodeoxyglucose positron emission tomography. J Clin Oncol 2005;23:4652–61.

68. Kostakoglu L, Goldsmith SJ, Leonard JP, et al. FDG-PET after 1 cycle of therapy predicts outcome in diffuse large cell lymphoma and classic Hodgkin disease. Cancer 2006;107:2678–87.

69. Picardi M, De Renzo A, Pane F, et al. Randomized comparison of consolidation radiation versus observation in bulky Hodgkin's lymphoma with post-chemotherapy negative positron emission tomography scans. Leuk Lymphoma 2007;48:1721–7.

70. Advani R, Maeda L, Lavori P, et al. Impact of positive positron emission tomography on prediction of freedom from progression after Stanford V chemotherapy in Hodgkin's disease. J Clin Oncol 2007;25: 3902–7.

71. Armitage JO, Weisenburger DD, Hutchins M, et al. Chemotherapy for diffuse large-cell lymphoma–rapidly responding patients have more durable remissions. J Clin Oncol 1986;4:160–4.

72. Front D, Bar-Shalom R, Mor M, et al. Hodgkin disease: prediction of outcome with 67Ga scintigraphy after one cycle of chemotherapy. Radiology 1999;210:487–91.

73. Hoekstra OS, Ossenkoppele GJ, Golding R, et al. Early treatment response in malignant lymphoma, as determined by planar fluorine-18-fluorodeoxyglucose scintigraphy. J Nucl Med 1993;34:1706–10.

74. Romer W, Hanauske AR, Ziegler S, et al. Positron emission tomography in non-Hodgkin's lymphoma: assessment of chemotherapy with fluorodeoxyglucose. Blood 1998;91:4464–71.

75. Humm JL, Rosenfeld A, Del Guerra A. From PET detectors to PET scanners. Eur J Nucl Med Mol Imaging 2003;30:1574–97.

76. Hall E, Giaccia A. Radiobiology for the radiologist. 4th edition. Philadelphia: Lippincott Williams & Wilkins; 2006.

77. Spaepen K, Stroobants S, Dupont P, et al. [(18)F]FDG-PET monitoring of tumour response to chemotherapy: does [(18)F]FDG uptake correlate with the viable tumour cell fraction? Eur J Nucl Med Mol Imaging 2003;30:682–8.

78. Yamane T, Daimaru O, Ito S, et al. Decreased 18F-FDG uptake 1 day after initiation of chemotherapy

for malignant lymphomas. J Nucl Med 2004;45: 1838–42.

79. Haioun C, Itti E, Rahmouni A, et al. [18F]fluoro-2-deoxy-D-glucose positron emission tomography (FDG-PET) in aggressive lymphoma: an early prognostic tool for predicting patient outcome. Blood 2005;106:1376–81.

80. Gallamini A, Hutchings M, Rigacci L, et al. Early interim 2-[18F]fluoro-2-deoxy-D-glucose positron emission tomography is prognostically superior to international prognostic score in advanced-stage Hodgkin's lymphoma: a report from a joint Italian-Danish study. J Clin Oncol 2007;25: 3746–52.

81. Gallamini A, Rigacci L, Merli F, et al. The predictive value of positron emission tomography scanning performed after two courses of standard therapy on treatment outcome in advanced stage Hodgkin's disease. Haematologica 2006;91:475–81.

82. Zinzani PL, Tani M, Fanti S, et al. Early positron emission tomography (PET) restaging: a predictive final response in Hodgkin's disease patients. Ann Oncol 2006;17:1296–300.

83. Spaepen K, Stroobants S, Dupont P, et al. Early restaging positron emission tomography with (18)F-fluorodeoxyglucose predicts outcome in patients with aggressive non-Hodgkin's lymphoma. Ann Oncol 2002;13:1356–63.

84. Shields AF, Grierson JR, Dohmen BM, et al. Imaging proliferation in vivo with [F-18]FLT and positron emission tomography. Nat Med 1998;4:1334–6.

85. Rasey JS, Grierson JR, Wiens LW, et al. Validation of FLT uptake as a measure of thymidine kinase-1 activity in A549 carcinoma cells. J Nucl Med 2002; 43:1210–7.

86. Wagner M, Seitz U, Buck A, et al. 3'-[18F]fluoro-3'-deoxythymidine ([18F]-FLT) as positron emission tomography tracer for imaging proliferation in a murine B-Cell lymphoma model and in the human disease. Cancer Res 2003;63:2681–7.

87. Buck AK, Kratochwil C, Glatting G, et al. Early assessment of therapy response in malignant lymphoma with the thymidine analogue [18F]FLT. Eur J Nucl Med Mol Imaging 2007;34:1775–82.

88. Herrmann K, Wieder HA, Buck AK, et al. Early response assessment using 3'-deoxy-3'-[18F]fluorothymidine-positron emission tomography in high-grade non-Hodgkin's lymphoma. Clin Cancer Res 2007;13:3552–8.

# Perspectives of Molecular Imaging and Radioimmunotherapy in Lymphoma

Andrei Iagaru, MD[a], Michael L. Goris, MD, PhD[a],
Sanjiv Sam Gambhir, MD, PhD[b],*

## KEYWORDS

- Lymphoma • Molecular imaging • Radioimmunotherapy

The American Cancer Society estimates 8220 new cases of Hodgkin lymphoma (HL) and 66,120 new cases of non-Hodgkin lymphoma (NHL) in the United States in 2008. The estimated number of deaths for the same year is 1350 from HL and 19,160 from NHL.[1] The classification of both HL and NHL continues to evolve and the World Health Organization incorporates in its current classification data derived from advances in the understanding of the pathogenesis of these disorders together with their distinguishing immunophenotypic, genotypic, clinical, and histopathological characteristics.[2] These advances allowed for significant improvements in survival of patients with HL and NHL through complex combinations of chemotherapy, radiation therapy, and immunotherapy capable of reducing long-term toxicity without sacrificing efficacy. However, successful treatment depends on accurate staging and prognostic estimations, as well as evaluation of response to therapy as early after initiation as possible to allow for identification of responders versus nonresponders. Thus, developing highly sensitive and specific imaging modalities has a paramount importance in the management of patients with cancer in general and HL/NHL in particular.

The basis of clinical molecular imaging is to provide functional information by imaging patients after they have been injected with a radiopharmaceutical that circulates within patients and is incorporated into various in vivo cellular processes.[3] This general principle has been applied for many years in nuclear medicine using various radiopharmaceuticals and gamma cameras. However, it is the more recent advent of positron emission tomography (PET) for oncology that has sparked a renewed interest in molecular imaging because of the greater resolution of this modality and also because of a radiotracer, $^{18}F$ Fluoro-2-Deoxyglucose ($^{18}F$ FDG), which has proven to be very accurate for imaging a wide variety of tumors. PET imaging technology advanced further after the introduction of the combined PET/CT scanner in 2001, which allowed merged visualization of complementary functional and anatomic information. Other molecular imaging techniques include single-photon emission computed tomography (SPECT), optical fluorescence, optical bioluminescence, magnetic resonance spectroscopy, molecular MR imaging, and targeted ultrasound.[4]

This review focuses on several aspects of molecular imaging and therapy that have an impact on the management of patients with

This work was supported in part by NCI ICMIC P50 CA114747 (SSG) and by the Doris Duke Foundation (SSG).

[a] Department of Radiology, Division of Nuclear Medicine, Stanford University Medical Center, 300 Pasteur Drive, Room H-0101, Stanford, CA 94305, USA

[b] Departments of Radiology and Bioengineering, Molecular Imaging Program at Stanford (MIPS), Stanford University School of Medicine, James H. Clark Center, 318 Campus Drive, East Wing, 1st Floor, Stanford, CA 94305-5427, USA

* Corresponding author.

*E-mail address:* sgambhir@stanford.edu (S.S. Gambhir).

Radiol Clin N Am 46 (2008) 243–252
doi:10.1016/j.rcl.2008.03.007

lymphoma. First, we review the prior use of gallium-67 citrate ($^{67}$Ga) for evaluation of lymphoma patients, mainly from a historical perspective, since it was the mainstream lymphoma functional imaging tracer for decades. Next, we dive into the current clinical uses of $^{18}$F FDG PET and PET/CT for evaluation of lymphoma patients, as well as into the use of radioimmunotherapy in lymphoma. Finally, we discuss advances in molecular imaging that may herald the next generation of PET radiotracers after $^{18}$F FDG.

## IMAGING LYMPHOMAS
### Gallium-67 Citrate and Gallium-67 Citrate Single-Photon Emission Computed Tomography

Historically, one of the first radiopharmaceuticals used in nuclear medicine to evaluate patients with lymphoma was $^{67}$Ga. Edwards and Hayes[5,6] describe the first uses of this radiopharmaceutical for scanning malignant neoplasms as early as 1969. After its introduction in 1969, $^{67}$Ga has become the most widely employed tumor-scanning agent in nuclear medicine. $^{67}$Ga citrate has been found to be of value in the staging and reevaluation of lymphomas as well as in detecting the extent and recurrence of lung tumors, breast tumors, malignant melanomas, testicular tumors, brain tumors, and malignant lesions involving the liver. Despite these promising initial reports, from the very beginning it was noted that $^{67}$Ga localizes in areas of inflammation as well, thus affecting its specificity.[7] Hodgkin lymphoma was one of the first neoplastic processes evaluated with this radiopharmaceutical.[8,9] Other reports that followed soon after included other non-Hodgkin lymphomas as potential indications for $^{67}$Ga imaging.[10] An example of $^{67}$Ga scintigraphy in a patient with NHL before and after therapy is presented in **Fig. 1.** Adler and colleagues[11] report a series of 108 patients with HL and NHL evaluated with $^{67}$Ga, suggesting 83% overall accuracy, with 87% accuracy for lymph node involvement, but only 48% accuracy for lesions of the lungs and liver. A report by Levi and colleagues[12] indicated that imaging lymphoma patients with $^{67}$Ga had the ability to detect involvement of intra-abdominal lymph nodes, thus sparing the patients from the morbidity associated with unnecessary staging laparotomies. Other reports from that era confirmed the role of $^{67}$Ga citrate imaging in HL and NHL, in particular for evaluation after therapy and for disease surveillance.[13–16] However, because of its hepatic clearance and subsequent bowel excretion, as well as the limitations of spatial

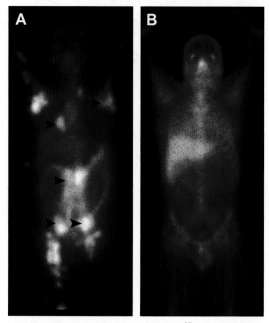

**Fig. 1.** A 28-year-old man with NHL. $^{67}$Ga citrate scintigraphy demonstrates (A) extensive disease involvement above and below the diaphragm (*arrowheads*) and (B) complete scintigraphic response to therapy. Normal $^{67}$Ga citrate uptake is seen in the lacrimary glands, liver, spleen, and bone marrow.

resolution of planar scintigraphy, $^{67}$Ga evaluation of abdominal lesions was a challenging task.

Advances in technology allowed for introduction of clinical SPECT, which led to significant improvements in the accuracy of $^{67}$Ga imaging of lymphoma. Tumeh and colleagues[17] concluded that SPECT was more accurate in depicting foci of gallium-avid lymphoma in the chest and abdomen and in excluding disease when planar imaging was equivocal. Kostakoglu and colleagues[18] suggested that $^{67}$Ga SPECT may prove particularly useful in detecting residual disease activity in patients in whom biopsy was positive but the interpretations of the CT scans were uncertain in regard to presence of tumors, with an overall accuracy of 93%.

One of the latest advances in medical imaging is image fusion, the combination of anatomic and functional information in a single image. Hybrid cameras combining SPECT and CT have become a clinical reality and this is reflected in the articles focusing on their use for imaging lymphoma. Palumbo and colleagues[19] report the use of $^{67}$Ga SPECT/CT in lymphoma, concluding that the hybrid system is able to provide information not obtained by SPECT alone, information that may cause a change in therapeutic strategy. A recent study of 74 patients with lymphoma suggested that [67]Ga SPECT/CT study improved the diagnostic yield over planar scintigraphy and SPECT alone, providing better anatomic localization of the lesions and detection of extranodal disease.[20] Despite these technical advances, the development of PET and more recently hybrid PET/CT technology, as well as their widespread acceptance and clinical use, have made [67]Ga imaging obsolete because of their improved spatial resolution and the less time required for imaging. [68]Ga, a positron emitter, may be useful in imaging lymphomas, but its role alone or in combination with [18]F FDG PET/CT remains to be investigated. The inherent superiority of PET imaging is a clear advantage compared with single-photon imaging, while the feasibility of a [68]Ge/[68]Ga generator (usable for more than a year) is extremely cost-effective, negating the need for an on-site cyclotron.[21]

## [18]F Fluoro-2-Deoxyglucose Positron Emission Tomography

As early as 1997, Hoh and colleagues[22] compared the staging results of [18]F FDG PET with staging using a combination of CT of the chest, abdomen, and pelvis; MR imaging scans; gallium scans; lymphangiograms; staging laparatomies; and bone scans. They concluded that a whole-body [18]F FDG PET–based staging algorithm may be an accurate and cost-effective method for staging or restaging HL and NHL. Kostakoglu and colleagues[23] compared [18]F FDG PET and [67]Ga scintigraphy in 51 patients with HL and NHL. Their study showed not only that [18]F FDG PET had significantly higher site and patient sensitivity than [67]Ga scintigraphy, but also that this change in disease stage by [18]F FDG PET may result in a change in therapy strategy. The findings of a study by Bar-Shalom and colleagues[24] support the fact that [18]F FDG PET allows a significantly more accurate definition of active disease compared with [67]Ga scintigraphy. Shen and colleagues[25] have also shown that [18]F FDG PET not only demonstrates more sites of disease than [67]Ga scintigraphy at initial staging of HL and NHL, but also this upstaging of the patients may result in a change in therapy strategy in 20% of their cases.

Currently, [18]F FDG is the standard PET radiopharmaceutical in clinical use. This radiopharmaceutical is taken up by cells in proportion to their rate of glucose metabolism and therefore acts as an indicator for malignancy. [18]F FDG PET and PET/CT is at least equivalent to CT for the initial staging of lymphomas.[26] However, the impact of combined PET/CT and fast-scanning CT with contrast has yet to be evaluated in the management of lymphoma patients. At this point, [18]F FDG PET and CT must be considered as giving complementary staging information. [18]F FDG PET also has high diagnostic accuracy for restaging lymphoma after initial treatment.[26,27] [18]F FDG PET has shown high accuracy in the early prediction of response to chemotherapy and in the evaluation of residual masses after chemotherapy or radiation therapy.[28] Therefore, PET is likely to play a major role in tailoring the intensity of the treatment to the individual patient. A pretreatment PET study is essential for accurate assessment of residual masses and early monitoring of response to the treatment. In addition, a baseline PET scan will help detect relapse or residual disease, because relapse occurs most often in the region of previous disease.

[18]F FDG PET is regarded as a superior modality, compared with CT, for assessing posttreatment response in lymphoma patients.[29,30] Its superiority lies in the ability to differentiate viable tumor from fibrosis. This is important, since up to 64% of patients with HL will present with a residual mass on CT following treatment, but only 18% will actually relapse.[31] It is desirable to assess response and predict prognosis as early as possible after treatment begins. Mid-treatment [18]F FDG PET scans have already been shown to be useful for early prediction of treatment response in both NHL and HL.[32–35] So far, Mikhaeel and colleagues[33] have provided the largest study on this subject. They included 121 patients with aggressive NHL and showed that [18]F FDG PET scans after 2 to three cycles of chemotherapy can predict progression-free and overall survival. Kostakoglu and colleagues[35] showed that interim [18]F FDG PET scans may be able to predict response as early as after one cycle of treatment. Currently, the optimal timing of the interim [18]F FDG PET/CT scan remains unclear as the predictive values of [18]F FDG PET/CT scans obtained at different mid-treatment periods have not been compared within a single study. Our previously reported results showed that [18]F FDG PET/CT scans obtained after both two and four cycles of chemotherapy correlated well (correlation coefficients of 0.98 and 0.80, respectively) with end-treatment response. Furthermore, scans performed at two cycles did not differ significantly from scans performed at four cycles in terms of [18]F FDG uptake from baseline to post-therapy.[36] This implies that patients who fail to respond to treatment can be identified by [18]F FDG PET as early as after two cycles, and that these patents can be spared additional cycles of an ineffective therapy and be offered an alternative chemotherapy regimen. Conversely, patients who respond after two cycles should complete the full course of chemotherapy, as they will likely

have an excellent prognosis. These results will have to be confirmed by larger, prospective trials. **Fig. 2** shows the [18]F FDG PET scans of a patient with HL who had complete response to therapy, while **Fig. 3** shows a patient with NHL with residual disease on [18]F FDG PET at the end of treatment.

## RADIOIMMUNOTHERAPY IN LYMPHOMAS

If radioimmunotherapy had to be initially validated, lymphomas would have been the malignancies of choice. This is because generally speaking lymphomas are radiosensitive. However, before reviewing radioimmunotherapy of (low grade) lymphomas, a more general review of radioimmunotherapy will be useful.

A first useful distinction is between the medical and surgical models in medicine. In medical models the therapeutic agent has an effect primarily only if it meets the target. For example, antibiotics, having effects on the bacteria they meet but not (one hopes) on other tissues. Immunotherapy is another good example, since in the absence of a receptor the antibody targeted for that receptor would have no effect. In the medical model, specificity resides in the mechanism (a specific interaction between agent and target). In the surgical model, the effect of the treatment is not specific to the target. The specificity originates in the precision of the anatomic aim toward the target. In radiation therapy, the goal of therapy planning is to concentrate the dose of radiation over a limited region near the target. The knife and the radiation are indifferent in their effect and work against the target only if well directed.

Second, if we consider radioimmunotherapy as a step beyond immunotherapy of cancer, the step was prompted by the (relative) failure of the latter. The conventional way to explain the failure is a lack of intrinsic killing effect and a lack of penetration into poorly vascularized tumor masses. The addition of a radioactive label (usually a β-emitter) to the antibody would improve both. Radiation is lethal and the type of radiation used (beta rays) has a sufficient range to overcome the lack of antibody penetration.

The introduction of radioimmunotherapy is transition from medical to surgical model: even those antibodies that have not reached their target (yet) are irradiating the tissues in which they are present. A quick and complete delivery of the antibody to the target(s) therefore becomes crucial. Additionally, if the goal of radioimmunotherapy is to increase the reach and killing effect, what should the range (and the energy) of the β-ray be? A higher energy and longer range would seem

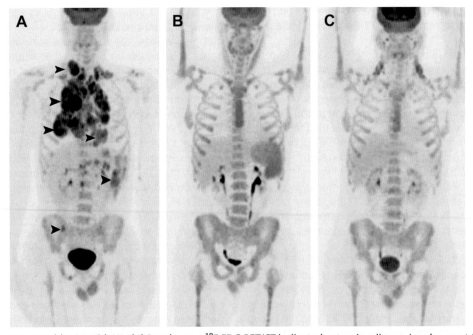

Fig. 2. A 19-year-old man with HL. (*A*) Pre-therapy [18]F FDG PET/CT indicated extensive disease involvement (*arrowheads*). (*B*) [18]F FDG PET/CT after four cycles of chemotherapy showed complete metabolic response to Stanford V therapy (Doxorubicin, Vinblastine, Mustargen, Etoposide, Bleomycin, Vincristine and Prednisone). (*C*) The scan at the end of therapy remained negative.

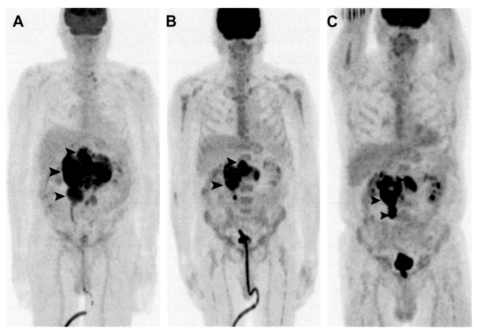

Fig. 3. A 75-year-old man with NHL. (*A*) Pre-therapy $^{18}$F FDG PET/CT showed extensive abdominal disease (*arrowheads*). (*B*) $^{18}$F FDG PET/CT after two cycles of chemotherapy indicated partial metabolic response to R-CHOP (Rituximab, Cyclophosphamide, Doxorubicin, Vincristine and Prednisolone) treatment (*arrowheads*). (*C*) At the end of therapy the scan remained positive (*arrowheads*).

advantageous in larger masses, but in submicroscopic disease, most of the energy would be dispensed to surrounding normal tissues. Finally, the fact that the specificity lies into location, combined with the fact that the target is not rapidly reached, suggests that the half-life of the label should be longer than the average time needed for an optimal accumulation in the tumor.

All available data, for all forms of disease, suggest that tumor doses are not high enough to have a curative effect and that measured tumor doses do not predict response.[37] Yet there is, at least in lymphomas, a curative effect. This discrepancy has preoccupied researchers for some time.[38] Some of the magnified effect of what is a relatively small radiation dose can be assigned to the continuous nature of the irradiation by radio-labeled antibodies.[39,40] More importantly, while in external beam irradiation an average dose to the tumor volume as a whole makes sense, the microscopic dose is very heterogeneous.[41] This heterogeneity may in fact increase the dose at a microscopic level to vital tumor elements.

Low-grade lymphomas are refractory to most treatments, and each subsequent treatment is less effective.[42] Radioimmunotherapy seemed a possibility to improve the treatment options. At present, the most successful (and approved by the Food and Drug Administration) radioimmunotherapy agents for lymphomas are anti-CD20 monoclonal antibodies. Rituximab (Rituxan) is a chimeric antibody, used as a nonradioactive antibody and to pre-load the patient when Zevalin is used. Zevalin is the Yttrium-90 ($^{90}$Y) or Indium-111 ($^{111}$In) labeled form of Ibritumomab Tiuxetan. Bexxar is the Iodine-131 ($^{131}$I) labeled form of Tositumomab. Ibritumomab Tiuxetan and Tositumomab are murine anti-CD20 monoclonal antibodies, not chimeric antibodies. The main characteristics of Bexxar and Zevalin are presented in **Table 1**.

The treatments with both tracers are very similar. In both cases the injection of the labeled antibody is preceded by the injection of a large amount of unlabeled antibody (Rituximab before Zevalin and Tositumomab before Bexxar).[43] This "pre-loading" occupies too easily reachable sites (bone marrow and spleen), and "forces" the labeled antibody to circulate longer and have a higher probability to reach the lymphoma sites. In the case of Zevalin, a biodistribution study with $^{111}$In-Zevalin precedes the therapeutic dose with the $^{90}$Y-labeled Zevalin. With Bexxar, the dosimetric and therapeutic phases of the study are performed with $^{131}$I-Bexxar (but with different doses). However, because of the large interpatient variability in whole-body retention of $^{131}$I, in the

**Table 1**
**Main characteristics of Bexxar and Zevalin**

|  | Bexxar | Zevalin |
|---|---|---|
| β-emitter | $^{131}$I (half-life: 8.01 days) | $^{90}$Y (half-life: 2.67 days) |
| Anti-CD20 antibody | Tositumomab | Ibritumomab Tiuxetan |
| Antibody type | Monoclonal murine | Monoclonal murine |
| Pre-dose injection | Unlabeled Tositumomab | Unlabeled Rituximab |
| Pre-therapy imaging | Yes (for dosimetry) | Yes (for biodistribution) |
| Pre-therapy dose | $^{131}$I-Tositumomab (5 mCi) | $^{111}$In-Ibritumomab Tiuxetan (5 mCi) |
| Treatment dose | 75 cGy (whole-body) | 0.4 mCi/kg (up to 32 mCi) |

case of Bexxar, an estimation of the amount that will deliver a dose of 75 cGy to the whole body is calculated. Our previously reported results showed that clinical practice of Bexxar and Zevalin radioimmunotherapy is an effective and safe adjunctive treatment for patients with NHL refractory/relapsed to conventional treatment. Both agents had comparable response rates and side effects.[44] Thus, the choice of one versus another appears to depend on the treating physicians' preferences and local logistics. **Fig. 4** shows the $^{18}$F FDG PET scans of a patient with NHL and complete response after Zevalin treatment. In **Fig. 5** the $^{18}$F FDG PET scans of a patient with

NHL indicate progressive disease after Zevalin treatment.

In neither case is the dose to the tumor calculated, because current in vivo imaging methods allow only the calculation of a macroscopic and average tumor dose, probably irrelevant in view of the microscopic heterogeneity. The administered quantity is limited by considerations of toxicity.

Horning and colleagues[45] reported on a series of 40 patients treated with Bexxar. The median number of prior treatments was 4. Most patients were low-grade lymphomas (70%). Some were transformed low grade (25%), a few were

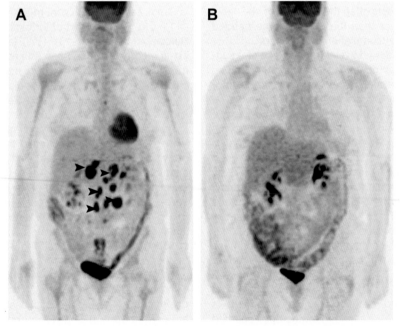

**Fig. 4.** A 60-year-old woman with NHL and complete response after Zevalin treatment. (*A*) Pre-therapy $^{18}$F FDG PET/CT shows lesions in the abdomen (*arrowheads*) and (*B*) resolution of the lesions noted before therapy.

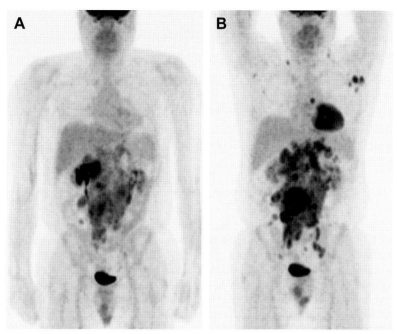

Fig. 5. A 45-year-old man with NHL and progressive disease after Zevalin treatment. [18]F FDG PET scans (A) before and (B) after therapy (3 months apart) show progression of disease.

intermediate grade. Thirty-five (88%) were Rituximab refractory. Overall response rate was 68%, with a median response duration of 16 months (1+ to 38+ months). A complete response was seen in 33% of the patients. The median duration was not reached. Similar results were reported by Kaminski and colleagues[46] about a series of 60 patients. Again, the group was handicapped by a median of 4 prior treatments. Low grade, transformed low grade, and intermediate grade were distributed as 56%, 38%, and 2% respectively. Overall response and complete response were 47% and 20%, with median duration of 12 and 47 months respectively. When the method was used as the first treatment, the complete response rate was higher than 72% and the 5-year survival higher than 55%.[47] In the context of other treatments and outcomes for low-grade B-cell lymphomas, these results are remarkable. Toxicity is primarily hematological, but rare and reversible with the actual clinical protocols. Interestingly, only one paper reports on a prospective and randomized study on the additional effect of the radioactive label.[48] In this study, with the same amount of antibody in identical regimens, but with one arm the addition of radioactivity, the complete response rate was 33% in the radioactive group and 8% in the unlabeled group. The overall response rate was 55% and 19% respectively. The same (positive) results should not be expected for all tumors.[49,50] However, improvement

will come by making the delivery more efficient by labeling the antibody, already joint to the target.[51]

## FUTURE DIRECTIONS

A multitude of new PET radiopharmaceuticals are currently being developed to complement [18]F FDG for use in cancer imaging. These can be categorized as nonspecific tracers, which take advantage of the increased metabolic activity and vascularity of malignant tumors, and specific agents that bind to tumor-specific antigens or receptors. Metabolic agents like [18]F FDG typically trace the enzymatic turnover of a parent compound. A promising radiopharmaceutical is the thymidine analog 3'-deoxy-3'-[[18]F] fluorothymidine (FLT), which provides a measure of DNA replication.[52] Herrmann and colleagues[53] conducted a trial of FLT PET in patients treated for NHL and concluded that FLT PET appeared to be promising for early evaluation of drug effects in lymphoma. Potential advantages of FLT over FDG include fewer false-positive lesions due to inflammation, increased sensitivity of detecting brain lesions due to decreased neuronal uptake, and theoretically greater reliability in monitoring response to selective (cytostatic) chemotherapies. PET radiopharmaceuticals that exploit the high vascularity of many tumors include pure perfusion tracers such as [15]O-labelled water or [13]NH$_3$, or measure

**Table 2**
Future approaches to molecular imaging of lymphomas may include a variety of new radiopharmaceuticals with various mechanisms of uptake

| Radiopharmaceutical | Radiotracer | Half-life | Mechanism of Uptake |
|---|---|---|---|
| 3'-deoxy-3'-[$^{18}$F]fluorothymidine (FLT) | $^{18}$F | 109 min | DNA Replication |
| $^{18}$F-galacto-RGD | $^{18}$F | 109 min | $\alpha_v\beta_3$-integrin expression |
| $^{18}$F Fluoromisonidazole ($^{18}$F MISO) | $^{18}$F | 109 min | Hypoxia |
| $^{64}$Cu-diacetyl-bis(N(4)-methylthiosemicarbazone) ($^{64}$Cu ATSM) | $^{64}$Cu | 12 hours | Hypoxia |
| $^{89}$Zr-Zevalin | $^{89}$Zr | 78 hours | Anti-CD20 antibody |

of angiogenesis such as the $^{18}$F-labeled glycosylated tripeptide $^{18}$F-galacto-RGD,[54] which targets $\alpha_v\beta_3$-integrin, a protein selectively expressed on activated endothelial cells. Hypoxia-sensitive radiopharmaceuticals include $^{18}$F Fluoromisonidazole (FMISO), an analog of 2-nitro-imidazole, and $^{64}$Cu diacetyl-bis (N(4)-methylthiosemicarbazone) ($^{64}$Cu-ATSM). Although nonspecific radiopharmaceuticals provide useful imaging of aggressive neoplasms, they typically exhibit decreased sensitivity in detecting tumors with low growth rates. It is therefore essential that PET radiopharmaceuticals be developed that bind selectively and with high tumor-to-background ratio to intracellular and cell-surface receptors up-regulated in cancer cells. A potentially useful class of tumor-imaging radiopharmaceuticals uses radio-chelated monoclonal antibodies labeled with relatively long half-life positron emitters $^{64}$Cu (12 hours) and $^{124}$I (4 days), which target tumor-specific antigens such as the CD-20 present on the surface of B-cells. The anti-CD20 monoclonal antibodies used for NHL therapy can potentially be used for imaging if labeled with a positron emitter. Perk and colleagues[55] labeled Zevalin with $^{89}$Zr and reported the first use in a human subject. Their PET images obtained after injection of $^{89}$Zr-Zevalin showed targeting of all known tumor lesions, but evaluation in prospective trials is required for validation of this type of imaging radiopharmaceuticals. From an imaging standpoint, plasma clearance of the bulky antibody molecule must be optimized to improve tumor-to-background activity, and so smaller engineered antibody fragments with rapid renal clearance are being developed.[56] **Table 2** summarizes the characteristics of these new molecular imaging agents.

## SUMMARY

Molecular imaging and PET in particular has gained widespread acceptance for the diagnosis, staging, assessing response to therapy and management of HL and NHL. The fundamental strength of PET over conventional CT imaging is the ability to convey functional information that even the most exquisitely detailed anatomic image cannot provide. Radioimmunotherapy has shown promising results in the therapy of advanced relapsed or therapy refractory NHL and may have even better results when introduced early, in combination with chemotherapy for the management of patients with NHL.

## REFERENCES

1. Jemal A, Siegel R, Ward E, et al. Cancer statistics, 2008. CA Cancer J Clin 2008;58(2):71–96.
2. Young GA, Iland HJ. Clinical perspectives in lymphoma. Intern Med J 2007;37(7):478–84.
3. Gambhir SS. Molecular imaging of cancer with positron emission tomography. Nat Rev Cancer 2002; 2(9):683–93.
4. Massoud TF, Gambhir SS. Molecular imaging in living subjects: seeing fundamental biological processes in a new light. Genes Dev 2003;17(5): 545–80.
5. Edwards CL, Hayes RL. Tumor scanning with 67Ga citrate. J Nucl Med 1969;10(2):103–5.
6. Edwards CL, Hayes RL. Scanning malignant neoplasms with gallium 67. JAMA 1970;212(7):1182–91.
7. Lavendar JP, Lowe J, Barker JR, et al. Gallium 67 citrate scanning in neoplastic and inflammatory lesions. Br J Radiol 1971;44(521):361–6.
8. Kay DN, McCready VR. Clinical isotope scanning using 67 Ga citrate in the management of Hodgkin's disease. Br J Radiol 1972;45(534):437–43.
9. Turner DA, Pinsky SM, Gottschalk A, et al. The use of 67 Ga scanning in the staging of Hodgkin's disease. Radiology 1972;104(1):97–101.
10. Palumbo R, Tonato M, Martelli MF, et al. Gallium-67 citrate in the staging of malignant lymphomas. J Nucl Biol Med 1973;17(3):100–3.
11. Adler S, Parthasarathy KL, Bakshi SP, et al. Gallium-67-citrate scanning for the localization and staging of lymphomas. J Nucl Med 1975;16(4):255–60.

12. Levi JA, O'Connell MJ, Murphy WL, et al. Role of 67gallium citrate scanning in the management of non-Hodgkin's lymphoma. Cancer 1975;36(5): 1690–741.

13. Horn NL, Ray GR, Kriss JP. Gallium-67 citrate scanning in Hodgkin's disease and non-Hodgkin's lymphoma. Cancer 1976;37(1):250–7.

14. Johnston GS, Go MF, Benua RS, et al. Gallium-67 citrate imaging in Hodgkin's disease: final report of cooperative group. J Nucl Med 1977;18(7):692–8.

15. Andrews GA, Hubner KF, Greenlaw RH. Ga-67 citrate imaging in malignant lymphoma: final report of cooperative group. J Nucl Med 1978;19(9):1013–9.

16. Herman TS, Jones SE. Systematic restaging in patients with Hodgkin's disease: a Southwest Oncology Group Study. Cancer 1978;42(4):1976–82.

17. Tumeh SS, Rosenthal DS, Kaplan WD, et al. Lymphoma: evaluation with Ga-67 SPECT. Radiology 1987;164(1):111–4.

18. Kostakoglu L, Yeh SD, Portlock C, et al. Validation of gallium-67-citrate single-photon emission computed tomography in biopsy-confirmed residual Hodgkin's disease in the mediastinum. J Nucl Med 1992;33(3): 345–50.

19. Palumbo B, Sivolella S, Palumbo I, et al. 67Ga-SPECT/CT with a hybrid system in the clinical management of lymphoma. Eur J Nucl Med Mol Imaging 2005;32(9):1011–7.

20. Fuertes Manuel J, Estorch Cabrera M, Camacho Martí V, et al. SPECT-CT 67Ga studies in lymphoma disease. Contribution to staging and follow-up. Rev Esp Med Nucl 2006;25(4):242–9.

21. Al-Nahhas A, Win Z, Szyszko T, et al. What can gallium-68 PET add to receptor and molecular imaging? Eur J Nucl Med Mol Imaging 2007;34(12):1897–901.

22. Hoh CK, Glaspy J, Rosen P, et al. Whole-body FDG-PET imaging for staging of Hodgkin's disease and lymphoma. J Nucl Med 1997;38(3):343–8.

23. Kostakoglu L, Leonard JP, Kuji I, et al. Comparison of fluorine-18 fluorodeoxyglucose positron emission tomography and Ga-67 scintigraphy in evaluation of lymphoma. Cancer 2002;94(4):879–88.

24. Bar-Shalom R, Yefremov N, Haim N, et al. Camera-based FDG PET and 67Ga SPECT in evaluation of lymphoma: comparative study. Radiology 2003; 227(2):353–60.

25. Shen YY, Kao A, Yen RF. Comparison of 18F-fluoro-2-deoxyglucose positron emission tomography and gallium-67 citrate scintigraphy for detecting malignant lymphoma. Oncol Rep 2002;9(2):321–5.

26. la Fougere C, Hundt W, Brockel N, et al. Value of PET/CT versus PET and CT performed as separate investigations in patients with Hodgkin's disease and non-Hodgkin's lymphoma. Eur J Nucl Med Mol Imaging 2006;33(12):1417–25.

27. Tatsumi M, Cohade C, Nakamoto Y, et al. Direct comparison of FDG PET and CT findings in patients with lymphoma: initial experience. Radiology 2005; 237(3):1038–45.

28. Kazama T, Faria SC, Varavithya V, et al. FDG PET in the evaluation of treatment for lymphoma: clinical usefulness and pitfalls. Radiographics 2005;25(1): 191–207.

29. De Wit M, Bumann D, Beyer W, et al. Whole-body positron emission tomography (PET) for diagnosis of residual mass in patients with lymphoma. Ann Oncol 1997;8(Suppl 1):S57–60.

30. Jerusalem G, Beguin Y, Fassotte MF, et al. Whole-body positron emission tomography using fluorine-18-fluorodeoxyglucose for post-treatment evaluation in Hodgkin's disease and non-Hodgkin's lymphoma has a higher diagnostic and prognostic value than classical computed tomography scan imaging. Blood 1999;94:429–33.

31. Radford JA, Cowan RA, Flanagan M, et al. The significance of residual mediastinal abnormality on CXR following treatment for Hodgkin's disease. J Clin Oncol 1988;6:940–6.

32. Hoekstra OS, Ossenkoppele GJ, Golding R, et al. Early treatment response in malignant lymphoma, as determined by planar fluorine-18-fluorodeoxyglucose scintigraphy. J Nucl Med 1993;34:1706–10.

33. Mikhaeel NG, Hutchings M, Fields PA, et al. FDG-PET after two to three cycles of chemotherapy predicts progression-free and overall survival in high-grade non-Hodgkin lymphoma. Ann Oncol 2005;16:1514–23.

34. Hutchings M, Loft A, Hansen M, et al. FDG-PET after two cycles of chemotherapy predicts treatment failure and progression-free survival in Hodgkin lymphoma. Blood 2006;107:52–9.

35. Kostakoglu L, Coleman M, Leonard JP, et al. PET predicts prognosis after 1 cycle of chemotherapy in aggressive lymphoma and Hodgkin disease. J Nucl Med 2002;43:1018–27.

36. Iagaru A, Wang Y, Mari C, et al. 18F FDG PET/CT prediction of response to chemotherapy in lymphoma: when is the optimal time for the first re-evaluation scan? Clin Nucl Med 2008;33(1):77.

37. Knox SJ, Goris ML, Trisler K, et al. 90-Y-labeled anti-CD20 monoclonal antibody therapy of recurrent B cell lymphoma. Clin Cancer Res 1996;2: 457–70.

38. Knox SJ, Goris ML, Wessels BW. Overview of animal studies comparing radioimmunotherapy with dose equivalent external beam irradiation. Radiother Oncol 1992;23:111–7.

39. Knox S, Levy R, Miller RA, et al. Determinants of the anti-tumor effect of radiolabelled monoclonal antibodies. Cancer Res 1990;50:4935–40.

40. Knox SJ, Sutherland W, Goris ML. Correlation of tumor sensitivity to low dose rate irradiation with G2/M-phase block and other radiobiological parameters. Radiat Res 1993;135:24–31.

41. Langmuir VK, Fowler JF, Knox SJ, et al. Radiobiology of radiolabeled antibody therapy as applied to tumor dosimetry. Med Phys 1993;20(2 Pt 2):601–10.

42. Johnson PW, Rohatiner AZ, Whelan JS, et al. Patterns of survival in patients with recurrent follicular lymphoma: a 20-year study from a single center. J Clin Oncol 1995;13:140–7.

43. Schiele J, Knox SJ, Ruehl W, et al. The effect of unlabelled monoclonal antibody (MAB) on the biodistribution of 131I-anti-idiotype MAB in murine B cell lymphoma. Radiother Oncol 1992;24:169–76.

44. Iagaru A, Zhu H, Mari C, et al. Comparison of efficacy and toxicity of bexxar and zevalin in the management of refractory non-Hodgkin's lymphoma. Eur J Nucl Med Mol Imaging 2007;34(10):S168.

45. Horning SJ, Younes A, Kroll S, et al. Efficacy and safety of tositumomab and iodine-131 tositumomab (bexxar) in b-cell lymphoma progressive after rituximab. J Clin Oncol 2005;23(4):712–9.

46. Kaminski MS, Zelenetz AD, Press OW, et al. Pivotal study of I-131 tositumomab for chemotherapy-refractory low-grade or transformed low-grade B-cell non-Hodgkin's lymphomas. J Clin Oncol 2001;19:3918–28.

47. Kaminski MS, Tuck M, Estes J, et al. 131I-tositumomab therapy as initial treatment for follicular lymphoma. N Engl J Med 2005;352(5):441–9.

48. Davis TA, Kaminsky MS, Leonard J, et al. The radioisotope contributes significantly to the activity of radioimmunotherapy. Clin Cancer Res 2004;10(23):7792–8.

49. Deb N, Goris ML, Trisler K. Treatment of hormone refractory prostate cancer with 90Y-CYT-356 monoclonal antibody. Clin Cancer Res 1996;2:1289–97.

50. Knox SJ, Goris ML, Tempero M, et al. Phase II trial of Yttrium-90-Dota-Biotin pretargeted by NR-LU-10 antibody/Streptavidin in patients with metastatic colon cancer. Clin Cancer Res 2000;6:406–14.

51. Forero A, Weiden PL, Vose JM, et al. Phase I trial of a novel anti-CD20 fusion protein in pretargeted radioimmunotherapy for B-cell non-Hodgkin's lymphoma. Blood 2004;104(1):227–36.

52. Yap CS, Czernin J, Fishbein MC, et al. Evaluation of thoracic tumors with 18F-fluorothymidine and 18F-fluorodeoxyglucose-positron emission tomography. Chest 2006;129(2):393–401.

53. Herrmann K, Wieder HA, Buck AK, et al. Early response assessment using 3'-deoxy-3'-[18F]fluorothymidine-positron emission tomography in high-grade non-Hodgkin's lymphoma. Clin Cancer Res 2007;13(12):3552–8.

54. Beer AJ, Haubner R, Goebel M, et al. Biodistribution and pharmacokinetics of the alphavbeta3-selective tracer 18F-galacto-RGD in cancer patients. J Nucl Med 2005;46(8):1333–41.

55. Perk LR, Visser OJ, Stigter-van Walsum M, et al. Preparation and evaluation of (89)Zr-Zevalin for monitoring of (90)Y-Zevalin biodistribution with positron emission tomography. Eur J Nucl Med Mol Imaging 2006;33(11):1337–45.

56. Cai W, Chen X. Anti-angiogenic cancer therapy based on integrin alphavbeta3 antagonism. Anticancer Agents Med Chem 2006;6(5):407–28.

# Cross-Sectional Evaluation of Thoracic Lymphoma

Young A Bae, MD[a,b], Kyung Soo Lee, MD[a,*]

**KEYWORDS**

- Lymphoma • CT • Hodgkin lymphoma
- Thoracic neoplasms

Lymphomas are a diverse group of neoplastic disorders. They are divided into Hodgkin lymphoma (HL) and non-Hodgkin lymphoma (NHL) and further subdivisions depend on the histologic types.[1]

The presence and distribution of thoracic involvement are important in both tumor staging and treatment, especially when radiation therapy is planned.[2] Intrathoracic involvement is commoner in HL than NHL.[3,4] Although HL represents only 10% to 15% of all cases of lymphomas, approximately 85% of patients with HL have intrathoracic disease at presentation.[5] NHL represents about 85% to 90% of all cases of lymphoma and approximately 40% to 45% of patients with NHL have intrathoracic disease at the initial presentation.[4]

Although HL and NHL may have overlapping imaging findings, there are some significant differences in their radiologic features. In this article, we demonstrate the diverse radiologic features of thoracic lymphomas.

## MEDIASTINAL INVOLVEMENT OF LYMPHOMAS

HL is the most common lymphoma presenting with mediastinal lymphadenopathy and most frequently involves lymph nodes in anterior mediastinal and paratracheal areas in a contiguous manner, and thus involves in decreasing order of frequency the nodes in the hilar, subcarinal, peridiaphragmatic, paraesophageal, and internal mammary areas (**Fig. 1**).[1] Nodular sclerosing HL, the commonest subtype, has a unique predilection for the nodes in the anterior mediastinum.

On CT, HL is characterized by the presence of a discrete anterior mediastinal mass with a lobulated contour. The tumor most commonly demonstrates homogeneous soft-tissue attenuation, although large lymph node masses may demonstrate heterogeneity with complex low attenuation representing necrosis, hemorrhage, or cystic degeneration (**Fig. 2**).[6] In the series by Hopper and colleagues,[7] necrotic and cystic-appearing mediastinal lymph nodes were noticed at presentation in 21% of cases of HL. Necrosis is observed most commonly in the nodular sclerosing and mixed cellularity cell types of HL and was not seen in the lymphocyte predominant variety.

In NHL, thoracic involvement is present in up to 45% of cases[8] and, most often, mediastinal lymphomatous involvement occurs as a disseminated or recurrent form of extrathoracic lymphoma. Generally, involved lymph nodes tend to be larger as compared with those in HL and have a predilection for noncontiguous or hematogenous spread to thoracic and distant nodal and extranodal sites.[9,10] Unlike HL, in which anatomic sites of involvement are important, the histologic subtype and tumor bulk are more important prognostic factors in NHL.

Nodes in the paratracheal and anterior mediastinal areas are still the most common sites for NHL

This study was supported by the SRC/ERC Program of MOST/KOSEF (R11-2002-103).

[a] Department of Radiology, Center for Imaging Science, Samsung Medical Center, Sungkyunkwan University School of Medicine, 50, Ilwon-Dong, Kangnam-Ku, Seoul 135-710, Republic of Korea

[b] Department of Radiology, Hallym University College of Medicine, Pyongchon, Kyungki-do 431-070, Republic of Korea

* Corresponding author.

*E-mail address:* kyungs.lee@samsung.com (K.S. Lee).

Radiol Clin N Am 46 (2008) 253–264
doi:10.1016/j.rcl.2008.03.006

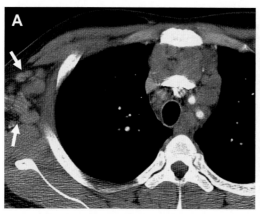
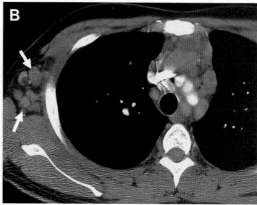

Fig. 1. Hodgkin lymphoma (nodular sclerosing type) in a 26-year-old man. (*A, B*) Transverse mediastinal-window CT (5.0-mm section thickness) scans obtained at levels of left innominate vein show conglomerated lymph node enlargement showing contiguous growth in prevascular (anterior mediastinal) and bilateral paratracheal areas. Also note enlarged lymph nodes (*arrows*) in the right axillary area.

involvement followed by those in the subcarinal, hilar, posterior mediastinal (para-aortic, paravertebral, and retrocrural), and pericardial areas.[8] It is difficult to differentiate HL from NHL on the basis of nodal distribution alone.[1] Although lymphoma is one of the commonest mediastinal tumors, it is uncommon for either NHL or HL to be limited to the mediastinum at the time of diagnosis. The sole mediastinum involvement occurs in only about 5% of lymphoma cases.[11] On CT, the majority of tumors have a relatively homogeneous soft tissue density; large tumors commonly contain areas of low attenuation due to hemorrhage or necrosis (**Fig. 3**). Enlarged nodes in contiguous lymph node groups are frequently present.

Although there are many subtypes of NHL, large B-cell lymphoma and lymphoblastic lymphoma are the most common subtypes, primarily involving the anterior mediastinum (**Table 1**). Primary mediastinal large B-cell lymphomas usually present with large and lobulated anterior mediastinal masses and occur predominantly in young adults with a median age of 26 years (see **Fig. 3**).[12] Low attenuation areas of necrosis (see **Fig. 3**) within the mass were seen in 50% and calcification in 5%.[13] Also they often directly invade adjacent structures. Lymphoblastic lymphomas are highly aggressive and high-grade lymphomas, arising from thymic lymphocytes.[14] They usually occur in patients in the first to second decades of life. The involvement of extrathoracic structures and bone marrow is commoner at presentation than in large B-cell lymphoma.[15]

Lymphoma is the third most common (12%, range; 1%–25%) malignant cause of superior vena cava syndrome following non–small cell lung cancer (50%, range; 43%–59%) and small cell lung cancer (22%, range; 7%–39%) (**Fig. 4**).

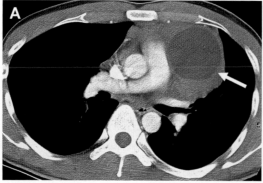
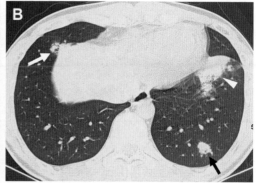

Fig. 2. Hodgkin lymphoma (nodular sclerosing type) in a 23-year-old man. (*A*) Transverse mediastinal-window CT (7.0-mm section thickness) scan shows left anterior mediastinal mass containing necrotic low-attenuation area (*arrow*) within mass. (*B*) Lung-window CT scan shows multiple poorly defined nodules (*arrows*) in both lower lobes and area of consolidation (*arrowhead*) in left lower lobe.

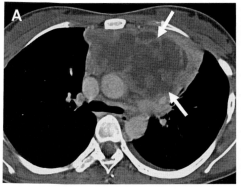
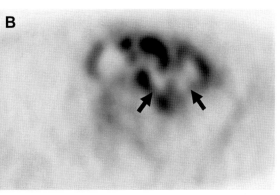

Fig. 3. Non-Hodgkin lymphoma (diffuse large B-cell type) in a 23-year-old woman. (*A*) Transverse mediastinal-window CT (3.0-mm section thickness) scan at the level of carina demonstrates large heterogeneous mass in anterior mediastinum containing large necrotic low attenuation areas (*arrows*). Also note small amount of left pleural effusion. (*B*) Transverse PET scan obtained at similar level to *A* demonstrates avid FDG uptake in peripheral portion of mass (maximum standardized uptake value = 16.9). Central portions of tumor are necrotic and show no significant FDG uptake (*arrows*).

Complete relief of symptoms is achieved with chemotherapy in approximately 80% of patients with NHL.[16]

Recurrent disease is common in the pericardial and internal mammary lymph nodes, since these nodes are usually not included in the radiation field.[1]

Dystrophic calcification may develop in involved lymph nodes following mediastinal radiation (**Fig. 5**).[17,18] The time interval between radiation and the appearance of calcification may be 1 to 9 years. Lymph node calcification before treatment is unusual, but has been associated with aggressive HL or NHL.[19]

When interpreting lymphomatous involvement of each nodal station based on CT images (**Table 2**), professional judgment should be used. A normal-sized lymph node may be involved with lymphoma and be PET (positron emission tomography) avid. Conversely, a lymph node could remain enlarged after successful treatment of lymphoma due to post-treatment changes.

$^{18}$F-fluorodeoxyglucose ($^{18}$F-FDG) PET or PET-CT provides whole body images that allow a comprehensive assessment of disease extent during staging workup and follow-up evaluation. PET or PET-CT helps detect more disease sites and involved organs than conventional staging

**Table 1**
**Frequent thoracic-primary lymphomas and their manifestations**

| Sites | Cell Types (WHO Classification) | Age/M:F Ratio | Common Imaging Findings |
|---|---|---|---|
| Mediastinum | | | |
| | Mediastinal (thymic) large B-cell lymphoma | Young adults/slightly F > M | Large lobulated anterior mediastinal mass ± low attenuation areas |
| | Lymphoblastic lymphoma | Young adults/M > F | |
| | Angioimmunoblastic lymphoma | Patients > 50 y/slightly M > F | Extensive hilar or mediastinal lymphadenopathy with enlargement of multiple nodal groups |
| Lung | | | |
| | Marginal zone lymphoma of BALT | Usually 6th and 7th decades/slightly F > M | Single or multiple nodule(s) and area(s) of consolidation |
| | Diffuse large B-cell lymphoma | Middle aged or elderly/slightly M > F | |

*Abbreviations:* BALT, bronchus-associated lymphoid tissue; F, female; M, male; WHO, World Health Organization.

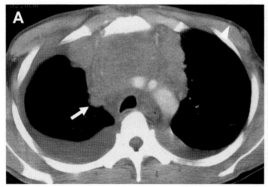
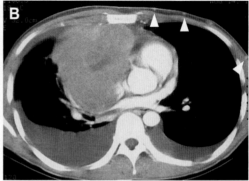

Fig. 4. Hodgkin lymphoma (nodular sclerosing type) in a 36-year-old man. Transverse mediastinal-window CT (5.0-mm section thickness) scans obtained at levels of aortic arch (A) and inferior pulmonary vein (B), respectively, show large anterior mediastinal mass. Also note total occlusion of superior vena cava (arrow) by mediastinal mass and collateral vessels (arrowheads) in left anterior chest wall. Bilateral pleural effusions are associated.

procedures including CT, and has a major impact on staging.[20] PET mostly upstaged disease when compared with CT.[21–23] Upstaging includes the detection of increased FDG uptake in normal-sized lymph nodes (usually < 10 mm in diameter) as well as in extranodal sites. In addition, PET or PET-CT is of value for monitoring the response to various therapeutic protocols, for prognostic stratification, and for detection for relapse during follow-up.[24]

PET or PET-CT is superior to CT in differentiation of viable tumor, necrosis, and fibrosis.[25] With anatomic imaging modalities only, it is difficult to differentiate viable tumor from post-therapy changes such as scarring or fibrosis. Residual abnormalities after therapy in lymphomas are often encountered. However, only a maximum of 10% to 20% of residual masses is reported to be

positive for lymphoma at the end of treatment.[26] In these situations of treatment completion or of partial cycle(s) of chemotherapy, [18]F-FDG PET has a high prognostic value as a valid imaging tool for post-treatment evaluation of malignant NHL and HL, as compared to conventional anatomic imaging techniques.[27]

## LUNG

Pulmonary involvement is identified more often in HL than in NHL. The lung is more frequently involved in disseminated or recurrent disease than in primary disease.[3,28,29] Pulmonary parenchymal involvement may present with variable patterns. The commonest feature of pulmonary involvement is a direct extension from hilar or mediastinal nodes toward the lungs (Fig. 6); however,

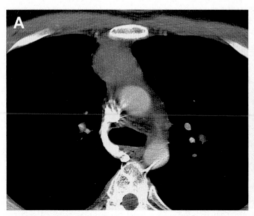
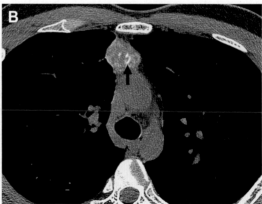

Fig. 5. Non-Hodgkin lymphoma (diffuse large B-cell type) in a 29-year-old man. (A) Transverse mediastinal-window CT (7.0-mm section thickness) scan obtained at level of azygos arch shows homogeneous soft tissue mass in anterior mediastinum. (B) CT scan obtained at same level as A 13 months after completion of radiation therapy demonstrates that tumor has decreased in size and contains dystrophic calcifications (arrow) within remaining tumor.

**Table 2**
**Recommendations for upper limits of normal lymph node size in a short-axis diameter at CT**

| Site | Location | Short-axis Nodal Diameter, mm |
|---|---|---|
| Axilla | | 10 |
| Mediastinum | Subcarinal | 12 |
| | Paracardiac | 8 |
| | Retrocrural | 6 |
| | All other sites | 10 |

*Data from* Hricak H, Husband J, Panicek DM. Oncologic imaging: essentials of reporting common cancers. Philadelphia: Saunders Elsevier; 2007.

recurrences in the lung may be seen without associated lymphadenopathy. Other appearances include pulmonary nodules (with or without cavitation) (**Fig. 7**), lobar or segmental consolidation with air bronchograms representing peribronchial tumor infiltration without destruction of bronchial wall (**Fig. 8**), reticular pattern with bronchovascular bundle and interlobular septal thickening (**Fig. 9**), disseminated small nodules, cavitating masses, endobronchial lesion per se, and atelectasis or obstructive pneumonia secondary to endobronchial or nodal obstruction (**Fig. 10**).[4,25,30–32] When these findings are seen in a patient with newly diagnosed lymphoma, pulmonary involvement of lymphoma should be considered. In treated patients, however, it is often difficult to differentiate between pulmonary involvement and other benign conditions such as infection,

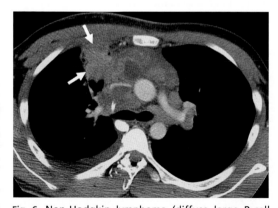

Fig. 6. Non-Hodgkin lymphoma (diffuse large B-cell type) showing direct lung involvement from adjacent mediastinal lymphadenopathy in a 17-year-old man. Transverse mediastinal-window CT (5.0-mm section thickness) scan obtained at level of main bronchi shows lymph node enlargement in anterior and middle mediastinal and left hilar areas. Note direct lung involvement from adjacent lymphadenopathy (*arrows*).

radiation pneumonia, or drug-induced lung disease.[33,34] It is important to determine whether the tumor originated from lung parenchyma (primary pulmonary lymphoma), whether it originated in nodal tissue and direct spread to the adjacent lung, or whether it originated in nodal tissue and hematogenously spread to extranodal sites.[35]

Primary pulmonary lymphoma is rare and is encountered usually in NHL. The frequency of lymphoma arising from the lung is estimated to be less than 1% of all lymphomas.[36] The disease usually takes the form of bronchus-associated lymphoid tissue (BALT) lymphoma. In the BALT lymphoma, tumor infiltration develops in multiple extranodal mucosal sites through the lungs.[37] According to a report,[38] BALT lymphoma may manifest diverse patterns of lung abnormality on CT, but single or multiple nodule (or nodules) and area (or areas) of consolidation are the main patterns that occur in a majority (**Fig. 11**). Other patterns include the findings of bronchiectasis and cellular bronchiolitis and diffuse interstitial lung disease. Pleural involvement is rare. Another important finding is the indolent nature of the lesions. On PET-CT, most tumors showed subtle FDG uptake (see **Fig. 11**). It should be noted that some cases of BALT lymphoma would show increased uptake of [18]F-FDG, whereas others would not.

Most cases of primary high-grade pulmonary lymphoma are of B-cell type (**Fig. 12**); occasional cases of anaplastic lymphoma or peripheral T-cell lymphoma have also been reported.[39–41] Some tumors appear to be derived from the low-grade B-cell lymphoma.[42] Others occur in patients who have organ transplants (post-transplant lymphoproliferative disorder [PTLD]) or occur in association with AIDS (AIDS-related lymphoma [ARL]). The most common type of lymphoma in PTLD and ARL is B-cell NHL. PTLD represents an abnormal proliferation of lymphoid cells that is induced by the Epstein-Barr virus and progresses because of a compromised immune system. Nearly all patients (approximately 90%) with PTLD are positive for Epstein-Barr virus.[36] ARL is the major cause of parenchymal nodule (or nodules) in AIDS patients, which often coexisted with a pleural effusion or axillary lymphadenopathy.[43]

On CT, lymphomas in patients with PTLD and ARL commonly manifest as multiple bilateral nodules (**Fig. 13**) or occasionally as a single nodule or mass. The nodules tend to have well-defined margins and do not show evidence of cavitation. Rarely, the lymphomas appear as a diffuse disease with numerous small nodules and thickening of interstitium.

High-grade lymphomas show avid FDG uptake; therefore PET imaging is useful for staging

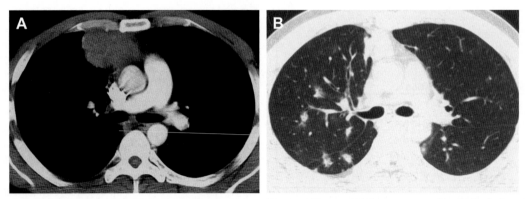

Fig. 7. Hodgkin lymphoma (nodular sclerosing type) in a 35-year-old man. (A) Transverse mediastinal-window CT (7.0-mm section thickness) scan obtained at level of right upper lobar bronchus shows homogeneous right anterior mediastinal mass. (B) Transverse lung-window CT scan shows multiple pulmonary nodules in both lungs with ill-defined margin.

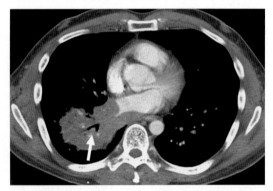

Fig. 8. Hodgkin lymphoma (nodular sclerosing type) in a 42-year-old man. Transverse mediastinal-window CT (5.0-mm section thickness) scan shows homogeneous soft-tissue mass in right lower lobe. Note air bronchograms (arrow) within tumor.

high-grade lymphoma[35,44] and to monitor response to therapy.

## THYMUS

Current staging and treatment methods consider the thymus as a nodal site, and thymic involvement does not change the stage of the disease.[45] In adults, the thymus is regarded enlarged if it is greater than 15 mm in the largest diameter. The two morphologic criteria that suggest the presence of an enlarged thymus are a triangular configuration of the thymus or the presence of cyst(s) within it.[2,45,46] Although thymic enlargement is seen in 30% to 56% of patients with intrathoracic involvement at presentation in HL,[3,5] it is often impossible to differentiate the thymic enlargement

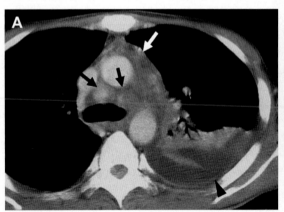
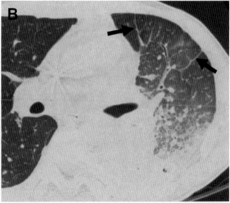

Fig. 9. Non-Hodgkin lymphoma (angioimmunoblastic type) in a 33-year-old man. (A) Transverse mediastinal-window CT (10-mm section thickness) scan obtained at level of azygos arch shows lymph node enlargement in anterior mediastinal and paratracheal areas (arrows). Also note left pleural effusion with pleural thickening (arrowhead). (B) Transverse lung-window CT scan demonstrates smooth interlobular septal thickening (arrows) with diffuse ground-glass opacity in left lung that represents lymphomatous infiltration with or without edema.

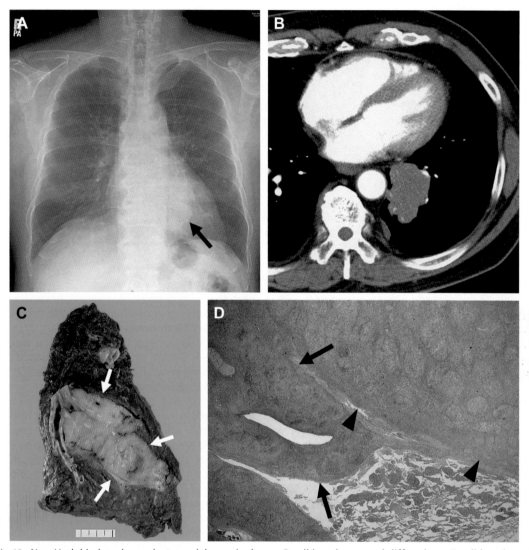

**Fig. 10.** Non-Hodgkin lymphoma (extranodal marginal zone B-cell lymphoma and diffuse large B-cell lymphoma) in a 72-year-old man. (*A*) Chest radiograph shows vertically oriented masslike lesion in left retrocardiac area (*arrow*). (*B*) Transverse mediastinal-window CT (1.0-mm section thickness) scan obtained at ventricular level shows a mass with homogeneous attenuation and lobulated contour in left lower lobe. (*C*) Gross pathologic specimen shows a gray tan and firm mass on left basal trunk and posterolateral basal segmental bronchus (*arrows*). (*D*) Low-magnification (hematoxylin-eosin stain; original magnification ×40) photomicrograph discloses monocytoid B-cell lymphocytic infiltration involving airways (*arrows*) and lung parenchyma (*arrowheads*).

from thymus infiltrated with tumor on the basis of CT appearance alone.

Post-therapeutic enlargement of the thymus may represent recurrent disease, thymic rebound (hyperplastic thymus), or development or persistence of thymic cysts.[3,45,46] The hyperplastic thymus is usually triangular, whereas the infiltrated thymus is quadrilateral with a lobulated border.[47] When thymic enlargement is present in adults, if the thymus was not the original site of disease or if there is no other evidence of disease relapse, it should be considered that this is due to hyperplasia rather than to tumor infiltration.[48,49]

Thymic cysts may occur in HL either at the initial presentation (21%–50%) or after treatment. Thymic cysts may persist or enlarge and this indicates neither residual or recurrent disease nor an increased risk of relapse.[45]

## PLEURA, PERICARDIUM, AND HEART INVOLVEMENT

Pleural effusions are observed at presentation in approximately 10% of patients in HL[4,5] and eventually develop in approximately 30%, most often in association with other intrathoracic

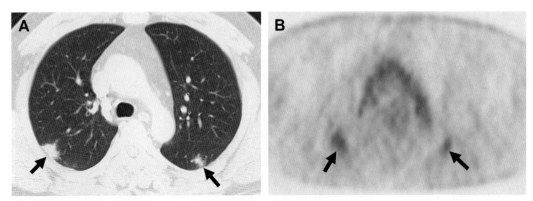

Fig. 11. Marginal zone B-cell lymphoma of bronchus-associated lymphoid tissue in a 47-year-old man. (*A*) Transverse lung-window CT (5.0-mm section thickness) scan shows two subpleural nodules (*arrows*) with poorly defined margin in right upper lobe and superior segment of left lower lobe. (*B*) Transverse PET scan obtained at similar level to *A* demonstrates subtle FDG uptake (*arrows*) (maximum standardized uptake value = 2.6 and 2.2, respectively).

manifestations of the disease.[30] They are not of prognostic significance unless associated with a pleural mass, because they rarely contain malignant cells and usually resolve following treatment.[2,3,5,33] Pleural effusions are often caused by lymphatic or venous obstruction by enlarged lymph nodes rather than from direct lymphomatous involvement.[50] The fluid can be serous, chylous, pseudochylous, or rarely serosanguinous.[51] However, NHL may rarely present with pleural effusion as a sole manifestation, most often occurs in the setting of immunodeficiency (primary effusion lymphoma, [PEL]; approximately 3% of AIDS-related lymphomas and < 1% of non–AIDS-related lymphomas).[52]

Pleural involvement by lymphoma may occur in both HL and NHL and represents a manifestation of systemic disease.[2,53–56] According to a report, approximately 16% of patients with NHL present with, or subsequently develop, pleural involvement

during the course of the disease.[57] They may manifest as a solitary nodule or multiple, broad-based pleural mass, or a combination of the two, and usually are associated with pleural effusion (**Fig. 14**). It is important to recognize the pleural involvement (which is frequently overlooked on conventional imaging), because that finding of pleural involvement may significantly affect patient management and because unrecognized pleural involvement increases the risk of treatment failure.

Pericardial effusion, by contrast with pleural effusion, is presumed to represent lymphomatous invasion of the pericardium. It may arise from lymphatic or hematogenous spread or by direct extension of mediastinal tumor.[49]

Cardiac and pericardial involvement (**Fig. 15**) of lymphoma may arise from retrograde lymphatic spread, hematogenous spread, or from direct extension of mediastinal lymphadenopathy. According to a report,[58] the prevalence of cardiac

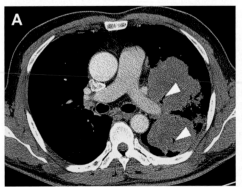

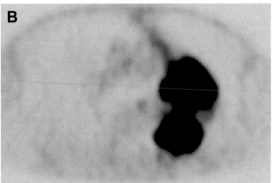

Fig. 12. Non-Hodgkin lymphoma (diffuse large B-cell type) in a 71-year-old man. (*A*) Transverse mediastinal-window CT (2.5-mm section thickness) scan obtained at subcarinal level shows large masslike consolidative lesions in left upper lobe and left lower lobe. Note these masses have internal air bronchograms (*arrowheads*). (*B*) Transverse PET scan obtained at similar level to *A* demonstrates high FDG uptake (maximum standardized uptake values = 20.5 in both lesions) within masses.

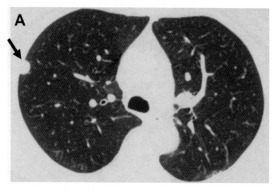

**Fig. 13.** AIDS-related (large B-cell type) lymphoma in a 56-year-old woman. Transverse lung-window CT (5.0-mm section thickness) scans obtained at levels of azygos arch (*A*) and bronchus intermedius (*B*), respectively, show two subpleural nodules (*arrows*), one each in right upper lobe and left upper lobe, with well-defined margins.

and pericardial involvement by malignant lymphoma (both HL and NHL) at autopsy is estimated at 8.7%.

The incidence of pneumothorax is increased in patients who have HL. In one study of 1977 patients who had the lymphoma, the complication was 10 times higher than expected, most patients being younger than 30 years of age.[59] Treatment with radiotherapy, lung involvement, radiation fibrosis, and infection appear to be risk factors.

## CHEST WALL AND THORACIC SKELETAL INVOLVEMENT

Chest wall involvement occurs in about 6.4% of cases in HL[5] and may represent an initial

manifestation of the disease or a site of recurrence in HL (**Fig. 16**). Detection of chest wall invasion is of clinical relevance, because it is associated with higher relapse rates and requires more aggressive therapy.[2] Most patients with chest wall involvement have associated intrathoracic disease.[3,60] Parasternal and thoracic spine involvements are often secondary to extension of anterior (especially internal mammary chain) and posterior mediastinal lymphadenopathy, respectively.[2,3,61] Isolated chest wall masses are uncommon and are usually a manifestation of NHL, especially large B-cell lymphoma.

Approximately 5% to 20% of patients with HL manifest bone involvement during the course. But, the bone involvement is seen in only 1% to

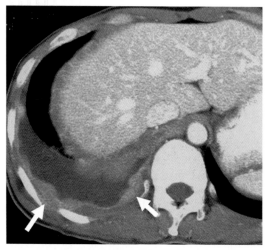

**Fig. 14.** Non-Hodgkin lymphoma (lymphoblastic type) in a 24-year-old man. Transverse mediastinal-window CT (10.0-mm section thickness) scan obtained at level of liver dome shows pleural effusion and enhancing uneven pleural thickening in right hemithorax (*arrows*).

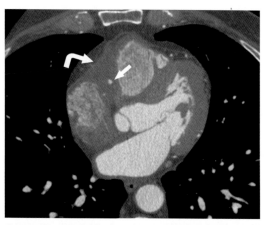

**Fig. 15.** Non-Hodgkin lymphoma (diffuse large B-cell type) in a 63-year-old woman. Transverse mediastinal window image of ECG-gated CT (2.5-mm section thickness) scan shows low-attenuation infiltrative mass lesion at right atrium/right heart border (*curved arrow*). Mass is indistinguishable from muscle and replaces epicardiac fat. There is encasement of right coronary artery (*arrow*) within lesion.

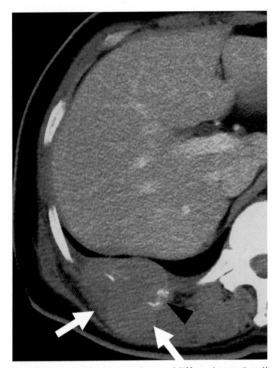

**Fig. 16.** Non-Hodgkin lymphoma (diffuse large B-cell type) in a 46-year-old woman. Transverse mediastinal-window CT (7.0-mm section thickness) scan shows well-defined solid mass in right posterior chest wall (*arrows*). Also note rib destruction (*arrowhead*).

4% at presentation.[33,62–64] The thoracic skeleton usually, but not invariably, is affected by direct extension of tumor from the mediastinum or lungs.

## BREAST

Breast lymphoma accounts for approximately 0.15% of all malignant breast tumors.[65] Primary breast lymphoma accounts for only 0.1% to 0.5% of all breast tumors;[66] approximately 2.0% of extranodal lymphomas involve the breasts. Most breast lymphomas are B-cell lymphomas and rarely, T-cell or histiocytic lymphomas.[67,68] The diagnosis of primary breast lymphoma depends on the absence of systemic lymphoma (with the exception of ipsilateral axillary nodes) and no previous diagnosis of extramammary lymphoma. Regardless of histologic subtype, breast lymphomas manifest most frequently as a single, lobular or irregular mass with indistinct margin at mammography and a solid, hypervascular irregular mass with indistinct margin or an echogenic boundary at ultrasound.[69,70]

## SUMMARY

Thoracic lymphomas most frequently involve mediastinal lymph nodes in the anterior mediastinum and paratracheal areas. The lymphomas may also involve lung, thymus, pleura, pericardium, chest wall, and the breast and their radiologic manifestations are diverse. Lymphomas (mostly BALT lymphoma and large B-cell lymphoma) may arise primarily from the lung with various imaging features including single or multiple nodule(s) and area(s) of consolidation. CT is currently the most important imaging modality for the evaluation of thoracic lymphoma but FDG PET also plays a crucial role in the clinical management of these cases.

## REFERENCES

1. Sharma A, Fidias P, Hayman LA, et al. Patterns of lymphadenopathy in thoracic malignancies. Radiographics 2004;24:419–34.
2. Guermazi A, Brice P, de Kerviler EE, et al. Extranodal Hodgkin disease: spectrum of disease. Radiographics 2001;21:161–79.
3. North LB, Libshitz HI, Lorigan JG. Thoracic lymphoma. Radiol Clin North Am 1990;28:745–62.
4. Filly R, Bland N, Castellino RA. Radiographic distribution of intrathoracic disease in previously untreated patients with Hodgkin's disease and non-Hodgkin's lymphoma. Radiology 1976;120:277–81.
5. Castellino RA, Blank N, Hoppe RT, et al. Hodgkin disease: contributions of chest CT in the initial staging evaluation. Radiology 1986;160:603–5.
6. Tateishi U, Müller NL, Johkoh T, et al. Primary mediastinal lymphoma: characteristic features of the various histological subtypes on CT. J Comput Assist Tomogr 2004;28:782–9.
7. Hopper KD, Diehl LF, Cole BA, et al. The significance of necrotic mediastinal lymph nodes on CT in patients with newly diagnosed Hodgkin disease. AJR Am J Roentgenol 1990;155:267–70.
8. Castellino RA, Hilton S, O'Brien JP, et al. Non-Hodgkin lymphoma: contribution of chest CT in the initial staging evaluation. Radiology 1996;199:129–32.
9. Castellino RA. The non-Hodgkin lymphomas: practical concepts for the diagnostic radiologist. Radiology 1991;178:315–21.
10. Keller AR, Kaplan HS, Lukes RJ, et al. Correlation of histopathology with other prognostic indicators in Hodgkin's disease. Cancer 1968;22:487–99.
11. Levitt LJ, Aisenberg AC, Harris NL, et al. Primary non-Hodgkin's lymphoma of the mediastinum. Cancer 1982;50:2486–92.
12. Lazzarino M, Orlandi E, Paulli M, et al. Primary mediastinal B-cell lymphoma with sclerosis: an aggressive tumor with distinctive clinical and pathologic features. J Clin Oncol 1993;11:2306–13.
13. Shaffer K, Smith D, Kirn D, et al. Primary mediastinal large-B-cell lymphoma: radiologic findings at presentation. AJR Am J Roentgenol 1996;167:425–30.

14. Thomas DA, Kantarjian HM. Lymphoblastic lymphoma. Hematol Oncol Clin North Am 2001;15:51–95.

15. Duwe BV, Sterman DH, Musani AI. Tumors of the mediastinum. Chest 2005;128:2893–909.

16. Wilson LD, Detterbeck FC, Yahalom J. Superior vena cava syndrome with malignant causes. N Engl J Med 2007;356:1862–9.

17. Fishman EK, Kuhlman JE, Jones RJ. CT of lymphoma: spectrum of disease. Radiographics 1991; 11:647–69.

18. Brereton HD, Johnson RE. Calcification in mediastinal lymph nodes after radiation therapy of Hodgkin's disease. Radiology 1974;112:705–7.

19. Apter S, Avigdor A, Gayer G, et al. Calcification in lymphoma occurring before therapy: CT features and clinical correlation. AJR Am J Roentgenol 2002;178:935–8.

20. Podoloff DA, Macapinlac HA. PET and PET/CT in management of the lymphomas. Radiol Clin North Am 2007;45:689–96.

21. Bangerter M, Moog F, Buchmann I, et al. Whole-body 2-[18F]-fluoro-2-deoxy-D-glucose positron emission tomography (FDG-PET) for accurate staging of Hodgkin's disease. Ann Oncol 1998;9: 1117–22.

22. Young CS, Young BL, Smith SM. Staging Hodgkin's disease with 18-FDG PET. Clin Positron Imaging 1998;1:161–4.

23. Foo SS, Mitchell PL, Berlangieri SU, et al. Positron emission tomography scanning in the assessment of patients with lymphoma. Intern Med J 2004;34: 388–97.

24. Bar-Shalom R. Normal and abnormal patterns of 18F-fluorodeoxyglucose PET/CT in lymphoma. PET Clinics 2006;1:231–42.

25. Rademaker J. Hodgkin's and non-Hodgkin's lymphomas. Radiol Clin North Am 2007;45:69–83.

26. Surbone A, Longo DL, DeVita VT, et al. Residual abdominal masses in aggressive non-Hodgkin's lymphoma after combination chemotherapy: significance and management. J Clin Oncol 1998;6: 1832–7.

27. Kostakoglu L, Coleman M, Leonard JP, et al. PET predicts prognosis after 1cycle of chemotherapy in aggressive lymphoma and Hodgkin's disease. J Nucl Med 2002;43:1018–27.

28. Brennan DD, Gleeson T, Coate LE, et al. A comparison of whole-body MRI and CT for the staging of lymphoma. AJR Am J Roentgenol 2005;185:711–6.

29. Radin AI. Primary pulmonary Hodgkin's disease. Cancer 1990;65:550–63.

30. Fisher AM, Kendall B, Van Leuven BD. Hodgkin's disease: a radiological survey. Clin Radiol 1962;13: 115–27.

31. Diehl LF, Hopper KD, Giguere J, et al. The pattern of intrathoracic Hodgkin's disease assessed by computed tomography. J Clin Oncol 1991;9:438–43.

32. Mentzer SJ, Reilly JJ, Skarin AT, et al. Patterns of lung involvement by malignant lymphoma. Surgery 1993;113:507–14.

33. Sandrasegaran K, Robinson PJ, Selby P. Staging of lymphoma in adults. Clin Radiol 1994;49:149–61.

34. Lewis ER, Caskey CI, Fishman EK. Lymphoma of the lung: CT findings in 31 patients. AJR Am J Roentgenol 1991;156:711–4.

35. Even-Sapir E, Lievshitz G, Perry C, et al. Fluorine-18 fluorodeoxyglucose PET/CT patterns of extranodal involvement in patients with Non-Hodgkin lymphoma and Hodgkin's disease. Radiol Clin North Am 2007; 45:697–709.

36. Lee KS, Kim Y, Primack SL. Imaging of pulmonary lymphomas. AJR Am J Roentgenol 1997;168: 339–45.

37. Cordier JF, Chailleux E, Lauque D, et al. Primary pulmonary lymphomas. A clinical study of 70 cases in nonimmunocompromised patients. Chest 1993; 103:201–8.

38. Bae YA, Lee KS, Han J, et al. Marginal zone B-cell lymphoma of bronchus-associated lymphoid tissue (BALT): imaging findings in 21 patients. Chest 2008;133:433–40.

39. Close PM, Macrae MB, Hammond JM, et al. Anaplastic large-cell Ki-1 lymphoma: pulmonary presentation mimicking military tuberculosis. Am J Clin Pathol 1993;99:631–6.

40. Cheng AL, Su IJ, Chen YC, et al. Characteristic clinicopathologic features of Epstein-Barr virus-associated peripheral T-cell lymphoma. Cancer 1993;72:909–16.

41. Harrison NK, Twelves C, Addis JB, et al. Peripheral T-cell lymphoma presenting with angioedema and diffuse pulmonary infiltrates. Am Rev Respir Dis 1988;138:976–80.

42. Koss MN. Pulmonary lymphoid disorders. Semin Diagn Pathol 1995;12:158–71.

43. Sider L, Gabriel H, Curry DR, et al. Pattern recognition of the pulmonary manifestations of AIDS on CT scans. Radiographics 1993;13:771–84.

44. Marom EM, McAdams HP, Butnor KJ, et al. Positron emission tomography with fluoro-2-deoxy-D-glucose (FDG-PET) in the staging of posttransplant lymphoproliferative disorder in lung transplant recipients. J Comput Assist Tomogr 2004;19:74–8.

45. Wernecke K, Vassallo P, Rutsch F, et al. Thymic involvement in Hodgkin disease: CT and sonographic findings. Radiology 1991;181:375–83.

46. Heron CW, Husband JE, Williams MP. Hodgkin disease: CT of the thymus. Radiology 1988;167:647–51.

47. Luker GD, Siegel MJ. Mediastinal Hodgkin disease in children: response to therapy. Radiology 1993; 189:737–40.

48. Kissin CM, Husband JE, Nicholas D, et al. Benign thymic enlargement in adults after chemotherapy: CT demonstration. Radiology 1987;163:67–70.

49. Fletcher BD, Xiong X, Kauffman WM, et al. Hodgkin disease: use of TI-201 to monitor mediastinal involvement after treatment. Radiology 1998;209: 471–5.

50. Rademaker J. Diagnostic imaging modalities for assessment of lymphoma with special emphasis on CT, MRI, and ultrasound. PET Clinics 2006;1: 219–30.

51. Strickland B. Intra-thoracic Hodgkin's disease. Part II. Peripheral manifestations of Hodgkin's disease in the chest. Br J Radiol 1967;40:930–8.

52. Pileri SA, Leoncini L, Falini B. Revised European-American lymphoma classification. Curr Opin Oncol 1995;7:401–7.

53. Schmutz GR, Fisch-Ponsot C, Regent D, et al. Computed tomography (CT) and magnetic resonance imaging (MRI) of pleural masses. Crit Rev Diagn Imaging 1993;34:309–83.

54. Manoharan A, Pitney WR, Schonell ME, et al. Intra-thoracic manifestations in non-Hodgkin's lymphoma. Thorax 1979;34:29–32.

55. Berkman N, Breuer R, Kramer MR, et al. Pulmonary involvement in lymphoma. Leuk Lymphoma 1996;20: 229–37.

56. Vega F, Padula A, Valbuena JR, et al. Lymphomas involving the pleura: a clinicopathologic study of 34 cases diagnosed by pleural biopsy. Arch Pathol Lab Med 2006;130:1497–502.

57. Das DK, Gupta SK, Ayyagari S, et al. Pleural effusions in non-Hodgkin's lymphoma. A cytomorphologic, cytochemical and immunologic study. Acta Cytol 1987;31:119–24.

58. McDonnell PJ, Mann RB, Bulkley BH. Involvement of the heart by malignant lymphoma: a clinicopathologic study. Cancer 1982;49:944–51.

59. Yellin A, Benfield JR. Pneumothorax associated with lymphoma. Am Rev Respir Dis 1986;134: 590–2.

60. Carlsen SE, Bergin CJ, Hoppe RT. MR imaging to detect chest wall and pleural involvement in patients with lymphoma: effect on radiation therapy planning. AJR Am J Roentgenol 1993;160:1191–5.

61. Cho CS, Blank N, Castellino RA. Computerized tomography evaluation of chest wall involvement in lymphoma. Cancer 1985;55:1892–4.

62. Gaudin P, Juvin R, Rozand Y, et al. Skeletal involvement as the initial disease manifestation in Hodgkin's disease: a review of 6 cases. J Rheumatol 1992;19: 146–52.

63. Edeiken-Monroe B, Edeiken J, Kim EE. Radiologic concepts of lymphoma of bone. Radiol Clin North Am 1990;28:841–64.

64. Sullivan WT, Solonick DM. Case report 414: nodular sclerosing Hodgkin disease involving sternum and chest wall. Skeletal Radiol 1987;16:166–9.

65. Rosen PP. Lymphoid and hematopoietic tumors. In: Rosen PP, editor. Rosen's breast pathology. Philadelphia: Lippincott-Raven; 1997. p. 757–78.

66. Giardini R, Piccolo C, Rilke F. Primary non-Hodgkin's lymphomas of the female breast. Cancer 1992;69: 725–35.

67. Arber DA, Simpson JF, Weiss LM, et al. Non-Hodgkin's lymphoma involving the breast. Am J Surg Pathol 1994;18:288–95.

68. Jeon HJ, Akagi T, Hoshida Y, et al. Primary non-Hodgkin malignant lymphoma of the breast. An immunohistochemical study of seven patients and literature review of 152 patients with breast lymphoma in Japan. Cancer 1992;70:2451–9.

69. Liberman L, Giess CS, Dershaw DD, et al. Non-Hodgkin lymphoma of the breast: imaging characteristics and correlation with histopathologic findings. Radiology 1994;192:157–60.

70. Yang WT, Lane DL, Le-Petross HT, et al. Breast lymphoma: imaging findings of 32 tumors in 27 patients. Radiology 2007;245:692–702.

# Imaging of Abdominal Lymphoma

Munazza Anis, MD*, Abid Irshad, MD

**KEYWORDS**

• Lymphoma • Abdominal • Pelvic

Lymphoma is a general term for a group of cancers that originate in the lymphatic system. The lymphomas are divided into two major categories: Hodgkin lymphoma (HL) and non-Hodgkin lymphoma (NHL). Most patients with NHL compared with less than half of the patients with HL have abdominal involvement. Para-aortic lymphadenopathy is the most common finding (**Figs. 1–4**). HL and NHL may present with involvement of one or more lymph nodal groups, of an isolated organ, or as widely disseminated disease. In general, there is a displacement of structures by enlarged lymph nodes without invasion (see **Fig. 1**B and **Fig. 2**A). This imaging feature distinguishes lymphomas from carcinomas. Although HL and NHL share similar radiologic features, there are some significant differences in their radiographic appearances.

## LYMPHOMA CLASSIFICATION AND STAGING

In 2001, the World Health Organization published a comprehensive classification system for lymphoid neoplasms incorporating entities like morphology, immunology, genetic features, and clinical features.[1–3] The three large groups are (1) the B-cell tumors, (2) the T-cell and natural killer cell tumors, and (3) HL.[2,3] Lymphomas have been historically staged by Ann Arbor staging system introduced in 1970. This system, however, was modified in 1989 because of the introduction of CT (Costwald staging classification).[4] The prognosis in NHL depends on many factors, such as stage, performance status, presence of B symptoms, age, and high lactate dehydrogenase (LDH), which limits the value of Ann Arbor classification in this group of patients.

## Non-Hodgkin Lymphoma

NHL represents a diverse group of cancers, with the distinctions between types based on the characteristics of the cancerous cells. It is the fifth most common cancer in men and women in the United States. In NHL, involved lymph nodes tend to be larger as compared with HL. Involvement of nodal groups is common but extranodal sites are also frequently involved. This includes extranodal lymphatic tissue (eg, Peyer's patches in the small bowel, spleen) and nonlymphatic organs, such as the liver, bone marrow, bone, and central nervous system. Patients who have had renal transplants, have AIDS, or are immunocompromised for other reasons are all at increased risk for developing NHL.

## Hodgkin Lymphoma

HL is characterized by the presence of an abnormal cell called the Reed-Sternberg cell (a large, malignant cell found in HL tissues). HL is comprised of two disease entities: nodular lymphocyte predominant HL and classical HL, which in turn consists of nodular sclerosis, mixed cellularity, lymphocyte-depleted, and lymphocyte-rich subtypes.

It is more common in adults in higher socioeconomic groups and peaks in both the third and the fifth decades of life. In HL, the most common sites of involvement are the cervical lymph nodes and intrathoracic lymphadenopathy (approximately 60%–80% of all patients with HL). Isolated infradiaphragmatic lymphadenopathy occurs in less than 10% of patients at diagnosis. HL spreads in a contiguous fashion from one lymph node group to the adjacent lymph nodes. Adjacent structures

Department of Radiology, Medical University of South Carolina, 169 Ashley Avenue, PO Box 250322, Charleston, SC 29425, USA
* Corresponding author.
*E-mail address:* anis@musc.edu (M. Anis).

Radiol Clin N Am 46 (2008) 265–285
doi:10.1016/j.rcl.2008.04.001

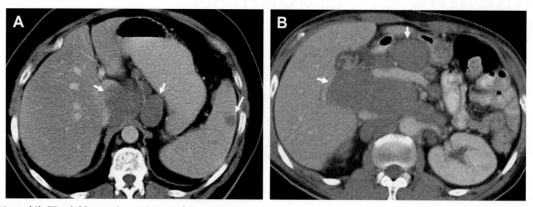

Fig. 1. (*A*) CT axial image in a 37-year-old man with newly diagnosed NHL demonstrating gastrohepatic ligament lymphadenopathy (*short arrows*) and splenic masses (*long arrow*). (*B*) Extensive para-aortic and peripancreatic lymphadenopathy (*short arrows*).

may be invaded, such as chest wall, lung, or bone. Extranodal involvement is less common in HL than in NHL (**Fig. 5**).

## IMAGING TECHNIQUES

Cross-sectional imaging (CT scan, MR imaging) is primarily used to detect lymphadenopathy and the pattern of nodal involvement. Anatomic imaging is limited in accurate lymphoma evaluation as small lymph nodes may harbor malignant cells, whereas large lymph nodes may be benign (**Table 1**).[5] Functional imaging, such as positron emission tomography (PET) with fluorodeoxyglucose (FDG), has shown promising results in the diagnosis of lymphoma and complete assessment of the extent

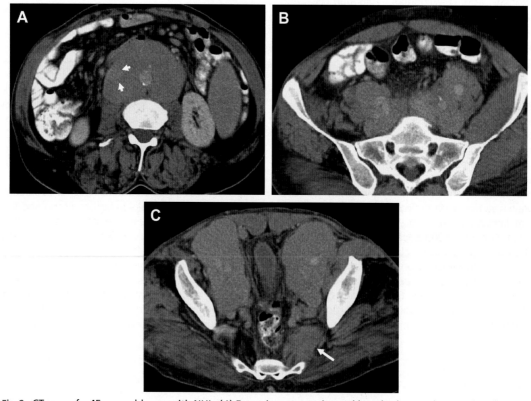

Fig. 2. CT scan of a 45-year-old man with NHL. (*A*) Extensive retroperitoneal lymphadenopathy encasing the aorta and branches of the inferior vena cava (*arrows*). The lymphadenopathy extends along the common iliac vasculature (*B*) and along bilateral external iliac and left internal iliac (*arrow*) vasculature (*C*).

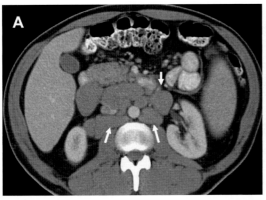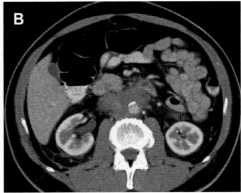

Fig. 3. (A) CT axial image in a 27-year-old woman with NHL demonstrating extensive retroperitoneal lymphadenopathy (arrows), which elevates the aorta from the spine. (B) CT axial image in a different patient with biopsy-proved retroperitoneal fibrosis, which is characterized by a mantle of soft tissue encircling the great vessels and ureters in the retroperitoneum. Differentiation from lymphoma, which appears identical in most cases, is made by biopsy.

of disease. It is also very useful in the follow-up of PET-avid lymphoma (see **Fig. 5**; **Fig. 6**).

## CT

Most clinical management decisions are currently based on either CT or PET. CT scan is the most commonly used imaging modality for the detection, staging, and follow-up of lymphoma. The role of CT scan in lymphoma is multifold. It is used to (1) define the full extent of disease to allow accurate staging; (2) assist in treatment planning (ie, determine the site of nodal biopsy, create radiation planning portals, and select chemotherapy protocols); (3) evaluate response to therapy; and (4) monitor patient progress and possible relapse. The diagnosis of abdominal organ involvement is aided by the use of intravenous contrast.

### Imaging pitfalls

Reporting of increased number of normal-sized lymph nodes in the initial, early staging CT is important. This finding should be reported explicitly because these normal-sized but increased number of lymph nodes may represent early abdominal disease, which may be relevant in staging; however, this finding is still of unknown significance. This is different in patients who have had multiple prior studies, which have established stable lymph nodes.

Comparison with the most recent CT study is often not sufficient because the growth becomes obvious only if serial studies are compared. Small difference in measurement (approximately 15%) in near normal-sized lymph nodes between two CT examination is often related to "plane of section" artifact (ie, related to slice section). A follow-up study in 3 months is not sufficient for follow-up of slow-growing lymphoma.

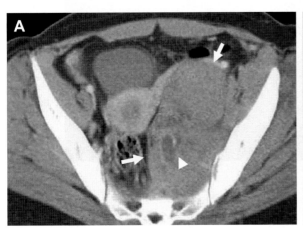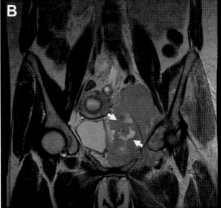

Fig. 4. (A) CT axial image in a 28-year-old woman with HL with extensive left pelvic wall lymphadenopathy (arrows) with areas of hypoattenuation centrally (arrowhead). (B) MR imaging T2 single shot fast spin echo (SSFSE) axial image demonstrates T2 hyperintense foci suggesting necrosis seen as areas of hypoattenuation on CT (arrows).

**Table 1**
**Recommendations for upper limits of normal lymph node size (short axis) at CT**

| Site | Location | Short Axis Nodal Diameter (mm) |
|------|----------|-------------------------------|
| Abdomen | Gastrohepatic ligament | 8 |
| | Porta hepatis | 8 |
| | Portacaval | 10 |
| | Celiac axis to renal artery | 10 |
| | Renal artery to aortic bifurcation | 12 |
| Pelvis | Common iliac | 9 |
| | External iliac | 10 |
| | Internal iliac | 7 |
| | Obturator | 8 |
| Inguinal region | | 10 |

Professional judgment should be used in applying these recommendations. A normal-sized lymph node could be involved with lymphoma and be PET avid. A lymph node could remain enlarged, however, after successful treatment of lymphoma because of posttreatment changes.
*Data from* Refs. [14–16].

## MR Imaging

The accuracy of MR imaging in detecting lymph node and organ involvement is similar to that of CT (see **Fig. 4; Fig. 7**). MR imaging reveals the lymphoma masses to be low to iso-signal intensity on T1-weighted images and moderately high signal on T2-weighted imaging, less than the high signal associated with cysts. Active untreated tumor tissue contains an excess of free water, which increases the signal intensity on T2-weighted imaging. With successful treatment, cellular elements and the water content of the tumor are reduced, whereas the collagen and fibrotic stroma of the original tumor account for the main component of the signal. Tumor masses are hyperintense on T2-weighted images, and chronic fibrosis or scar is often hypointense. The sensitivity of these findings is low, however, because of necrosis, immature fibrotic tissue, edema, and inflammation that can simulate the high T2 signal intensity of a viable tumor. The mean gadolinium enhancement of residual masses after treatment is often substantially weaker than that observed before treatment in patients in complete remission.[6,7]

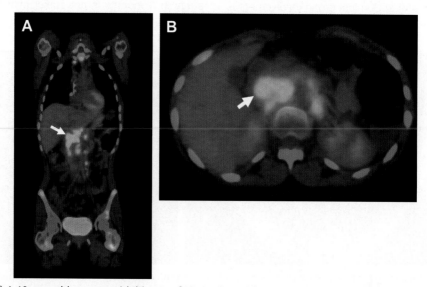

**Fig. 5.** (*A, B*) A 19-year-old woman with history of HL staging with PET scan before allogenic stem cell transplant. Extensive retroperitoneal lymphadenopathy as marked by arrows.

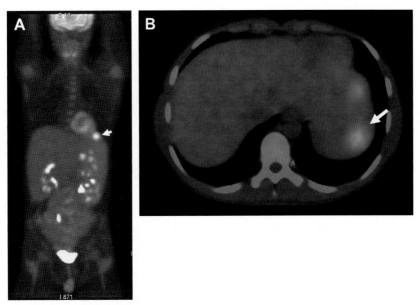

Fig. 6. (*A, B*) A 20-year-old man with history of NHL presenting with hepatosplenomegaly and multiple PET-avid splenic masses (*arrows*); three-dimensional and axial image.

## Other uses

Other uses of MR imaging in lymphoma include out-of-phase images, which might help to differentiate unilateral or bilateral adrenal lymphoma from lipid-rich adenoma (**Fig. 8**). MR imaging is more sensitive than CT for the detection of bone marrow involvement. It can be used in the patients with CT contrast allergy.

## Future potential role of MR imaging in lymphoma

Preliminary studies have suggested a potential role of diffusion MR imaging in oncologic patients by allowing the detection of water motion over small distances. The development of body MR imaging using multichannel phased-array surface coils combined with parallel imaging techniques could enable whole body MR diffusion imaging in cancer patients. No study has yet been published assessing the impact of such techniques in staging and monitoring lymphoma. Diffusion-weighted imaging and apparent diffusion coefficient mapping in the radiologic diagnosis of neoplasms was initially suggested as useful for analysis of the central nervous system.[8–11] Among the neoplasms, lymphomas were shown to have characteristically low apparent diffusion coefficient values. Nakayama and colleagues[8] showed the apparent diffusion coefficient values of retroperitoneal lymphomas to be significantly lower than those of other malignant and benign mesenchymal tumors arising from the retroperitoneum.

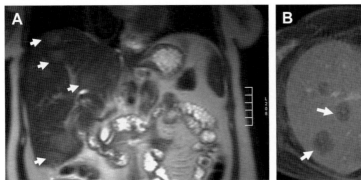
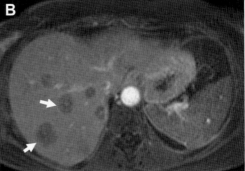

Fig. 7. A 50-year-old woman with diffuse large B-cell lymphoma. Cor SSFSE T2 image (*A*) demonstrates multiple large T2 hyperintense hepatic masses (*arrows*) of varying sizes, which demonstrate hypointense SI on postgadolinium sequence (*arrows*) (*B*).

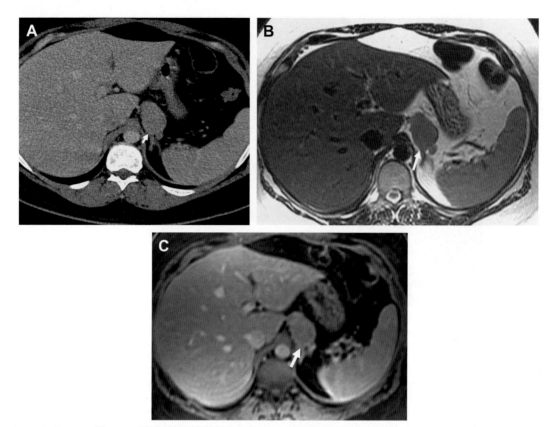

**Fig. 8.** A 40-year-old man with history of NHL. (*A*) CT axial slice demonstrates a homogeneous, well-circumscribed mass (*arrow*) in the left adrenal gland genu. (*B*) The in- and out-of-phase images demonstrated no signal drop out excluding a lipid-containing adenoma. (*C*) The left adrenal mass is slightly T2 hyperintense on T2 SSFSE sequences.

Carcinomas (retroperitoneal nodal metastases), however, also showed low apparent diffusion coefficient values, and these values were indistinguishable from those obtained for lymphomas. Further studies with newer MR imaging techniques including perfusion analysis are going to provide an interesting comparison with FDG-PET.[12]

## Ultrasound

Ultrasound (US) is useful for the evaluation of the genitourinary tract, including possible testicular involvement, and for the evaluation of superficial lymph nodes. US-guided biopsies of focal lesions (eg, in the liver and spleen) are useful for tissue sampling. US is also useful for the initial evaluation of symptoms in the abdomen (eg, gallbladder, kidney).

## ASSESSMENT OF RESPONSE TO THERAPY

Patients require routine follow-up to assess tumor shrinkage in response to therapy and to decide on treatment modification if required.[13]

Measurements of lesions should be bidimensional (biperpendicular measurement in the axial plane, longest axial dimension × perpendicular dimension). **Table 1** provides recommendations for the upper limits of the size of the abdominal and pelvic lymph nodes.[14–16] Most of these measurements are relatively easy but might be difficult in cases of irregular edges or rare infiltrating lesions. In some patients, lymph node attenuation values may decrease as a response to treatment with or without overall reduction in lymph node size.

CT-based criteria of response were defined for NHL but are also often used for HL (**Box 1**).[17] Recommendations include separate definitions for complete remission; complete remission (unconfirmed or uncertain); partial response; stable diseases; and progressive disease. Progressive disease, for example, includes the appearance of new lesions or an increase of more than 50% in known lesions. An increase of more than 50% in the greatest diameter of any previously identified node that was greater than 1 cm also represents progressive disease. The main limitations of CT criteria are (1) the limited accuracy of CT at initial staging for assessing lymphoma in small nodes (<1–1.5 cm), bone marrow, or various extranodal sites; (2) the inability of CT to differentiate active disease within a residual mass; and (3) the limited ability of CT to assess early response to treatment.

FDG-PET is superior to CT in differentiation of viable tumor, necrosis, and fibrosis.[6] New PET-based criteria were published in 2007 to assess treatment response in selected NHL and HL. These criteria are also going to be used for the assessment of abdominal and pelvic lymphoma. A simplified version of these criteria is summarized in **Box 2**. A patient with a PET-avid lymphoma in the baseline evaluation has progressive-relapsed disease if there is a greater than or equal to 50% increase in disease or new lesions that are PET positive. Cheson[18] describes the new response criteria and measurement of the lesions in previously mentioned publications (see article on new staging and response criteria for NHL and HL by Cheson in this issue).

## SPECTRUM OF IMAGING FEATURES

In the abdomen and pelvis, lymphoma may present as unifocal, multifocal masses; lymphadenopathy; or diffuse infiltration. On US, these masses often appear markedly homogeneous and hypoechoic resembling cysts except for the fact that the posterior acoustic enhancement seen with cysts is lacking in lymphoma. On CT scan, these masses often appear slightly hyperattenuating on noncontrast images related to inherent hypercellularity of the lymphoma masses. Masses are typically very homogeneous and show homogenous attenuation. Lymphoma often shows a lower degree of enhancement than the involved organ (eg, liver, spleen, kidney). With increasing size, there may be central necrosis causing heterogeneous enhancement. Calcification is rare without treatment. MR imaging is comparable with CT in detection of lymphoma masses and more specific for differentiating them from microabscesses; however, it is less available and less practical than CT.

The following section summarizes the most common and important imaging findings of abdominal and pelvic solid organs involved with lymphoma. Solid organs from the gastrointestinal section and the genitourinary and gynecologic systems are discussed further.

### Liver

Hepatic lymphoma usually occurs in the setting of systemic lymphoma in both HL and in NHL. Rarely, it may be a primary lesion, almost always of the

easily overlooked on cross-sectional images because of homogenous appearance of the liver.

2. Multifocal hepatic masses resemble metastatic disease (see **Fig. 7**; **Fig. 9**). Differentiation is based on the homogeneous appearance of the lymphoma masses. Metastases tend to be heterogeneous and demonstrate ring-like or target-like enhancement pattern.

3. Miliary lesions (<1 cm in diameter) mostly seen in Hodgkin disease, which need to be differentiated from fungal abscesses. Fungal microabscesses (**Fig. 10**) are characterized by the rim-enhancement pattern and are favored in the clinical setting of fever and immunocompromised status.

4. Lymphomatous infiltration (**Figs. 11 and 12**) may be seen extending from the porta hepatis along the margins of the portal veins resulting in periportal patchy, irregular areas.

Hepatic lymphoma is found more frequently in middle-aged white immunocompromised individual, such as after organ transplant or in patients with AIDS (see **Fig. 11**). HL of the liver is often associated with splenic involvement. In both HL and NHL, the portal area is typically involved initially because this is the region where lymphatic tissue is present.

### Gallbladder

Lymphoma of the gallbladder is very rare and not widely reported in the literature. Lymphoma of the gallbladder is seen most often with multisystem involvement; isolated involvement of the gallbladder may be difficult to differentiate from acute or chronic cholecystitis. Lymphoma may present as homogeneous thickening of the gallbladder wall without a hypoechoic edematous middle layer within the gallbladder wall (eg, no halo sign). This

NHL large cell type. There are several patterns of hepatic involvement including[19]

1. Hepatomegaly, which is suggestive of diffuse liver infiltration, mainly in NHL. This pattern is

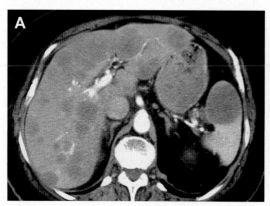
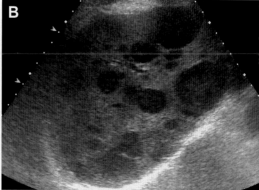

**Fig. 9.** (*A*, *B*) CT axial slice in 54-year-old man with NHL presenting as multiple hypodense masses in the liver and spleen. Spleen is almost always involved with hepatic lymphoma. Sagittal ultrasound image of the liver shows multiple hypoechoic masses studding the liver parenchyma.

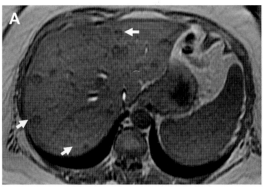 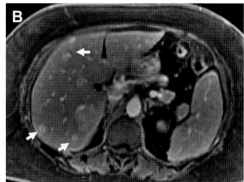

Fig. 10. Hepatic fungal abscesses in a patient with NHL status postchemotherapy presenting with fever and right upper quadrant pain. (A) T1 gradient echo sequence demonstrating multiple T1 hypointense subcentimeter hepatic lesions (arrows) in this patient with NHL on chemotherapy presenting with fever. (B) Postgadolinium image shows these lesions to be rim enhancing (arrows).

appearance may aid in the ultrasonographic diagnosis of gallbladder lymphoma and differentiation from cholecystitis.

## Spleen

A staging laparotomy performed more commonly in the past showed splenic involvement in 30% to 40% of patients at presentation.[19,20] NHL is the most common tumor of the spleen.[19–21] The imaging appearance of lymphoma of the spleen consists of

1. Splenomegaly: Homogeneous enlargement without a discrete mass (Fig. 13). Marked splenomegaly is consistent with splenic lymphoma. Isolated splenomegaly is the classic finding in mantle cell lymphoma. Splenomegaly with splenic hilar lymphadenopathy also suggests splenic lymphoma. Mild splenomegaly alone may or may not be related to lymphomatous involvement.

2. Solitary mass (Fig. 14): A single splenic mass is commonly found to represent a large cell lymphoma, especially with necrosis or invasion beyond the splenic capsule. In the setting of indolent lymphoma, a splenic mass should raise the suspicion of transformation, especially in the setting of high FDG uptake by PET (see Fig. 6).

3. Multifocal nodules (Figs. 15 and 16): Usually seen in NHL or in immunocompromised states. It needs to be differentiated from fungal microabscesses or splenic infarcts. Fungal microabscesses of the spleen are seen in the immunocompromised, are typically smaller than lymphoma masses, and occur in the absence of lymphadenopathy. Splenic infarctions, which may occur in association with lymphoma, display mass-like features on CT and MR imaging but have a characteristic wedge shape and peripheral location.

4. Diffuse infiltration: Diffuse involvement of the spleen is difficult to detect with US, CT, and

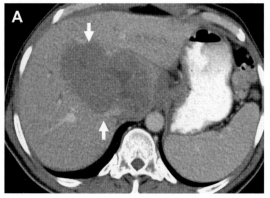 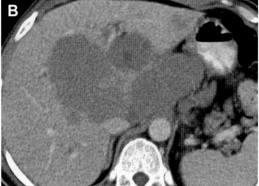

Fig. 11. AIDS-related lymphoma in a 39-year-old man presenting as large central hypodense mass (A, arrows) with associated peripancreatic and porta hepatis lymphadenopathy (B).

MR imaging. Splenic size often decreases after chemotherapy and this should not be misinterpreted as initial splenic involvement.

## Pancreas

Pancreatic lymphoma is a rare extranodal manifestation of NHL; the B-cell type of NHL predominantly involves the pancreas. Involvement of the pancreas occurs in more than 30% of patients with NHL and is most likely attributable to direct infiltration from adjacent lymphadenopathy. Two distinct morphologic patterns of pancreatic involvement are seen. One is a well-circumscribed focal mass (see **Fig. 16**). In patients with pancreatic lymphoma, pancreatic ductal dilation may be absent, even with ductal invasion.[22,23] In addition, there is no evidence of atrophy of the pancreatic parenchyma. The combination of a bulky localized tumor in the pancreatic head without significant dilatation of the main pancreatic duct strengthens a diagnosis of pancreatic lymphoma over adenocarcinoma. The second is diffuse enlargement infiltrating or replacing most of the pancreatic gland (**Fig. 17**). This pattern involves organ enlargement and irregular peripancreatic fat infiltration, which may resemble acute pancreatitis on imaging.[22] Patients with this pattern, however, never show the typical clinical signs of acute pancreatitis even if the serum amylase is elevated. **Table 2** summarizes the imaging features of pancreatic lymphoma versus the more common pancreatic adenocarcinoma. Lymphadenopathy below the level of renal veins is virtually never seen with pancreatic adenocarcinoma. In addition, lymphoma is known for envelopment rather than encasement or obstruction of the vasculature.

## Gastric, Small Bowel, and Colon

The stomach is the most commonly involved organ, followed by the small bowel (**Fig. 18**) (see the article by Gollub in this issue for a detailed discussion).

## Mesentery

Lymphoma is the most common cause of mesenteric masses and adenopathy. Most cases of mesenteric lymphadenopathy are associated with NHL rather than with epithelial tumors. Mesenteric involvement is the predominant finding in 4% to 5% of patients with HL and in 30% to 50% of patients with NHL. Mesenteric masses caused by lymphoma may involve the small bowel by means of direct extension or indirectly by displacement.

### Nodal disease

Lymphoma of the mesentery can range in size from small to bulky and in shape from round or oval to irregular masses and can appear as multiple round, mildly enhancing, homogenous masses that often surround mesenteric arteries and veins. Lymphoma can grow so large that it encases the mesenteric vasculature without causing ischemia. The sandwich sign is a hallmark of lymphoma characterized by lobulated, confluent mesenteric soft tissue masses that resemble two halves of a sandwich and the mesenteric vessels in between represent the filling (**Fig. 19**).[24] Alternatively, lymphoma of the mesentery can also appear as a large, lobulated, cake-like heterogeneous mass with areas of low attenuation representing necrosis that displaces bowel loops.

### Peritoneal disease

Mesenteric or peritoneal infiltration by lymphoma is seen almost exclusively in NHL. Lymphoma

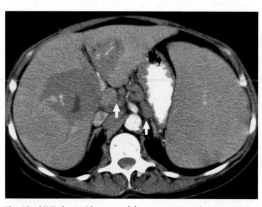

**Fig. 12.** NHL in a 40-year-old man presenting as an infiltrative mass emanating from the porta hepatis and splenomegaly. Celiac axis lymphadenopathy (*arrows*) is also evident.

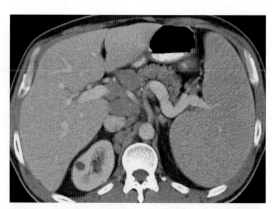

**Fig. 13.** CT axial image in a 27-year-old woman with NHL with extensive porta hepatis lymphadenopathy and splenomegaly.

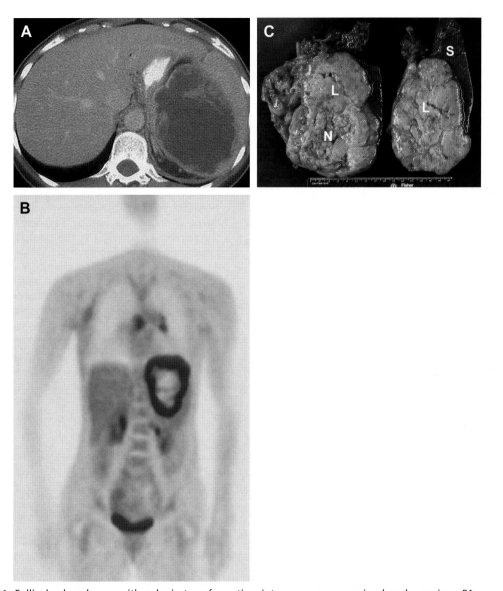

**Fig. 14.** Follicular lymphoma with splenic transformation into a more aggressive lymphoma in a 51-year-old woman with an enlarged spleen and subcarinal, axillary, and hilar lymphadenopathy. (*A*) Axial CT scan shows a single large low-attenuation mass occupying most of the spleen. (*B*) PET image shows increased FDG uptake in the spleen with maximum standardized uptake value 18, but essentially no uptake in the center of the spleen. Biopsy of an axillary lymph node had revealed follicular lymphoma. (*C*) Gross pathology demonstrates a large necrotic mass (N) surrounded by a thick rind of tissue consistent with lymphoma (L) replacing most of the spleen (S). Further evaluation revealed diffuse large B-cell lymphoma with extensive necrosis (transformed follicular lymphoma). (*Courtesy of* C. Portlock and M.E. Burkard, New York, NY.)

typically spreads in sheets along the peritoneal surface causing a rigid pleating of thickened mesenteric leaves. This stellate appearance may also be seen in ovarian, colonic, and pancreatic carcinoma. Ascites is more common than in carcinomatosis. Imaging findings may mimic peritoneal carcinomatosis, with peritoneal nodules, ascites, and mesenteric infiltration. Omental caking, hallmark of metastatic ovarian cancer, can also be seen (**Fig. 20**). Alternatively, misty mesentery[25–27] may be the presentation; however, this is more common after therapy.

## Genitourinary System

### Kidneys
Renal involvement by lymphoma is usually seen in systemic disease, because the kidney does not

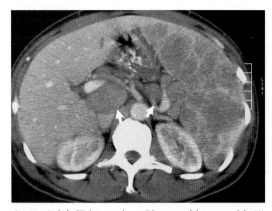

**Fig. 15.** Axial CT image in a 50-year-old man with HL presenting as multiple hypodense masses in the spleen. Multiple large porta hepatis and mesenteric nodes are also evident (*arrows*).

contain lymphoid tissue. Renal lymphoma is most often seen in advanced NHL. There are five patterns of renal involvement in lymphoma described by different authors with slight differences in frequency.[28–31] Most common pattern of renal involvement is the infiltration of kidney by multiple masses and the diffusely enlarged lobular kidneys. The renal arteries and veins remain patent despite tumor envelopment, a finding that is characteristic for lymphoma.

1. Diffuse renal infiltration (**Fig. 21**): This pattern may present as enlarged kidneys. The renal parenchyma remains relatively hypodense in the early postcontrast study. Parenchymal enhancement is exhibited in the nephrographic phase and normal excretion is evident on the excretory phase. Differential diagnosis includes epithelial tumors, such as renal cell cancer; medullary tumors, such as collecting duct carcinoma and renal medullary carcinoma;

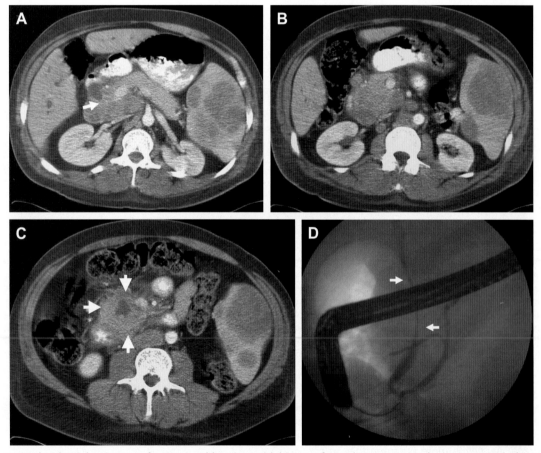

**Fig. 16.** (*A–C*) Axial CT images of a 37-year-old patient with history of NHL demonstrates splenic masses and a large solid mass in the head of the pancreas without any associated pancreatic duct dilatation. (*D*) Endoscopic retrograde cholangiopancreatography image demonstrates smooth extrinsic compression and stretching of the mid common bile duct (*arrows*) related to lymphadenopathy. Of note is the absence of the double duct sign associated with pancreatic adenocarcinoma.

**Table 2**
**Features of pancreatic lymphoma versus adenocarcinoma**

| CT and MR Imaging Appearance | Pancreatic Lymphoma | Pancreatic Carcinoma |
|---|---|---|
| Pancreatic duct dilatation | Rare | Present |
| Pancreatic parenchymal atrophy | Rare | Present |
| Density of the involving mass | Homogeneous | Heterogeneous |
| Enhancement of the mass | Homogeneous | Heterogeneous |
| Calcification | Rare | Present |
| Vascular invasion | Rare | Present |
| Lymph nodes | Extensive retroperitoneal and mesenteric lymph nodes | Peripancreatic and porta hepatic lymph nodes |

*Data from* Leite N, Kased N, Rana R, et al. Cross-sectional imaging of extranodal involvement in abdominopelvic lymphoproliferative malignancies. Radiographics 2007;27:1613–34.

transitional cell carcinoma of the renal pelvis; and inflammatory diseases, such as bacterial pyelonephritis, xanthogranulomatous pyelonephritis, and renal parenchymal malakoplakia.
2. Multiple renal masses (**Fig. 22**): These tend to be hyperdense on CT scans before contrast administration relating to the hypercellualrity of the lymphomas. Otherwise, these are characterized by multiple, bilateral, focal intraparenchymal, and hypoattenuating masses. Differential diagnosis includes metastases. Sometimes this form also presents as bilateral diffuse areas of nonenhancing hypodensities

in the kidneys. Differential diagnosis includes renal infarcts.
3. Renal invasion from contiguous retroperitoneal disease (**Fig. 23**): Renal involvement from retroperitoneal lymphoma commonly occurs either by invasion through the renal capsule or by extension through the renal sinus. Retroperitoneal adenopathy is invariably present, and many patients show obstructive hydronephrosis. Retroperitoneal tissue secondary to treated lymphoma can be difficult to differentiate from retroperitoneal fibrosis, which typically does not elevate the aorta from the spine (see **Fig. 3**).

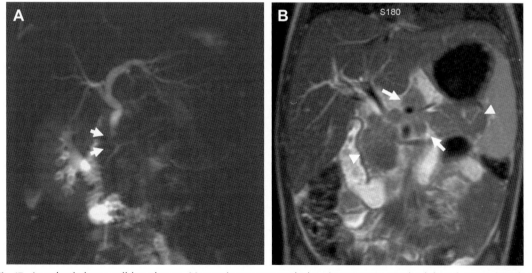

**Fig. 17.** Anaplastic large cell lymphoma. Magnetic resonance cholangiopancreatography (*A*) and coronal T2 fast spin echo (*B*) sequences. MRCP image (*A*) shows a narrowing in the distal common bile duct related to extrinsic compression and is slightly enlarged with minimal intrahepatic biliary dilatation; the pancreatic duct is normal. T2 coronal sequence demonstrates pancreatic enlargement (*arrowheads*) and peripancreatic lymphadenopathy (*arrows*) without associated pancreatic duct dilation.

4. Solitary masses: Seen as a single, focal, intra-parenchymal, hypoenhancing hypoattenuating mass. Differential diagnosis includes renal cortical tumors.

5. Perirenal infiltrates (**Fig. 24**): Perirenal or capsular involvement is often associated with retroperitoneal lymphomatous masses. Differential diagnosis includes perirenal hematoma. Rarely, however, this form may present as nodular perirenal soft tissue thickening (**Fig. 25**).

### Adrenal

Adrenal glands are an unusual site for primary lymphoma (see **Fig. 8**). The adrenal gland is involved in 4% of patients with NHL. At autopsy, however, the adrenal gland has been found to be involved in 25% of the cases of disseminated NHL. In all age groups, involvement of the adrenal glands occurs more often in patients with NHL than in those with HL. Adrenal involvement is often (50%) bilateral and may cause adrenal insufficiency.

Lymphoma of the adrenal glands may present as a solid mass or masses; however, the most common presentation is of diffuse bilateral enlargement of the adrenal gland. In addition, there may be associated retroperitoneal lymphadenopathy and extranodal disease. Nonlymphomatous bilateral adrenal hyperplasia has been described in association with lymphoma and should be differentiated from tumoral involvement, which is possible with FDG-PET.

### Urinary bladder

Lymphoma of the bladder is extremely rare. It can be seen in the setting of widespread nodal and extranodal disease, recurrent lymphoma, or as primary lymphoma limited to the bladder (**Fig. 26**). Specific radiologic appearances are not described in the literature; the universal features of lymphoma including homogeneity, uniform wall thickness, are described in case reports.

### Testes

Lymphoma accounts for 5% of testicular tumors, but it is the most common testicular tumor in patients older than 60 years. It is practically nonexistent in Hodgkin disease. Bilateral involvement is even rarer, constituting 23% of all cases of primary testicular lymphoma. Lymphoma appears as a diffuse, symmetric enlargement of the entire organ with involvement of epididymis and spermatic cord but without invasion through the tunica vaginalis. The testis seems to provide a sanctuary for lymphoma cells, because of the "gonadal barrier" that inhibits crossing of the chemotherapeutic agents. A patient can get lymphoma relapse in the testis even sometime after remission. Rarely, recurrence may also be seen in the spermatic cord or the inguinal canal.

The radiologic appearances available in the literature are primarily with US because of the superficial placement and lack of radiation. The sonographic pattern of involvement includes focal or diffuse areas of decreased echogenicity in an enlarged testis. Differential diagnosis includes metastases, primary testicular tumors, or sarcoidosis.

### Prostate

Primary lymphoma of the prostate is rare (**Figs. 27 and 28**). It represents 0.09% of prostate neoplasms and 0.1% of all NHL.[32–34] Multifocal involvement of the gland is the most common presentation in such cases. Lymphoma of the prostate occurs on average in men over 60 years.

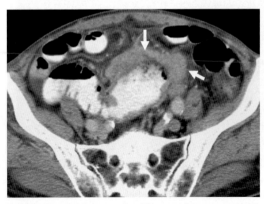

Fig. 18. CT axial image of a 52-year-old woman with NHL presenting as aneurysmally dilated small bowel loops (*arrows*) and mesenteric lymphadenopathy.

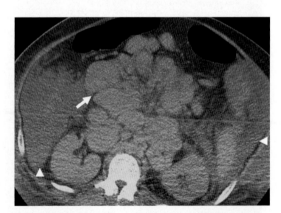

Fig. 19. A 43-year-old man with large cell NHL presenting with bulky mesenteric lymphadenopathy; the arrow points to the sandwich sign marked by large lymph nodes denoting the buns with mesenteric vessels traversing in between without any obstruction or compression. Arrowheads mark the ascites.

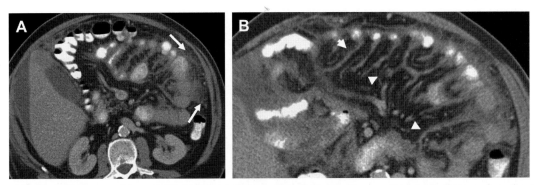

**Fig. 20.** (*A, B*) A 40-year-old man with NHL presenting as mesenteric lymphoma, which typically spreads as sheets along the peritoneal surface causing a rigid pleating of thickened mesenteric leaves (*arrowheads*). Arrows mark the omental disease.

The digital rectal examination can reveal an extremely enlarged prostate with normal consistency, with an unaltered prostate-specific antigen.[33] On imaging, there is diffuse, homogeneous enlargement of the prostate gland with or without extension to adjacent tissues (see **Figs. 27 and 28**).[34]

### Gynecologic System

#### Ovaries

NHL may involve the gynecologic tract, and the ovary is one of the more common anatomic sites to be involved.[35,36] Ovarian involvement by NHL usually occurs as a part of systemic disease. Localized NHL of the ovary is rare.[37,38] A common

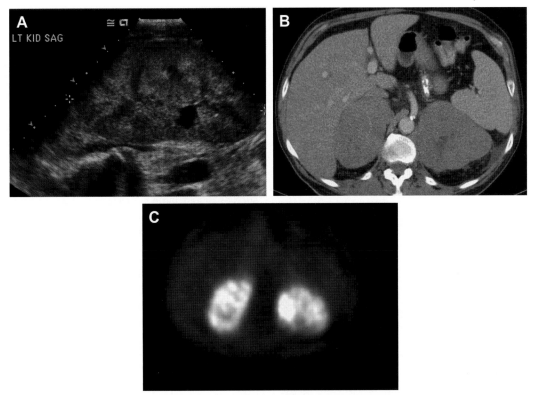

**Fig. 21.** US, CT axial image, and PET axial scan of a 55-year-old man with history of NHL. (*A*) US image demonstrates enlargement of the kidney with loss of corticomedullary differentiation. (*B*) CT image demonstrates diffuse infiltration of both kidneys and marked hypoenhancement, which demonstrates marked uptake on PET scan (*C*).

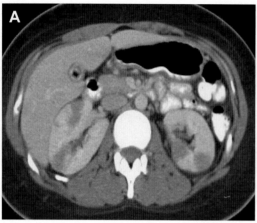
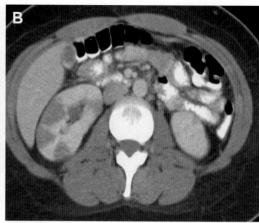

Fig. 22. (*A, B*) Axial CT images in a patient with NHL presenting as multiple hypodense masses in both kidneys.

pattern of involvement is diffuse bilateral homogeneous enlargement, usually associated with retroperitoneal or extranodal manifestations of lymphoma elsewhere. Ovarian lymphoma demonstrates a propensity to be bilateral (**Fig. 29**). Differential diagnoses in ovarian lymphoma include granulosa cell tumors, dysgerminoma, and metastatic cancer.

### Uterus

Uterine involvement by lymphoma is rare and is usually observed in the cervix. Its frequency in Western countries was reported to be 0.008% of primary cervical tumors and 2% of extranodal lymphomas in women.[35,36,39]

US and CT evaluation demonstrates diffuse homogeneous enlargement of the uterus. On MR imaging, lymphoma tends to be hypointense on T1-weighted images and relatively hyperintense on T2-weighted images.[36] MR imaging findings of uterine cervical lymphoma closely resemble

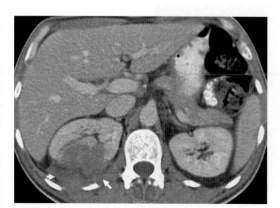

Fig. 23. CT axial image in a 54-year-old man with B-cell lymphoma presenting as a focal right kidney (*arrows*) with extension into the retroperitoneum.

those of carcinoma of the cervix. Preserved cervical epithelium in the presence of extensive involvement of the cervical stroma may be a clue to the diagnosis of malignant lymphoma. Diffuse enlargement of the uterus without disruption of the endometrial epithelium is also reported to be a characteristic finding for lymphoma involving the uterine body.

## MISCELLANEOUS

Certain important aspects of lymphoma, such as malignant transformation, and some specific features in immunocompromised patients are discussed in the preceding paragraphs.

### Malignant Transformation of Lymphoma

Malignant transformation is a phenomenon whereby low-grade lymphomas such as chronic lymphocytic leukemia or follicular lymphoma transition into intermediate- or high-grade cell types, such as diffuse large B-cell lymphomas. Clinically, this is suspected when the patient develops sudden enlargement of the lymph nodes or development of B-cell symptoms. In addition, new nodes or group of nodes with significantly increased FGD avidity in comparison with other involved nodes with lower SUV is also another indication of malignant transformation. Biopsy is needed for final diagnosis.

### Immunocompromised Patients

There is an increased incidence of NHL in patients with HIV infection or secondary to organ transplantation. In particular, cyclosporine therapy may be associated with NHL or posttransplantation lymphoproliferative disorders (PTLD).[40] Unlike lymphoma in the general population, immune

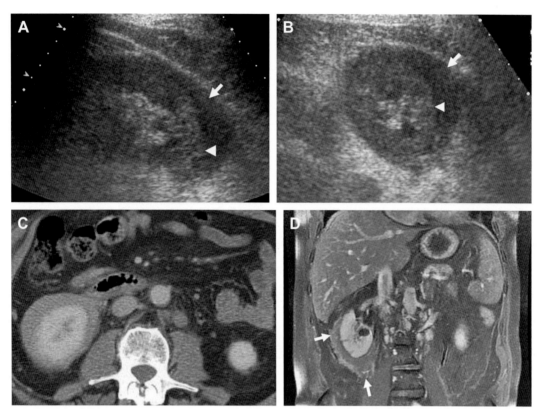

**Fig. 24.** Multimodality perirenal lymphoma. Sagittal (*A*) and transverse (*B*) US images of the inferior pole of the kidney, which demonstrate a small perirenal hypoechoic mass; arrowheads marking the cortex, the arrows mark the perirenal soft tissue mass. (*C*) CT axial image demonstrates curivilinear perirenal hypodense mass at the inferior pole of the right kidney. (*D*) Coronal postgadolinium image outlines the extent of the inferior pole perirenal lymphoma (*arrows*) involvement.

deficiency–related lymphoma is often of extranodal origin, with the central nervous system, bone marrow, gastrointestinal tract, lung, and liver being the most common sites of disease.[40–42]

## Posttransplantation Lymphoproliferative Disorders

PTLDs are an uncommon complication of solid organ transplantation (**Fig. 30**). A transient lymphoproliferative disorder occurs when a primary infection with Epstein-Barr virus occurs in an immunocompetent host; however, this proliferation of infected B lymphocytes is controlled by cytotoxic and suppressive T lymphocytes. The proliferation of B cells is not controlled in an immunodeficient Epstein-Barr virus infected host resulting in PTLD. It includes a spectrum of disease ranging from polyclonal B-cell hyperplasia to monoclonal B-cell lymphoma.

The reported incidence of PTLD varies from 12% in pancreas transplant recipients, to 9% in heart and lung transplant recipients, and to 1% to 2% in renal and liver transplant recipients.[40]

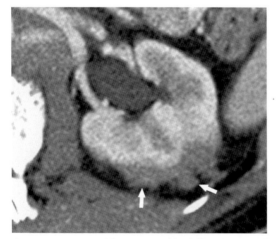

**Fig. 25.** A 48-year-old woman with diffuse large cell lymphoma presenting as nodular growth of perirenal (*arrows*) lymphoma.

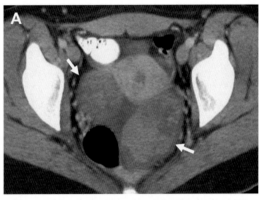
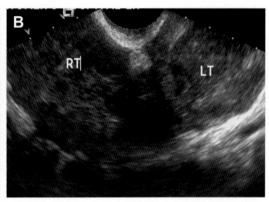

Fig. 26. (*A*) CT axial image of the pelvis demonstrates bilateral enlarged ovaries (*arrows*) with diffuse homogeneous enhancement in a rare case of ovarian lymphoma. (*B*) US image also demonstrates the lymphomatous involvement as large hypoechoic somewhat homogeneous enlargement of the ovaries.

Early diagnosis of PTLD is important because reduction of immunosuppression improves the clinical outcome (see **Fig. 30**). The anatomic region of the transplant organ is the most common site of involvement in lung and liver transplant recipients.[42] There is a relatively high incidence of extranodal disease in PTLD to almost 81% in comparison with NHL. On CT, PTLD is similar to NHL with predominant involvement of solid abdominal organs and hollow viscous. The most common sites of involvement are the liver, small bowel, and kidney, but virtually any organ within the abdomen and pelvis can be affected.

Although the CT appearance of gastrointestinal involvement in PTLD mimics that of lymphoma, PTLD has a propensity for ulceration and perforation of the alimentary tract.

### AIDS-associated Lymphoma

The diagnosis of NHL in a patient with HIV infection fulfils the criteria for the diagnosis of AIDS. In general, HIV-related NHL is characterized by exuberant lymph node enlargement. Abdominal visceral organ involvement (resulting in hepatic, splenic, and gastrointestinal tract masses) and omental disease are much more commonly seen than in other lymphoma patients (see **Fig. 11**). AIDS-related lymphomas tend to be poorly differentiated and aggressive. Advanced disease is often present at the time of diagnosis and the prognosis is poor. AIDS-related lymphoma often manifests with multiple sites of abdominal involvement.

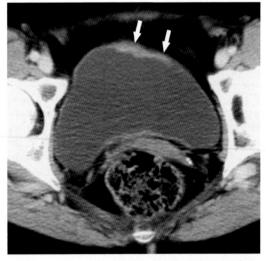

Fig. 27. A 63-year-old woman with lymphoma of the bladder (concurrent low-grade mucosa-associated lymphoid tissue lymphoma and aggressive diffuse large cell lymphoma) presenting as focal thickening of the anterior wall of the urinary bladder (*arrows*).

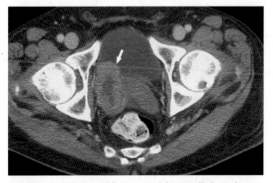

Fig. 28. A 70-year-old man with B-cell lymphoma. Patient has supra and infradiaphragmatic lymphadenopathy. Image depicts infiltration of both seminal vesicles (*arrow*) from prostatic lymphoma.

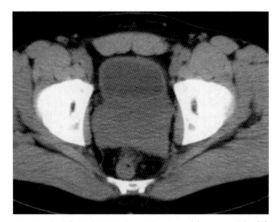

Fig. 29. Axial CT image in a 35-year-old man with diffuse large cell lymphoma of the prostate presenting as marked enlargement of the prostate gland.

Focal splenic lesions are more common in patients with lymphoma related to AIDS than in patients with lymphoma unrelated to AIDS. A significant number of primary manifestations (5%) in AIDS-related lymphoma arise in the pancreas.

### Primary Effusion Lymphoma

Primary effusion lymphoma is a malignancy of B cells that is caused by Kaposi's sarcoma–associated herpes virus commonly arising in patients with underlying immunodeficiency, such as AIDS. It is generally resistant to cancer chemotherapy drugs that are active against other lymphomas, and carries a very poor prognosis.[43] Primary effusion lymphoma is unusual in that most cases arise in body cavities, such as the pleural space or the pericardium; another name for primary effusion lymphoma is "body cavity lymphoma." It is a heterogeneous group of rare NHLs that proliferate within the serous body cavities and result in recurrent effusions.

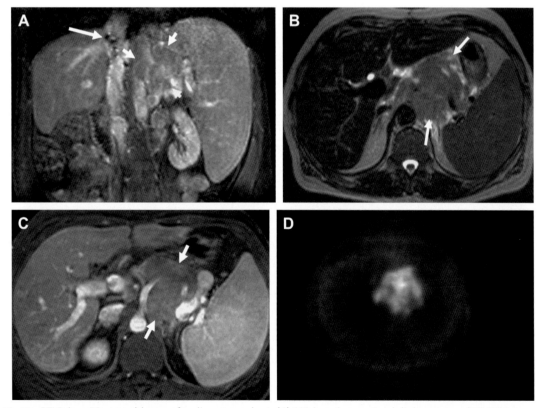

Fig. 30. PTLD in a 50-year-old man after liver transplant. (*A*) MR imaging postgadolinium coronal T1-VIBE image demonstrates susceptibility artifact (*long arrow*) related to surgical clips in the region of intrahepatic IVC presenting with extensive lymphadenopathy in the lesser sac (*short arrows*). (*B, C*) MRI T2 SSFSE and postgadolinium axial T1-VIBE images with extensive lymphadenopathy in the gastrohepatic ligament (*arrows*). (*D*) PET axial image showing increased uptake in the lesser sac. Follow-up PET examination 6 months after cessation of chemotherapy shows complete resolution.

## SUMMARY

The radiologic appearances of solid organ with HL and NHL involvement in the abdominopelvic region are discussed in this article. The most common radiologic patterns of involvement are illustrated. The imaging characteristics of lymphomatous involvement of abdominal organs overlap with several other disorders and the specific features pertaining to lymphoma are highlighted. In patients with known lymphoma, other important management considerations, such as staging, response to therapy, malignant transformation, and identification of recurrent disease, are also discussed. The emerging role of FDG-PET is briefly outlined.

## REFERENCES

1. Fisher RI. Overview of non-Hodgkin's lymphoma: biology, staging, and treatment. Semin Oncol 2003; 30:3–9.
2. Harris NL, Jaffe ES, Diebold J, et al. The World Health Organization classification of neoplastic diseases of the hematopoietic and lymphoid tissues. Report of the Clinical Advisory Committee meeting, Airlie House, Virginia, November, 1997. Ann Oncol 1999;10:1419–32.
3. Jaffe ES, Harris NL, Stein H, et al. World Health Organization classification of tumours. Pathology and genetics of tumours of haematopoietic and lymphoid tissues. Lyon (France): IARC Press; 2001.
4. Cheson BD, Horning SJ, Coiffier B, et al. Report of an international workshop to standardize response criteria for non-Hodgkin lymphomas. NCI Sponsored International Working Group. J Clin Oncol 1999;17: 1244–53.
5. Rademaker J. Diagnostic imaging modalities for the assessment of lymphoma with special emphasis on CT, MRI and US. PET Clinics 2006;1(3):219–30.
6. Moog F, Bangerter M, Diederchs CG, et al. Lymphoma: role of whole-body 2-deoxy-2-{F-18} fluoro-D-glucose (FDG) PET in nodal staging. Radiology 1997;203:795–800.
7. Rahmouni A, Divine M, Lepage E, et al. Mediastinal lymphoma: quantitative changes in gadolinium enhancement at MR imaging after treatment. Radiology 2001;219:621–8.
8. Nakayama TMD, Yoshimitsu KMD, Irie JH. Usefulness of the calculated apparent diffusion coefficient value in the differential diagnosis of retroperitoneal masses. Magn Reson Imaging 2004;20:735–42.
9. Chen S, Ikawa F, Kurisu K, et al. Quantitative MR evaluation of intracranial epidermoid tumors by fast fluid-attenuated inversion recovery imaging and echo-planar diffusion-weighted imaging. AJNR Am J Neuroradiol 2001;22:1089–96.
10. Guo AC, Cummings TJ, Dash RC, et al. Lymphomas and high grade astrocytomas: comparison of water diffusibility and histologic characteristics. Radiology 2002;224:177–83.
11. Stadnik TW, Chaskis C, Michotte A, et al. Diffusion-weighted MR imaging of intracerebral masses: comparison with conventional MR imaging and histologic findings. AJNR Am J Neuroradiol 2001; 22:969–76.
12. Rahmouni A, Luciani A, Itti E, et al. MRI and PET in monitoring response in lymphoma. Cancer Imaging 2005;5(Spec No A):S106–12.
13. Rankin SC. Assessment of response to therapy using conventional imaging. Eur J Nucl Med Mol Imaging 2003;30(Suppl 1):S56–64.
14. Dorfman RE, Alpern MB, Gross BH, et al. Upper abdominal lymph nodes: criteria for normal size determined with CT. Radiology 1991;180: 319–22.
15. Hricak H, Husband J, Panicek DM. Oncologic imaging: essentials of reporting common cancers. Philadelphia: Saunders Elsevier; 2007. p. 12.
16. Vinnicombe S, Norman A, Husband J, et al. Normal pelvic lymph nodes: documentation by CT scanning after bipedal lymphangiography. Radiology 1995; 194:349–55.
17. Lister TA, Crowther DM, Sutcliffe SB, et al. Report of a committee convened to discuss the evaluation and staging of patients with Hodgkin's disease: Cotswold's meeting. J Clin Oncol 1989; 7:1630–6.
18. Cheson BD, Pfistner B, Juweid ME, et al. Revised response criteria for malignant lymphoma. J Clin Oncol 2007;25:579–86.
19. Leite N, Kased N, Rana R, et al. Cross-sectional imaging of extranodal involvement in abdominopelvic lymphoproliferative malignancies. Radiographics 2007;27:1613–34.
20. Ahmann DL, Kiely JM, Harrison EG, et al. Malignant lymphoma of the spleen. Caner 1996;19:461–9.
21. Rabhuska LS, Kawashima A, Fishman EK. Imaging of the spleen: CT with supplemental MRI examination. Radiographics 1994;14:307–32.
22. Merkle ME, Bender NG, Brambs H. Imaging findings in pancreatic lymphoma: differential aspects. AJR Am J Roentgenol 2000;174:671–5.
23. Glass AG, Karnell LH, Menck HR. The national cancer database report on non-Hodgkin's lymphoma. Cancer 1997;80:2311–20.
24. Mueller PR, Ferrucci JT Jr, Harbin WP, et al. Appearance of lymphomatous involvement of the mesentery by ultrasound and body computed tomography: the sandwich sign. Radiology 1980; 134:467–73.
25. Horton KM, Lawler LP, Fishman EK. CT findings in sclerosing mesenteritis (panniculitis): spectrum of disease. Radiographics 2003;23:1561–7.

26. Hardy SM. The sandwich sign. Radiology 2003;226: 651–2.

27. Mindelzun RE, Jeffrey RB Jr, Lane MJ, et al. The misty mesentery. AJR Am J Roentgenol 1996;167:61–5.

28. Urban AB, Fishman K. E. Renal lymphoma: CT patterns with emphasis on helical CT. Radiographics 2000;20:197–212.

29. Sheth S, Ali S, Fishman E. Imaging of renal lymphoma: patterns of disease with pathologic correlation. Radiographics 2006;26:1151–68.

30. Semelka RC, Kelekis NL, Burdeny DA, et al. Renal lymphoma: demonstration by MR imaging. Am J Roentgenol 1996;166:823–7.

31. Sheeran SR, Sussman SK. Renal lymphoma: spectrum of CT findings and potential mimics. Am J Roentgenol 1998;171:1067–72.

32. Sarris A, Dimopoulos M, Pugh W, et al. Primary lymphoma of the prostate: good outcome with doxorubicin-based combination chemotherapy. J Urol 1995;153:1852–4.

33. Bostwick DG, Mann RB. Malignant lymphomas involving the prostate: a study of 13 cases. Cancer 1985;56:2932–8.

34. Fukutani K, Koyama Y, Fujimori M, et al. [Primary malignant lymphoma of the prostate: report of a case achieving complete response to combination chemotherapy and review of 22 Japanese cases]. Nippon Hinyokika Gakkai Zasshi 2003;94:621–5 [in Japanese].

35. Vang R, Medeiros LJ, Fuller GN, et al. Non-Hodgkin's lymphoma involving the gynecologic tract: a review of 88 cases. Adv Anat Pathol 2001; 8:200–17.

36. Fox H, More J. Primary malignant lymphoma of the uterus. J Clin Pathol 1965;18(6):723–8.

37. Monterroso V, Jaffe ES, Merino MJ, et al. Malignant lymphomas involving the ovary. Am J Surg Pathol 1993;17:154–70.

38. Osborne BM, Robboy SJ. Lymphomas or leukemia presenting as ovarian tumors: an analysis of 42 cases. Cancer 1983;52:1933–43.

39. Aozasa K, Saeli K, Ohsawa M, et al. Malignant lymphoma of the uterus: report of seven cases with immunohistochemical study. Cancer 1993;72: 1959–64.

40. Scarsbrook AF, Warakaulle DR, Dattani M, et al. Post-transplantation lymphoproliferative disorder: the spectrum of imaging findings. Clin Radiol 2005;60:47–55.

41. Claudon M, Kessler M, Champigneulle J, et al. Lymphoproliferative disorders after renal transplantation: role of medical imaging. Eur Radiol 1998;8: 1686–93.

42. Pickhardt PJ, Siegel MJ. Post transplantation lymphoproliferative disorder of the abdomen: CT evaluation of 51 patients. Radiology 1999;213: 73–8.

43. Cesarman E, Chang Y, Moore PS, et al. Kaposi's sarcoma-associated herpesvirus-like DNA sequences in AIDS-related body-cavity-based lymphomas. N Engl J Med 1995;332(18): 1186–91.

# Imaging of Gastrointestinal Lymphoma

Marc J. Gollub, MD[a,b]

**KEYWORDS**

- Stomach • Small intestine • Colon • Lymphoma • Imaging
- CT scan • Barium fluoroscopy

The gastrointestinal (GI) tract is the most common extranodal location for non-Hodgkin lymphoma (NHL) and accounts for up to 20% of cases. The incidence is increasing, mainly because of various environmental and exogenous factors, especially the increasing incidence of HIV infection. A world standardized incidence of 1.0 case in 100,000 individuals has been estimated.[1] Involvement may be seen from the pharynx to the rectum. Primary GI tract lymphoma is defined as:

> A tumor that predominantly involves the GI tract with lymph node involvement confined to the drainage area of the primary tumor site
> No liver or spleen involvement or palpable lymph nodes
> Normal chest radiography
> Normal peripheral white blood cells[2]

In the GI tract, primary lymphoma accounts for only 0.9% of all GI tract tumors.[1] The GI tract more commonly is involved secondarily in patients who have generalized lymphoma because of the frequent origination of lymphomas in the mesenteric and retroperitoneal lymph nodes.

The clinical definition predates the development of high-quality cross-sectional imaging modalities, but still applies. Differentiation between primary GI lymphoma and systemic lymphoma with GI tract involvement has important implications, because the prognosis is better in the primary form when diagnosed early on, with 5-year survival rates as high as 62% to 90%. Systemic lymphoma with involvement of the GI tract represents a more advanced stage of lymphoma with lower 5-year survival rates. One investigation attempted to distinguish radiologically between primary GI tract lymphoma and systemic lymphoma with GI tract involvement using a retrospective review of fluoroscopic images in 90 patients who had NHL of the GI tract. These investigators found the predictive value of a single lesion on barium studies for primary GI lymphoma was 76%, and the predictive value of multifocal disease for systemic lymphoma with GI lymphoma was 91%.[3]

In the western world, GI tract lymphoma—whether primary or systemic with GI tract involvement—most often involves the stomach (50%) followed by the small intestine (33%), the colon (10% to 16%), and the esophagus (1%).[4,5] With population migration and the increasing incidence of HIV infection, small intestinal involvement has increased in western series.[1]

Lymphoid tissue exists in the GI tract in the mucosa, the lamina propria, and the submucosal layers. The lymphocytes in these regions are more numerous than in all other immune system organs combined.[4,6] The epithelial cell layer contains numerous lymphocytes, mainly T cell. T cell and B cell lymphocytes are located in the lamina propria mucosae along with approximately 80% of the body's immunoglobulin-producing plasma cells, some arranged in lymphoid follicles. Clusters of five or more of these follicles in the small intestine are known as Peyer's patches and are most numerous in the distal ileum on the mesenteric border (**Fig. 1**). Most GI tract lymphoid tissue is referred to as mucosa-associated lymphoid tissue

a Weill Medical College of Cornell University, 525 E. 68th Street, New York, NY 10065, USA
b Department of Radiology, Memorial Sloan-Kettering Cancer Center, 1275 York Avenue, New York, NY, USA
*E-mail address:* gollubm@mskcc.org

Radiol Clin N Am 46 (2008) 287–312
doi:10.1016/j.rcl.2008.03.002

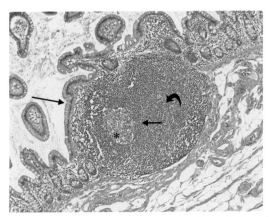

**Fig. 1.** Histologic section (H and E stain) through ileum showing a lymphoid follicle in a Peyer's patch subjacent to ileal mucosal lining (*long arrow*). Germinal center (*asterisk*), mantle zone (*short arrow*), and marginal zone (*curved arrow*) are demonstrated.

or MALT. This is a specially adapted component of the immune system that evolved to confer immunity upon the freely permeable surface of the GI tract and other mucosae that are exposed directly to the external environment.[7] It is found in various concentrations from Waldeyer's ring to the rectum. In response to immune stimulation, it may arise where not normally present, as in the stomach, in response to infection by *Haemophilus pylori* (*H pylori*). Under such circumstances, a lymphoproliferative disorder may arise and become monoclonal, leading to lymphoma.

Most lymphomas of the GI tract are NHLs arising mainly from native MALT (**Box 1**). These B cell lymphomas are referred to as marginal zone B cell MALT lymphomas (indicating their histologic similarity to the marginal zone of the lymphoid follicle as opposed to the follicle center (see **Fig. 1**). Paradoxically, the stomach is the most frequent site of GI tract lymphoma, and yet normally it does not contain MALT. MALT lymphoma arises here in response to *H pylori* infection.[4]

T cell lymphomas are uncommon, comprising only 0.5% to 3.0% of all GI tract NHLs.[8] They form a heterogeneous group with the exception of the specific subtype known as enteropathy-associated T cell lymphoma complicating celiac disease (CD).[6] Unlike B cell lymphomas, they tend to: involve the jejunum, be multifocal, have minimal bowel wall thickening, and have minimal associated lymphadenopathy. Another distinguishing characteristic is their higher tendency toward perforation, thought to be caused by their angioinvasive behavior.[8]

NHL of the GI tract has a better prognosis than GI tract adenocarcinoma because of its tendency to remain confined to the bowel wall for prolonged

---

**Box 1**
**Common gastrointestinal lymphoma (primary gastrointestinal lymphoma and systemic lymphoma with gastrointestinal involvement)**

**B cell**

MALT type (including immunoproliferative small intestine disease)

    Includes transformation of MALT to diffuse large B cell lymphoma (DLBCL)

Mantle

Burkitt

Systemic lymphoma with GI tract involvement

    Follicular

    Lymphocytic

    Large B cell lymphoma (DLBCL)

Immunodeficiency-related

    After stem-cell transplant (therapeutic immunosuppression)

    HIV/AIDS

    Congenital

**T Cell**

Enteropathy-associated

Peripheral T cell lymphoma, not otherwise specified with GI involvement.

*Modified from* Mendelson RM, Fermoyle S. Primary gastrointestinal lymphomas: a radiological–pathologic review. Part 1: stomach, esophagus and colon. Australasian Radiology 2005;49:354; with permission.

---

periods of time before the tumor spreads and because of more effective chemotherapy. The prognosis depends, not only on depth of bowel wall involvement and nodal involvement (stage), but also on cell type (classification).[4] Poor prognostic factors include advanced stage, involvement of para-aortic nodes, large tumor bulk, serosal penetration, and intestinal rather than gastric origin.[9] NHL of the GI tract is more common in men than women (3:2). Although predominantly a disease of middle-aged persons, there is a double peak with the first peak in patients less than 10 years of age and the second peak at a mean age of 53. Although rare in children, these tumors constitute the most common GI tumor in childhood.[1] Symptoms will depend on site of involvement, but may include dysphagia, abdominal pain, nausea, vomiting, anorexia, weight loss, diarrhea, and GI bleeding—all of which are nonspecific.

As with nodal lymphoma, extranodal GI tract lymphoma may be classified and also may be staged. The classification system addresses the cell type and can be derived from the World Health Organization (WHO) classification.[6] The staging system addresses the severity of bowel wall, nodal, and distant involvement (**Box 2**).

Lymphoma, like other malignancies, may be seen in association with infections and immunodeficiency states. Some examples include AIDS, *H pylori* infection, *Campylobacter jejuni*,[10] Epstein Barr virus (EBV) infection after bone-marrow or stem cell transplant, and complicating CD. Other conditions that predispose to NHL of the GI tract include systemic lupus erythematosus[4] and inflammatory bowel disease.[11]

Treatment modalities for GI tract lymphomas include chemotherapy, radiation therapy, stem cell transplant, and antibiotic treatment for *H pylori*. Details of treatment are presented elsewhere in this issue.

This article focuses on the typical appearances of GI tract lymphoma seen at barium fluoroscopy and CT. Newer modalities such as CT enterography also will be discussed. MR imaging and ultrasound (US), not as frequently used in the diagnosis, are mentioned briefly with some examples.

## PHARYNX

In the oropharynx, Waldeyer's tonsillar ring of lymphoid tissue, which includes the adenoids, palatine tonsils, and lingual tonsil, may be the site of origin of NHL. Here, lymphoma comprises 10% to 15% of tumors. Multiple sites may be involved in 25% of patients. Cervical lymph nodes are involved in more than 50% of patients. Pharyngeal lymphomas typically appear on barium studies as lobular masses near the base of the tongue in the palatine fossae. The overlying mucosa may be nodular. The appearance can be hard to differentiate from the more common pharyngeal carcinoma (**Fig. 2**).

## ESOPHAGUS

The esophagus is the least common site of involvement of lymphoma of the GI tract, accounting for less than 1% of cases. Most cases arise as secondary extension from cervical or mediastinal nodes or contiguous extension from the gastric fundus (**Fig. 3**). Transhiatal spread of gastric

---

**Box 2**
**Staging of gastrointestinal non-Hodgkin lymphoma**

*Stage I*

Tumor confined to GI tract

Single primary site or multiple noncontiguous lesions

*Stage II*

Tumor extending in abdomen from primary GI site

Nodal involvement:

   II₁ local (paragastric or paraintestinal)

   II₂ distant (mesenteric, para-aortic, paracaval, pelvic, inguinal)

*Stage IIIE*

Penetration of serosa to involve adjacent organs or tissues

*Stage IV*

Disseminated extranodal involvement or a GI tract lesion with supradiaphragmatic nodal involvement

*Data from* Rohatiner A, d'Amore F, Coiffier B, et al. Report on a workshop convened to discuss the pathologic and staging classifications of gastrointestinal tract lymphoma. Ann Onc 1994;5:399.

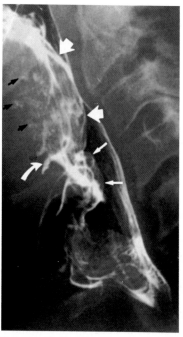

Fig. 2. Pharyngeal lymphoma involving base of tongue and epiglottis. Lateral view of pharynx from double-contrast barium study shows flat mass involving base of tongue (*large straight white arrows*). Note barium in interstices of tumor (*black arrows*). Also note lobulated mass (*small straight white arrows*) involving epiglottis and obliteration of valleculae (*curved arrow*) by tumor. (*From* Rubesin SE. The pharynx: structural disorders. Radiol Clinics of North Am 1994;32:1098; with permission.)

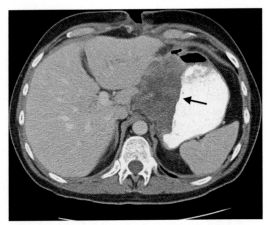

Fig. 3. Multidetector contrast-enhanced helical CT demonstrating bulky esophagogastric junction lymphoma involving distal esophagus and cardia region of stomach (*arrow*).

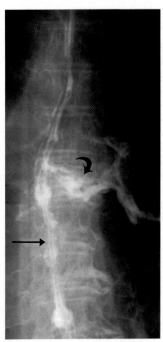

Fig. 4. Esophagobronchial fistula. Gastrografin esophagogram, magnified frontal view, demonstrating collapsed esophageal lumen (*long arrow*), left lower lobe bronchus (*short arrow*), and fistulous tract through necrotic lymph nodes in the mediastinum (*curved arrow*).

lymphoma occurs in 10% of cases. Occasionally, this can mimic carcinoma and present with a picture of secondary achalasia.[5] Primary esophageal non-Hodgkin B cell lymphoma without extraesophageal involvement is rare and comprises less than 0.1% of all lymphomas.[12] Patients may be asymptomatic or complain of dysphagia. Signs occasionally can include upper GI bleed, hematemesis, or melena. Biopsies can be falsely negative in 25% to 35% of cases, because the tumor may be confined to the submucosa.[5]

MALT is not known to occur normally in the esophagus, but may arise in cases of Barrett's esophagus.[13] MALT lymphomas of the esophagus recently have been reported.[12–14] The cases of MALT demonstrated invasion of esophageal glands forming characteristic lymphoepithelial lesions. Interestingly, *H pylori* and reflux esophagitis/Barrett's esophagus were notably absent.

There is no characteristic appearance of lymphoma in the esophagus, and when present, the much more common carcinoma first must be considered. Extrinsic mediastinal adenopathy can narrow the esophageal lumen. These nodes eventually may erode into the esophagus and cause ulceration. Esophagobronchial fistulae may result, especially after radiation treatment (**Fig. 4**). Intrinsic disease, whether primary or synchronous with systemic lymphoma, may have various appearances on esophagography, including an annular, polypoid or ulcerated mass, or an irregular or smooth stricture (**Fig. 5**) or thickened tortuous, submucosal folds mimicking varices. Rarely, multiple submucosal nodules can be seen (**Fig. 6**).[1,4] The appearance of esophageal lymphoma at CT also will mimic other more common tumors such as esophageal carcinoma. CT

will assess the extent of wall thickening better (**Fig. 7**), extraluminal mass, and fistula to the airways.

## STOMACH

The stomach is the most common extranodal location for either primary GI tract lymphoma or systemic lymphoma with GI tract involvement, accounting for approximately 50% of cases. Involvement of the GI tract in systemic lymphoma is far more common than the primary form.[15] Nearly all cases are B cell non-Hodgkin type. Lymphoma of the stomach is the second most common gastric malignancy after adenocarcinoma and accounts for 1% to 7% of gastric neoplasms.[9,16]

### Mucosa-Associated Lymphoid Tissue Lymphoma

MALT lymphoma first was described by Isaacson and Wright[17] in 1983. MALT tissue is present throughout the GI tract and also in the lung. Lymphomas arising in MALT comprise less than 8% of all types of NHLs[18] and exhibit a biologic behavior different from nodal lymphoma. These

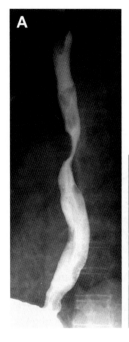

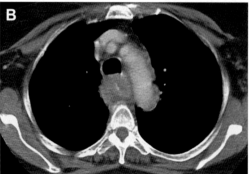

Fig. 5. Esophageal lymphoma. (A) Right posterior oblique barium esophagogram demonstrating smooth stricture above midesophagus, indicating circumferential tumor narrowing the lumen. (B) Axial contrast-enhanced thoracic CT demonstrating markedly concentrically thickened esophagus with uniform iso-attenuated density of esophageal wall, and narrow slit-like lumen.

lymphomas arise in sites normally devoid of organized lymphoid tissues such as the stomach, lung, breast, skin, salivary gland, ocular adnexa, and thyroid gland in the setting of chronic infectious conditions (eg, H pylori) or autoimmune conditions (eg, Sjögren's syndrome). The histologic features of MALT lymphomas closely resemble normal MALT, the tissue that has evolved to protect permeable mucosal surfaces as exemplified by the Peyer's patches of the ileum. MALT lymphomas are notable for their generally indolent course and good prognosis.[10,19]

Gastric MALT is the prototype of these tumors. Antigenic stimulation of B cells by H pylori is essential. This stimulation leads first to chronic gastritis (Fig. 8). This in turn leads to selective expansion of a monoclonal B cell population as a precursor to MALT lymphoma. In the disseminated state, however, the tumor likely has transformed to a more aggressive form that is antigen-independent. it is unclear, however whether all gastric lymphomas follow the sequence of H pylori infection, MALT, low-grade lymphoma, focal high-grade-lymphoma, high-grade lymphoma. It can be assumed that there is a subgroup that consists of primary blast cell gastric lymphoma that arises de novo. These may be independent of H pylori.[20]

Most patients present with nonspecific symptoms like dyspepsia or epigastric pain. Symptoms can be of several years' duration and mimic those of peptic ulcer disease.[18] Often a definitive mass is absent at endoscopy, whereas gastritis or ulceration is seen commonly.[10]

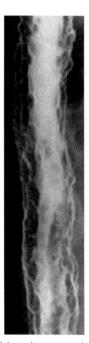

Fig. 6. Esophageal lymphoma, nodular type. Double-contrast esophagogram revealing multiple submucosal nodular defects indicating widespread submucosal tumor nodules. (From Levine MS, Rubensin SE, Pantongrag-Brown L, et al. Non-Hodgkin's lymphoma of the gastrointestinal tract: radiographic findings. AJR 1997;168:167; with permission.)

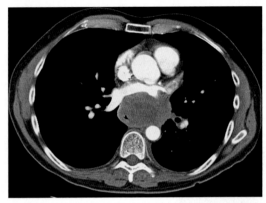

Fig. 7. Esophageal lymphoma. Multislice helical thoracic CT with intravenous contrast demonstrating bulky esophageal mass with uniform iso-attenuation to muscle and narrowed lumen.

Endoscopic biopsy provides adequate material for most patients to make a diagnosis using a combination of morphology, immunophenotyping, and molecular studies. This technique, however, has limitations.[9]

Certain characteristic histologic features are seen in MALT, including infiltrative centrocyte-like cells that invade glands to form prominent lymphoepithelial lesions, moderate cytologic atypia of neoplastic lymphocytes, and plasma cells with Dutcher bodies. The absence of these,

however, does not exclude this type of lymphoma. Also, monoclonality is not absolute proof of MALT lymphoma. Premalignant *H pylori* chronic gastritis also may demonstrate monoclonal B cells. Furthermore, 50% of normal gastric biopsies in patients after complete tumor regression show monoclonality. The similarity of this tumor to reactive-type lymphoid follicles led to the term pseudo-lymphoma in the older radiologic literature.[21]

Gastric MALT in specific may be staged using a modification of the Ann Arbor classification by Mushoff (**Box 3**).[22] Endoscopic US (EUS) is an imaging modality that is essential to the staging of gastric lymphoma. EUS is required to determine the extent of mural invasion and involvement of adjacent lymph nodes. Further details of EUS are beyond the scope of this article, but are available.[23]

The clinical course of MALT lymphomas differs from nodal lymphoma. It is the only NHL that regresses after antibiotic treatment. It tends to remain confined a long time to the initial location as opposed to even low-grade nodal lymphoma, which is a disseminated process at the time of diagnosis. Finally, when spread does occur, it tends to home to other MALT-containing organs (eg, other portions of the intestine, salivary glands), which may be because of the expression of homing receptors by the lymphocytes.[18]

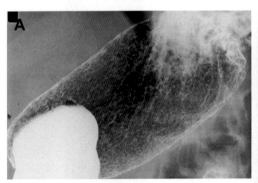
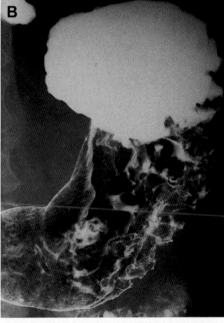

Fig. 8. *Helicobacter pylori* infection of the stomach. (*A*) double-contrast left posterior oblique view of stomach demonstrating prominent areae gastrica mucosal pattern in patient with proven *H pylori* infection. (*B*) Double contrast frontal view of stomach revealing severe fold thickening in the fundus and body, mimicking a neoplasm in another patient with biopsy proven *H pylori* gastritis.

First-line treatment of patients who have *H pylori*-positive MALT confined to the stomach should be antibiotic therapy and a proton pump inhibitor. This leads to durable remission in 60% to 80% of patients. *H pylori*-negative MALT lymphomas generally do not respond to antibiotics, and instead, other treatments, including radiation (for stage I$_E$)[24] and chemotherapy, are recommended.[10]

MALT lymphomas previously were classified by Isaacson and Wright[25] into low-grade and high-grade. The understanding of lymphoma is evolving rapidly, and future studies are likely not going to make this distinction (see **Box 1**). Transformation of MALT to DLBCL of the stomach was recognized, and future studies are likely going to distinguish between MALT lymphoma and diffuse large B cell lymphoma of the stomach (transformation of MALT to DLBCL). Significant numbers, if not all of the previously reported high-grade MALT lymphomas, were probably DLBCL. Prior studies about high-grade types of gastric MALT lymphomas have to be reviewed with caution.

One small study of fluoroscopy investigated the ability to distinguish the low-grade from the high-grade types of MALT. Although statistical analysis of individual findings was not discussed, there was a tendency for earlier lesions to show superficial spreading lesions with nodularity and shallow ulcers, and for late lesions to be more polypoid with deeper ulcerations.[19]

## Fluoroscopy

The art of fluoroscopy is fading rapidly.[26] The relatively lower cost and lower radiation from digital examinations, however, remain obvious advantages over endoscopy and CT respectively. Therefore, typical fluoroscopic appearances of GI lymphoma will be reviewed here.

Overall, the appearance of gastric lymphomas at barium fluoroscopy varies. Patterns may include solitary (nodular form) or multiple submucosal nodules (polypoid form) with or without ulcerations, larger exophytic masses with necrosis and ulceration (ulcerative form), and diffuse infiltration leading to fold thickening (infiltrative form). A sharp distinction between these forms is uncommon, and the terms are purely descriptive. Even though 90% to 95% of gastric lymphomas are detected on barium studies, that specific diagnosis is made less than 20% of the time because of the similarity in appearances to the more common carcinoma and the other differential diagnostic considerations like hypertrophic gastritis or Menetrier's disease. However these latter conditions tend involve the proximal half of the stomach, whereas lymphoma is more likely to involve the distal half.[4] Disease may be early (involving the mucosa and submucosa only) or advanced. Early lesions may be seen on well-performed double-contrast studies and may appear as depressed lesions with shallow irregular ulcers and nodular surrounding mucosa (**Fig. 9**), or small nodules or masses that are ulcerated and appear as bull's-eye lesions or as enlarged rugal folds. These patterns, however, may be indistinguishable from early gastric cancer. Advanced gastric lesions are usually 10 cm more in diameter on average. They tend to involve the antrum and body of the stomach.

The nodular form of disease consists of multiple submucosal masses measuring from millimeters to centimeters, which can umbilicate to form the bulls-eye or target lesions (**Fig. 10**). The central umbilication collecting barium tends to be large in comparison with the surrounding elevation. Others can present as multiple discrete polyps similar in appearance to various polyposis syndromes. The differential diagnosis of bulls-eye lesions also includes carcinoid, metastatic melanoma, lung and breast cancers, or Kaposi's sarcoma.[4,5]

The polypoid form consists of one of more lobulated intraluminal masses, which may be indistinguishable from polypoid carcinoma (**Fig. 11**). This can coexist with an infiltrative/ulcerative form.

The infiltrative form appears as a focal or diffuse enlargement of the rugal folds because of spreading submucosal tumor. The folds can become massively enlarged, distorted, and nodular (**Fig. 12**). Despite this, pliability usually is maintained, and peristaltic waves may pass through the area, unlike in the infiltrative form of carcinoma, called linitis plastica. Although case reports of linitis plastica caused by NHL exist,[27] it is a distinctly uncommon appearance and would

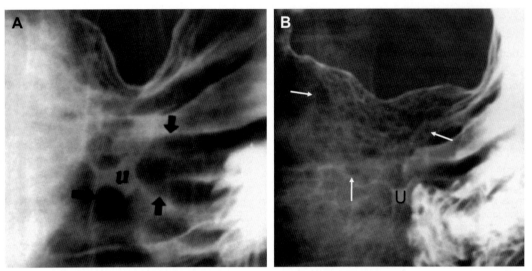

Fig. 9. 48 year-old-woman with low-grade gastric mucosa-associated lymphoid tissue lymphoma with combined pattern. (*A*) spot radiograph of upper gastrointestinal tract shows discrete ulcer (u) with convergence of surrounding rugae (*arrows*) in posterior wall of gastric body, which looks like early gastric carcinoma. (*B*) Spot radiograph shows multiple nodules (*arrows*) of varied sizes in a large area of gastric body and antrum, which are located distal to the ulcer (U) in Fig. 9A. (*From* Park MS, Kim KW, Yu JS, et al. Radiographic findings of primary B cell lymphoma of the stomach: low-grade versus high-grade malignancy in relation to the mucosa-associated lymphoid tissue concept. AJR Am J Roentgenol 2002;179:1301; with permission.)

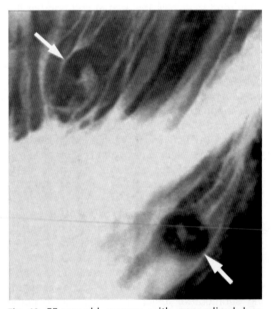

Fig. 10. 55-year-old woman with generalized lymphoma involving stomach. Double-contrast barium study shows two centrally ulcerated submucosal masses (*arrows*), or bull's-eye lesions, in body of stomach. (*From* Levine MS, Rubensin SE, Pantongrag-Brown L, et al. Non-Hodgkin's lymphoma of the gastrointestinal tract: radiographic findings. AJR 1997;168:18; with permission.)

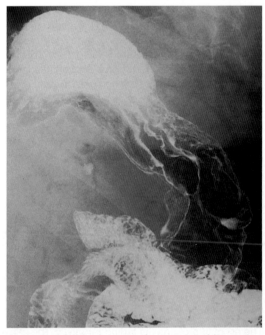

Fig. 11. Gastric lymphoma. Left posterior oblique view from double-contrast gastrointestinal series reveals nodular mass involving the midstomach. The smooth mucosal surface and widening of mucosal folds are suggestive of lymphoma, but carcinoma can appear similarly.

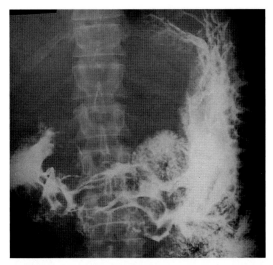

Fig. 12. Gastric lymphoma. Single-contrast frontal image of stomach revealing markedly thickened gastric rugal folds, indicating submucosal tumor infiltration.

necessitate a consideration of primary gastric adenocarcinoma.

The ulcerative form consists of one or more ulcers that are irregular with nodular surrounding mucosa and irregular thickened folds (**Fig. 13**). Occasionally more regular ulcers can exist and be surrounded by a smooth mound or symmetric radiating folds appearing like a benign ulcer. Other tumors may appear as giant cavitated lesions from necrosis and excavation of the tumor (**Fig. 14**).[5] The differential diagnosis of these cavitated lesions includes gastric metastases (especially melanoma) and malignant GI stromal tumors (GIST).

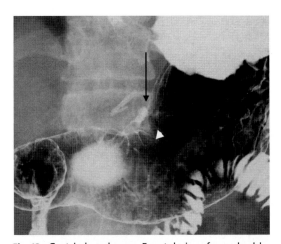

Fig. 13. Gastric lymphoma. Frontal view from double-contrast gastrointestinal series reveals lesser curvature malignant-appearing ulcer (*long black arrow*), surrounded by irregular blunt surrounding folds ending short of ulcer base (*white arrowhead*).

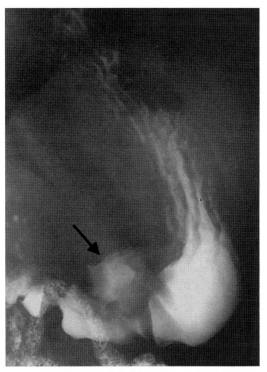

Fig. 14. Gastric lymphoma. Left posterior oblique view from single-contrast gastrointestinal series reveals large irregular ulceration along lesser curvature of stomach. A large lesser curvature ulcerated mass was present at CT scan (*arrow*).

Gastric lymphoma may spread to the esophagus in 10% of cases and to the duodenum in 5% to 13% of cases. This latter spread has led to the maxim that a tumor in the stomach that has spread to the duodenum favors a diagnosis of lymphoma over carcinoma; however, because carcinoma is far more common, that is not a reliable maxim.

As in other parts of the GI tract, the success of chemotherapy in achieving cell kill may lead to rapid necrosis, hemorrhage, and bowel wall perforation (**Fig. 15**). Other changes that can occur after chemotherapy or radiation include narrowing and deformity caused by scarring and fibrosis.[4]

## CT

CT is easy to perform, not operator-dependent like fluoroscopy, and accurate for the evaluation and staging of GI tract lymphoma. It provides information on tumor location, morphology, extension, and involvement of lymph nodes and other organs. Excellent visualization of true gastric wall thickening and ulcerations can be achieved with the use of positive (barium), neutral (eg, water, or 0.1% weight/volume barium), or negative (effervescent $CO_2$) oral contrast agents (**Fig. 16**). Agents that temporarily paralyze peristalsis, such as glucagon

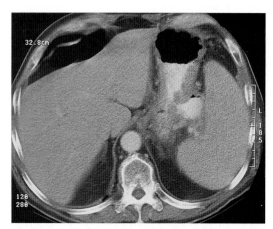

Fig. 15. Perforated gastric lymphoma. Axial contrast-enhanced CT reveals focal interruption in wall of greater curvature of stomach with contrast extravasation into gastrosplenic ligament in patient being treated with chemotherapy for gastric lymphoma.

or Buscopan, have become less critical with the ultrafast scanning capabilities of multidetector CT, in which the entire insufflated stomach can be imaged in 1 to 3 seconds and then reformatted in multiple planes (**Fig. 17**) with submillimeter slice thickness or maximum intensity projection reconstructions. Virtual gastroscopic views also can be created.[28] There is a common tendency for lymphoma of the intestinal wall, irrespective of where it is located, to have a very bland, hypo- or iso-attenuated (to muscle) homogeneous appearance in all but the most aggressive forms (**Fig. 18**). In the small intestine, the appearance is practically pathognomonic without a tissue diagnosis, because epithelial tumors tend to be heterogeneous with areas of necrosis or hyperattenuation caused by greater vascularity. The bi- or trilayer appearance

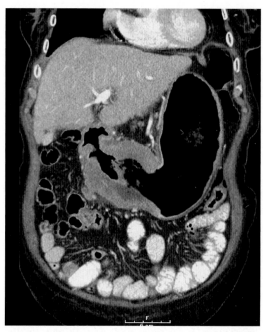

Fig. 17. Gastric lymphoma. Multislice helical CT scan after oral and intravenous contrast with isotropic coronal reformation demonstrating marked thickening of the gastric antrum.

seen in dynamic high-resolution studies of the normal wall may be obliterated in lymphoma because of tumor infiltration of the submucosa.[29] **Table 1** summarizes the CT findings of common GI lymphomas. Typical CT findings include mild-to-moderate circumferential thickening. Luminal constriction, dilatation (small bowel mainly), or cavitation may be observed. Because gastric adenocarcinoma is a far more common tumor than lymphoma, certain general differentiating features must be kept in mind that can be helpful but not

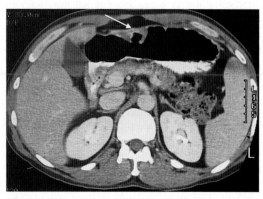

Fig. 16. HIV-associated gastric lymphoma. Axial CT scan with intravenous contrast, oral contrast, and after administration of effervescent $CO_2$, showing excellent distention of the stomach with an ulcerated mass along the anterior wall (*arrow*).

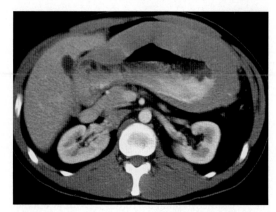

Fig. 18. Gastric advanced mucosa-associated lymphoid tissue lymphoma. Axial CT scan with oral and intravenous contrast demonstrating marked gastric wall thickening with uniform iso-attenuation to muscle.

**Table 1**
**CT features of common gastrointestinal tract lymphoma involvement**

| Histologic Type | Most Common Location | CT Features |
|---|---|---|
| Burkitt | Ileocecal region | Bulky mass right lower quadrant, uniform iso-attenuation |
| Enteropathy T cell | Jejunum, diffuse | Thickened nodular folds, ulcerations, perforation, obstruction |
| Large B cell | Distal ileum or other small bowel | Forms: polypoid (single or multiple nodules), infiltrating (homogeneous, marked circumferential wall thickening, aneurysmal dilatation), endoexoenteric with ulceration/fistulae, mesenteric. Can see intussusception |
| Mucosa-associated lymphoid tissue | Stomach | Early: lack of mass or subtle wall thickening |
| | | Advanced: smooth homogeneous, iso-attenuated (minimal enhancement), moderate circumferential wall thickening or mass in body/antrum, perigastric adenopathy |
| Mantle | Terminal ileum, jejunum, colon | Wall thickening, multiple lymphomatous polyposis (conglomerate mass at ileocecum unlike in familial adenomatous polyposis) |

sufficiently specific to make the diagnosis of lymphoma, including:

The tendency of lymphoma to show diffuse, extensive, or severe wall thickening (**Fig. 19**)

Minimal or mild tumor enhancement; preservation of the perigastric fat plane

Distensibility of the gastric lumen

Bulky, well-marginated lymphadenopathy;

Lymphadenopathy below the renal pedicle, particularly if there is no associated perigastric lymphadenopathy

The following findings favor a diagnosis of adenocarcinoma: milder, more focal wall thickening; greater tumor enhancement; direct infiltration beyond the gastric wall; mural rigidity; and luminal narrowing (linitis plastica), which may result in obstruction. As an isolated finding, perigastric lymphadenopathy (**Fig. 20**) is seen in 50% to 60% of cases of both lymphoma and adenocarcinoma and is thus not a helpful differentiating feature.[15] Other diseases that can be confused with lymphoma at CT include benign inflammatory conditions such as gastritis (see **Fig. 8B**), Crohn's disease and peptic ulcer disease.[30]

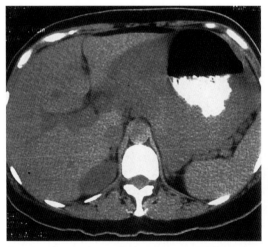

**Fig. 19.** Advanced gastric lymphoma. Axial noncontrast CT scan reveals severe gastric wall thickening up to 7 cm.

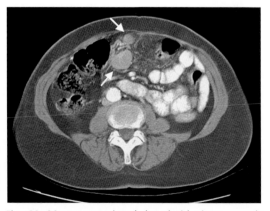

**Fig. 20.** Mucosa-associated lymphoid tissue gastric lymphoma with adenopathy. Axial CT scan with oral and intravenous contrast reveals enlarged perigastric well-marginated lymph nodes.

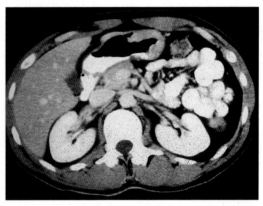

**Fig. 21.** Gastric mucosa-associated lymphoid tissue lymphoma. Axial CT scan reveals focal thickening of gastric body, indicating tumor location.

Several publications have specifically investigated the different appearances between low-grade and high-grade MALT lymphomas at CT.[19,21] These studies have to be read with caution, because significant numbers of their high-grade lymphomas might have been diffuse large B cell lymphomas. In each study, more than 50 patients underwent single-slice helical scanning after ingestion of 400 to 1200 mL of water or dilute meglumine diatrizoate and without a paralytic agent. The investigators found that in patients who had known MALT lymphoma, 50% of cases with low-grade disease showed normal gastric wall thickness (less than 5mm) and that in a patient who had suspected MALT, this absence of findings was highly predictive of low-grade disease. All patients who had high-grade MALT had either gastric wall thickening or mass formation (**Fig. 21**). There was a statistically significant difference between mean thickening for low-grade (5.8 mm, range 2 to 18 mm) and high-grade (14.1 mm, range 7 to 40mm) MALT. Furthermore, ulcer and lymphadenopathy were more frequent in the high-grade group. Tumor locations were not a distinguishing feature, with most tumors residing in the body or body and antrum. Fundal-only tumors were not found.

## SMALL INTESTINE

The small intestine is the second most common site of GI tract lymphoma after the stomach and accounts for about one third of cases. Approximately 20% of primary malignant tumors in the small bowel are lymphomas.

Clinically, patients may present with pain, nausea, vomiting, anemia, weight loss, and fever. There may be a palpable mass. Uncommonly, there may be small bowel obstruction. Bleeding, fever, and small bowel obstruction are poor prognosticators. Rarely, patients may present with malabsorption and diarrhea, symptoms more common with Mediterranean lymphoma and forms complicating CD.[5]

Four major forms of small bowel involvement may be seen: a primary form, lymphoma complicating CD, a mesenteric nodal form, and a disseminated form.[4]

Histologically, the types of lymphoma affecting the small intestine are more heterogeneous than is the case for the stomach. Distinctive histologic presentations include MALT lymphoma, diffuse large cell lymphoma, enteropathy-associated T cell lymphoma, mantle cell lymphoma (MCL), follicular lymphoma, and immunoproliferative small intestinal disease (IPSID).[9]

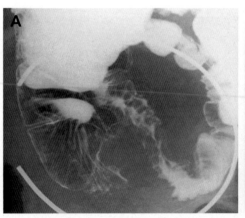
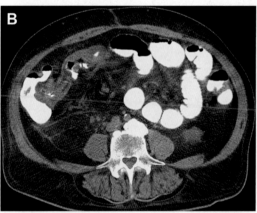

**Fig. 22.** Ileal lymphoma. (*A*) Spot radiograph from small bowel follow-through examination reveals markedly nodular thickened folds involving terminal ileum and cecal caput. Note small bowel fold separation from wall thickening also. (*B*) Axial CT scan from CT enteroclysis. Catheter-administered high-attenuation contrast reveals marked narrowing and ulceration of long segment of terminal ileum, indicating lymphomatous infiltration.

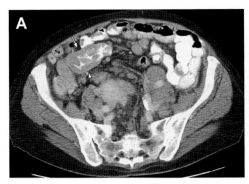
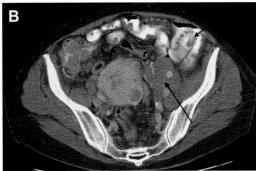

Fig. 23. Mantle cell lymphoma. Multiple lymphomatous polyposis. (*A*) axial CT scan in midpelvis reveals multiple nodular masses along with wall thickening in the terminal ileum (*arrows*). (*B*) Axial CT scan in midpelvis reveals multiple additional lymphomatous nodules in other loops of small bowel (*short arrows*). Note also external iliac lymphadenopathy (*long arrow*).

IPSID, also known as alpha chain disease, is a subtype of MALT lymphoma occurring in the small intestine. It is characterized by plasma cell infiltration of the bowel wall. Patients may have alpha-heavy chain immunoglobulins in their serum. The infiltration leads to malabsorption and protein-losing enteropathy. Transformation to high-grade Mediterranean lymphoma can occur. This condition usually is found in young adults in the Mediterranean basin, the Middle East, Africa, the Far East, and in Mexican Americans. In the Middle East, it accounts for one third of GI lymphomas. Recently, an association with *C jejuni* was identified in intestinal biopsy specimens of patients who had this disease, and they responded well to antibiotics paralleling the type of association seen with *H pylori* in gastric MALT.[10,31] IPSID occurs almost exclusively in developing countries where *C jejuni* infection is hyperendemic, often chronic, and asymptomatic. Histologically, this is an immunoblastic NHL and differs from western lymphoma in that patients may be in their mid- 20s (versus older than 40) with a proximal small intestinal predilection and may present with malabsorption and diarrhea, clinically uncommon in the western form unless associated with CD.[5]

MCL first was described by Cornes in 1961 as multiple lymphomatous polyposis.[32] The median age is 65 with a male predominance. It arises in the terminal ileum and jejunum most commonly,

Fig. 24. Enteropathy-associated T cell lymphoma. Small bowel series demonstrating multiple nodular defects (*arrows*) in proximal jejunum in a patient without associated celiac disease.

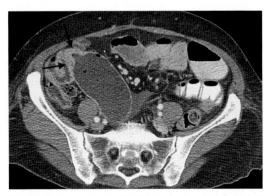

Fig. 25. T cell small intestinal lymphoma. Axial CT scan in midpelvis demonstrating small bowel obstruction by mild-to-moderate small bowel wall thickening (*arrows*).

but any part of the GI tract can be affected, including the colon. It may appear radiologically and pathologically as numerous polyps; thus the descriptive term sometimes used is lymphomatous polyposis. It has been recognized that the histology of this lymphoma resembles that of the mantle zone of the lymph node follicle (see **Fig. 1**). There is also a predilection for involvement of Waldeyer's ring, mesenteric lymph nodes, and blood and bone marrow involvement such that a greater percentage of patients who have MCL have stage IV disease at presentation, compared with other histologic subtypes of GI tract NHL.

Burkitt's lymphoma is associated with EBV. It is one of the fastest growing human malignancies and usually occurs in children, primarily in Africa. It is sporadic in western countries, with a less than 20% association with EBV; it also can be associated with HIV. It too most commonly affects the ileocecal region.

Rarely, certain types of lymphoma that usually present as systemic disease (eg, follicular, lymphocytic, large B cell) can appear as primary GI tract lymphomas. Occasionally these can cause numerous polyps in the small or large bowel.

GI tract lymphomas may be associated with HIV. These tend to be aggressive, small-cleaved

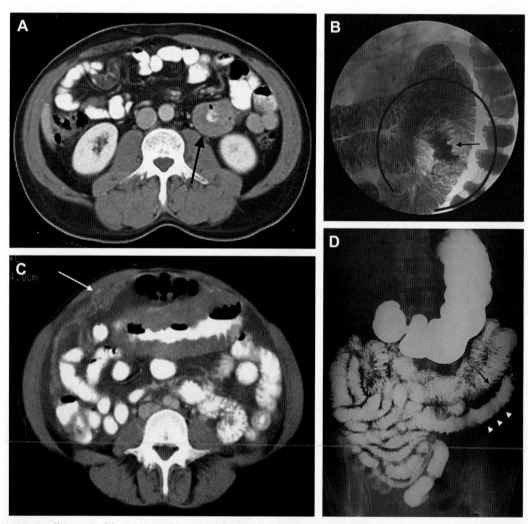

**Fig. 26.** Small intestinal lymphoma. (*A*) Axial CT scan demonstrating markedly thickened loop of jejunum with homogenously iso-attenuated appearance of wall (*arrow*). No small bowel obstruction is noted. (*B*) Spot radiograph from small bowel series reveals fold thickening (*arrow*) and separation of bowel loops in short segment corresponding to CT abnormality. (*C*) Additional example of long segment loop of jejunum with uniform iso-attenuated marked wall thickening without small bowel obstruction. Also note peritoneal lymphomatosis with ascites and thickening of omentum by lymphomatous mass (*arrow*). (*D*) Small bowel series demonstrating corresponding abnormality for part (*C*) with thickened valvula conniventes (*arrowheads*) and separation from adjacent loops (*arrow*).

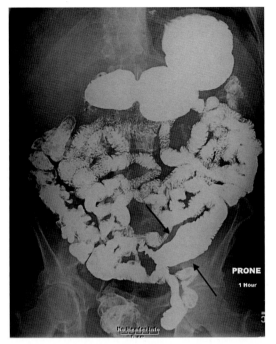

**Fig. 27.** Small intestinal lymphoma. Small bowel follow-through demonstrating aneurysmal dilatation and complete loss of normal fold pattern in a loop of distal jejunum (*arrows*).

cell Burkitt's or non-Burkitt's or large-cell immunoblastic-type lymphoma. GI tract involvement is seen in one fourth to one third of patients who have AIDS. Malignant lymphoma is the second most common malignancy in individuals who have HIV infection. The success of antiretroviral agents allows prolonged survival for these patients. This has resulted in an increased incidence of lymphoma, such that the risk of developing lymphoma at 3 years now approaches 30%. Most patients present with stage IV disease and B symptoms. NHL has been reported with an equal distribution between the stomach and small and large intestines.[9]

Patients who have allograft organ/marrow transplants have a 45 to 100 times higher risk of getting lymphoma. These usually are associated with EBV, known as EBV post-transplant lymphoproliferative disorder, and tend to be high-grade, large-cell multifocal B cell tumors. They often transform into an immunoblastic form of lymphoma.

T cell lymphomas of the small intestine account for approximately 10% to 25% of primary intestinal lymphomas[9] and primarily occur as enteropathy-associated T cell lymphoma, most often complicating CD. CD is much more common than previously thought and affects up to 1% of the United States population. It often goes undetected until complications ensue.[33] It is associated with an increased risk of T cell lymphoma of the small intestine. CD is characterized not only by villous atrophy but also by an increase in the presence of intraepithelial lymphocytes. Refractory CD, the form showing no improvement with a gluten-free diet, is associated with an increase in these lymphocytes and also in 30% is associated with the condition of chronic jejunoileitis (CJI), an otherwise rare condition. CJI manifests as multiple small bowel ulcers that may bleed or perforate or form strictures, and it is associated with high mortality. The ulcers rarely are seen radiologically, and more often the resulting strictures are noted.[34] Some feel CJI is a form of low-grade enteropathy-associated T cell lymphoma. Enteropathy-associated T cell lymphoma

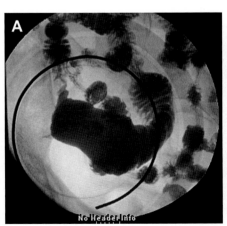
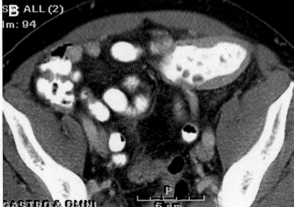

**Fig. 28.** Aneurysmal dilatation in small bowel lymphoma. (*A*) Spot radiograph from small bowel series demonstrates mild-to-moderate dilatation of a segment of jejunum with complete loss of fold pattern. (*B*) Axial CT scan through midpelvis corresponding to loop in part (*A*) demonstrating aneurysmal dilatation with moderate-to-marked increase in caliber of small bowel loop and thickened wall indicative of lymphoma with aneurysmal dilatation.

occurs in adults, with a peak in the sixth decade. The disease has not been found in children who have CD, indicating a long latency period. It remains a rare disease in western countries, with an annual incidence of 0.5 to 1 cases per 1 million population.[33] The disease also may occur in the stomach and colon, liver, spleen, thyroid, skin, nasal sinus, and brain. T cell lymphoma of the GI tract also may occur unassociated with CD.[8] Nonetheless, there is still an association with malabsorption.

The jejunum is the most common site involved, because it is the site of greatest villous damage and inflammation.[4] Findings include thickened, nodular folds or multiple ulcerative lesions, but the disease may be multifocal. These findings may be subtle and best appreciated at enteroclysis.[4,8] There is a higher frequency of intestinal perforation than in B cell NHL.[9] This is felt to be caused by angiocentric and angioinvasive infiltration of the vascular walls by lymphoid cells, leading to vascular occlusion and ischemic necrosis. In fact, approximately 50% of patients require laparotomy for complications of hemorrhage, perforation, or obstruction.[33] One study also found that this type was distinguished from B cell lymphoma on CT by minimal bowel wall thickening and less bulky adenopathy. The CT attenuation of the masses was similar, however.[8] The 5-year survival for T cell lymphomas is only 25% compared with 75% for B cell types.[9]

B cell small intestinal lymphomas mainly occur in the distal small intestine (whereas adenocarcinomas more commonly occur proximally) and especially in the terminal ileal region, where the greatest concentration of lymphoid tissue exists (**Fig. 22**). Lesions are typically solitary but may

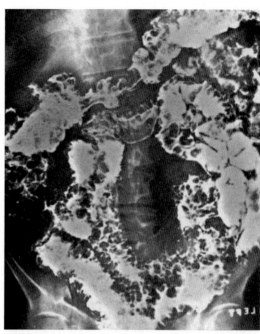

**Fig. 30.** Mantle cell lymphoma. Small bowel series demonstrating innumerable polypoid lesions throughout the small bowel indicative of multiple lymphomatous polyposis. (*From* Levine MS, Rubesin SE, Brown-Pantongrag L, et al. Non-Hodgkin's lymphoma of the gastrointestinal tract: radiographic findings. AJR Am J Roentgenol 1997;168:165–72; with permission.)

be multiple in 10% to 25% of patients.[4,34] Numerous patterns exist, and involvement may be multifocal.

Traditionally described radiographic patterns appreciable both at barium fluoroscopy and well-performed CT include: a polypoid form, multiple nodules, an infiltrating form, an endoexoenteric

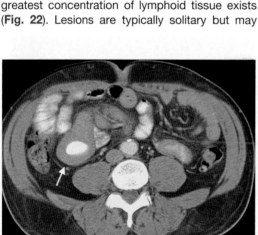

**Fig. 29.** Small intestinal lymphoma. Axial CT scan demonstrating moderate thickening of loop of small bowel with attenuation of bowel wall identical to that of muscle, highly characteristic of lymphomatous infiltration (*arrow*).

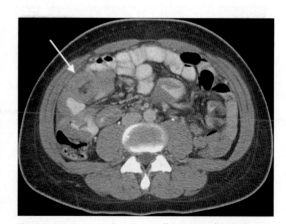

**Fig. 31.** Intussusception in small intestinal lymphoma. Axial CT scan in adult with Burkitt lymphoma demonstrating mesenteric fat and vessels within a thickened loop of ileum, consistent with intussusception (*arrow*). Note multiple areas of wall thickening.

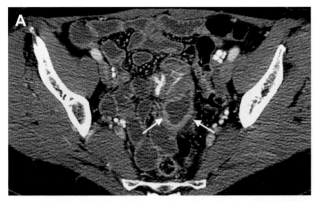
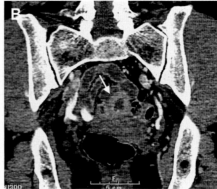

Fig. 32. Low-grade marginal B cell lymphoma. (*A*) Axial CT enterography demonstrating optimal distension of pelvic loops of ileum with 0.1 % barium solution. Note segmental bowel wall thickening of involved loop (*arrows*). (*B*) Coronal reformatted CT enterography demonstrating segmentally thickened (*arrow*) loop of ileum involved by lymphoma.

form with excavation and fistulization, and a mesenteric invasive form with extraluminal masses.

In general, there is poor correlation between cell type and radiographic pattern, but certain patterns do correlate with lymphoma type. MCL but also follicular cell lymphoma and rarely MALT lymphoma may produce a distinctive pattern of multiple polyps (**Fig. 23**) (multiple lymphomatous polyposis). IPSID tends to be proximal with a disseminated nodular pattern leading to mucosal fold thickening, irregularity, and spiculation. Enteropathy-associated T cell lymphoma is usually proximal or diffuse and shows nodules (**Fig. 24**), ulcers, or strictures (**Fig. 25**). Nodular GI tract lymphoma may present as multiple submucosal nodules, sometimes with ulceration to form the bulls-eye appearance. In the small intestine, several common differential diagnostic possibilities to consider for this appearance include metastatic melanoma, Kaposi's sarcoma, and Crohn's disease.

### Infiltrative Form

The infiltrative form is the most common and causes bowel wall thickening (**Fig. 26**), distortion or loss of the fold pattern (**Fig. 27**), nodularity, and either luminal narrowing or aneurysmal dilatation (**Fig. 28**). At fluoroscopy, submucosal infiltration by tumor may cause effacement of mucosal folds to produce a smooth featureless appearance (see **Fig. 27**). Generally, narrowing is less common than for other tumors, and aneurysmal dilatation is more common because of infiltration of the submucosal myenteric plexus and the muscularis propria with loss of tonicity of the bowel wall. As such, obstruction is less common than might be expected with other tumors. At CT, bowel wall thickening of a markedly bland, homogeneous

attenuation lower than or equal to that of muscle (**Fig. 29**) is common and may be greater than 2 cm in diameter and involve a long segment of bowel circumferentially. Wall thickening leads to a greater separation of bowel loops than that normally caused by mesenteric fat.[5] This form of lymphoma thus usually can be differentiated easily from carcinoma because of the length of involvement, the degree of narrowing, and the absence of obstruction. Remarkably, these findings can revert to normal after chemotherapy.

### Polypoid Form

The polypoid form manifests as single or multiple filling defects (**Fig. 30**), most often seen in MCL. This is the form that may cause intussusception (**Fig. 31**). Other conditions that can appear this way include nodular lymphoid hyperplasia, intestinal polyposis syndromes, GIST, lipomas, adenomas, or metastases.

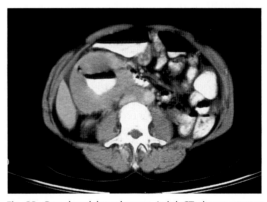

Fig. 33. Duodenal lymphoma. Axial CT demonstrates marked thickening of second portion of duodenum with aneurysmal dilatation.

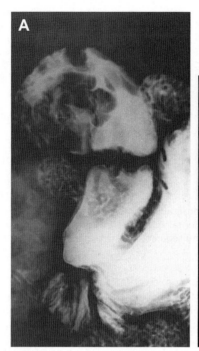
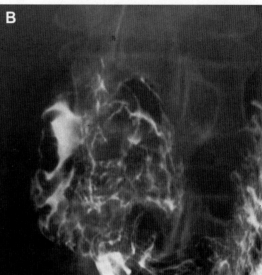

**Fig. 34.** Duodenal mucosa-associated lymphoid tissue lymphoma. (*A*) Spot radiograph from upper gastrointestinal series single-contrast view demonstrating nodularity of duodenal bulb. (*B*) Air contrast spot radiograph of duodenal bulb demonstrating markedly nodular mucosal pattern.

### Endoexoenteric Form

The endoexoenteric form may cause bowel wall thickening and excavating ulcerations. Similar findings, however, can be caused by GIST and metastases, especially metastatic melanoma. This process can form fistulas to other abdominal viscera or sinus tracts into the mesentery with sterile abscesses. Barium studies may reveal a large cavity along the mesenteric border of the affected bowel. CT may show extraluminal contrast material extending into the cavity, which often contains fluid and debris. The differential diagnosis includes a cavitated GIST or metastasis.

### Mesenteric Invasive Form

The mesenteric invasive form is thought to be caused by direct extension from affected nodes in the mesentery and may be seen as contiguous wall thickening adjacent to bulky mesenteric nodal enlargement with tethering of folds and angulation.[4] It is this form that most commonly is associated with obstruction.[35] There may also be a sandwich appearance at CT, where the mesenteric vessels form the middle of the sandwich surrounded by conglomerate nodal/intestinal masses. Barium fluoroscopy may not be able to distinguish between primary small intestinal lymphoma and the systemic form invading from

mesenteric lymph nodes. The differential diagnosis for this pattern includes tuberculosis, carcinoid tumor, metastases, and carcinoma.

In general, the differential diagnosis for small bowel lymphoma based on fluoroscopy includes Crohn's disease, carcinoma, and nodular lymphoid hyperplasia. In Crohn's disease, however,

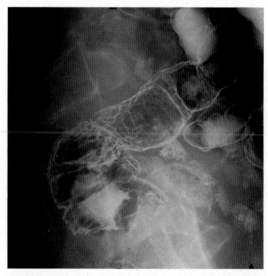

**Fig. 35.** Colonic lymphoma. Lateral view from double-contrast barium enema reveals mucosal nodularity involving rectum.

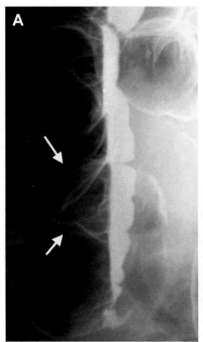
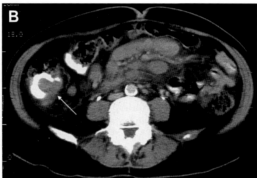

Fig. 36. Colonic lymphoma. (A) Spot radiograph from double-contrast barium enema revealing nodular mass at ileocecal valve region (*arrows*). (B) Axial CT scan demonstrating nodular mass projecting into cecal lumen (*arrow*). Note also bulky mesenteric lymphadenopathy in the midline.

it is more common to see thickened valvulae conniventes, fistulae, and ulcers (which may be more linear). In cancer, apple-core lesions are more typical, an appearance far less common in lymphoma. In nodular lymphoid hyperplasia, the nodules are distributed more evenly and of uniform size. The nodules in lymphoma are larger, variable in size, and irregular in distribution.[5]

Lower-grade lymphomas with more subtle bowel wall thickening or nodularity may be detected with more robust cross-sectional imaging techniques such as CT enteroclysis and CT

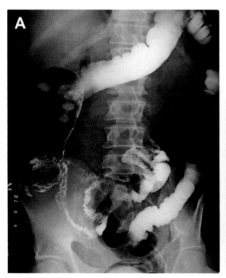
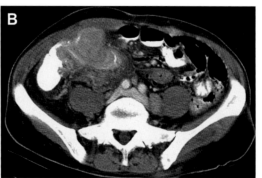

Fig. 37. Ileocecal lymphoma. (A) Double-contrast barium enema reveals bulky mass involving cecum and nodular thickening of distal ileal loops. (B) Axial CT scan demonstrates bulky mass involving both terminal ileum and cecal lumen with mesenteric infiltration.

enterography. In the latter examination, a large volume of neutral density fluid is ingested, either consisting of water, methylcellulose or 0.1% w/v barium to maximize luminal distension. CT is performed with a power-injected high rate of intravenous contrast infusion to maximize mural enhancement for detection of masses. Scanning begins at the enteric phase (approximately 55 seconds) (**Fig. 32**).

## Duodenal Lymphoma

Duodenal lymphoma usually occurs from contiguous spread from the distal stomach or proximal jejunum. It also may occur by encasement from peri-duodenal lymph nodes. Primary duodenal lymphoma is rare because of a paucity of lymphoid tissue here and accounts for less than 5% of all small intestinal lymphoma. Radiographic forms include infiltrative (**Fig. 33**), ulcerative, polypoid, and nodular forms (**Fig. 34**). MALT lymphoma[36] and lymphoma complicating CD (enteropathy-associated T cell lymphoma) also can occur here.

## COLON

Lymphoma infrequently involves the colon. It more commonly represents generalized lymphoma with associated colorectal involvement than primary lymphoma. It accounts for 6% to 12% of GI tract lymphoma, but only 0.4% of primary colonic malignancies. Interestingly, at autopsy, the colon is involved in 44% of patients who have systemic disease.[5] Most cases are non-Hodgkin B cell in origin. Symptoms are nonspecific and may include change in bowel habit, abdominal pain, weight loss, rectal bleeding, and diarrhea. Types that are seen in the colon include conventional large-cell lymphoma, MALT lymphoma, MCL, and T cell lymphoma.[1] Two risk factors may predispose patients, including immunosuppression (after organ or marrow transplant, AIDS, or immune disorder) and long-standing ulcerative colitis.[37] Although the various forms may occur anywhere in the colon, there is a propensity for the rectum and ascending colon/cecum to be affected most often or most severely.[4,13]

At CT and contrast enema examination, patients can have polypoid, infiltrative, endoexoenteric cavitary lesions, mucosal nodularity (**Fig. 35**), and fold thickening.

Polypoid lesions are the most common form and can be solitary; they most often are found at the ileocecal valve region with extension to the ileum (**Fig. 36**). Masses tend to be larger than adenocarcinomas and are reported up to 20 cm (**Fig. 37**).[38]

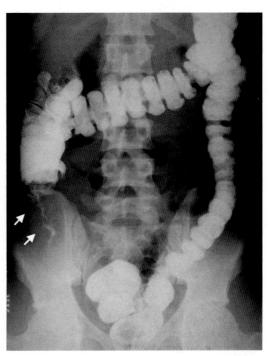

Fig. 38. Colonic lymphoma. Single-contrast enema view demonstrates infiltrative form of lymphoma causing luminal narrowing (*arrows*).

## Infiltrative Form

Infiltrative lesions are characterized by long segment concentric wall thickening resulting in narrowing (**Fig. 38**). There may be a smooth overlying mucosa from submucosal infiltration by tumor cells. Haustral folds may be thickened. The narrowing rarely results in obstruction, because desmoplasia is not characteristic of lymphoma. The length of involvement can be used to distinguish this from the shorter annular lesions of carcinoma. Other differential diagnostic

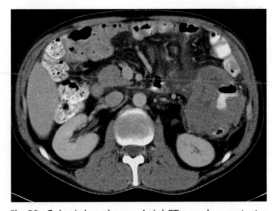

Fig. 39. Colonic lymphoma. Axial CT scan demonstrates predominately iso-attenuated marked wall thickening of descending colon with some mesenteric infiltration.

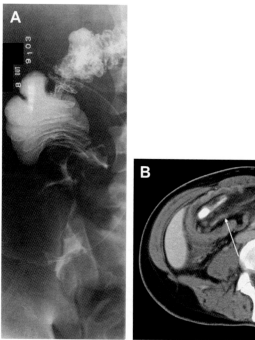

Fig. 40. Intussusception in lymphoma. (*A*) single-contrast barium enema spot radiograph of right colon demonstrates intussuscepting colonic mass with classic coil spring appearance in the middle right colon indicating intussusception. (*B*) Axial CT scan demonstrating two separate areas of colonic intussusception in the proximal and distal transverse colon (*long arrows*).

considerations for haustral fold thickening include hemorrhage, edema, and ischemia. Other features that can help to differentiate lymphoma from adenocarcinoma include extension into the terminal ileum, well-defined margins with preservation of fat planes, no invasion into adjacent structures, and perforation.[1] Wall thickening is reported up to 8.5 cm in some series. Bulky lymphadenopathy also may be more common in lymphoma.[15] As with lymphoma elsewhere in the GI tract, the tumors are densely cellular, but not particularly vascular. As such, on CT they show homogeneous, hypo- or iso-attenuation to muscle (**Fig. 39**).[13] Furthermore, mural stratification is atypical, because necrosis or submucosal edema usually is not found. As in small intestinal lymphoma,

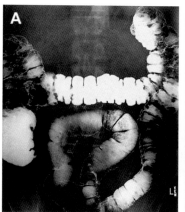
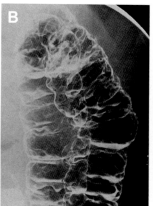
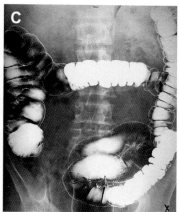

Fig. 41. Multiple lymphomatous polyposis. (*A*) Double-contrast barium enema demonstrating multiple polyps throughout the colon. (*B*) Spot radiograph of splenic flexure demonstrating innumerable polypoid masses of lymphoma in the colon. (*C*) Postchemotherapy double-contrast barium enema demonstrating complete resolution of multiple lymphomatous polyps.

obstruction is not common, but intussusception (**Fig. 40**) may occur, especially in the ileocecal region.

Large tumors of the colon can ulcerate and excavate and be similar in appearance to a malignant stromal tumor or perforated carcinoma.[4]

### Polypoid Form (Multiple Lymphomatous Polyposis)

A distinct, diffuse polypoid form of colonic lymphoma also exists, sometimes called multiple lymphomatous polyposis, in which there are over 100 polyps (**Fig. 41**). The polyps may be distributed evenly throughout the colon and range in size from 2 to 25 mm. Polyps are generally sessile and can be elongated, umbilicated, or filiform.[5] This form of the disease can be confused with familial polyposis coli (FAP) and is usually a manifestation of MCL. The pattern of lymphomatous polyposis also may be caused by follicular and by MALT lymphomas.[39] The presence of a conglomerate mass at the ileocecal valve/cecal region may help to distinguish this from FAP (**Fig. 42**).

MCL is a distinct clinical entity with an aggressive course. Patients are often male and have a median age of 65 years, unlike the younger presentation for FAP.[9]

Peripheral T cell lymphomas of the colon also have been reported. These may be diffuse or focal and segmental, with a propensity for ulcerated lesions and perforation as is commonly seen in T cell small intestinal lymphoma.[8] The differential diagnosis is carcinoma. Because there can be aphthous ulcers, segmental involvement, mucosal pseudopolyps, and ileocecal deformity, differentiation from inflammatory bowel disease may be difficult.[38]

Focal mucosal nodularity similar in appearance to the gastric form recently has been reported in low-grade B cell lymphoma arising from colonic MALT.[40]

### Rectal Lymphoma

Primary rectal lymphoma is rare and may be indistinguishable from adenocarcinoma. It only accounts for 0.1% of primary rectal tumors.[37] Patients present with rectal bleeding or alteration of bowel habits. At contrast enema lesions can present simply as fold thickening indistinguishable from hemorrhoids.[38] At CT, marked wall thickening with the typical homogenous, hypo- to isoattenuated appearance can be seen as in other intestinal sites (**Fig. 43**).[37]

### Appendiceal Lymphoma

Primary appendiceal lymphoma is also rare and more commonly occurs as extension of disease from the cecum. Only 11 cases were found in a review of 71,000 appendectomy specimens, for an

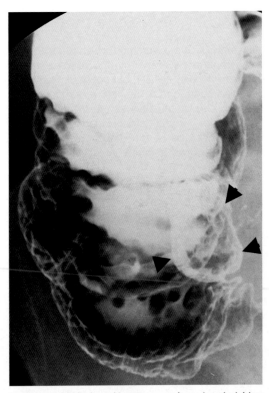

**Fig. 42.** Multiple lymphomatous polyposis mimicking familial polyposis coli. Double-contrast barium enema spot radiograph of cecum demonstrating differentiating feature of dominant mass at ileocecal valvulae (*arrowheads*).

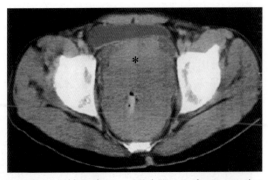

**Fig. 43.** Rectal lymphoma. Axial CT scan demonstrating marked wall thickening of rectum with uniform iso-attenuated appearance (*asterisk*). (*From* Bilsel Y, Balik E, Yamaner S, et al. Clinical and therapeutic considerations of rectal lymphoma: a case report and literature review. World J Gastroenterol 2005;11(3):460–1; with permission.)

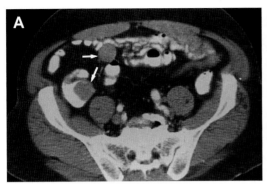
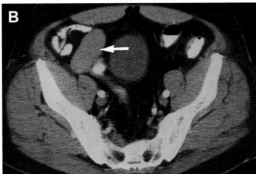

Fig. 44. Appendiceal lymphoma. (*A*) Axial CT scan reveal marked distension of the appendix (*arrows*), which measures 3 cm in diameter and coils in and out of the transverse axial plane. (*B*) Markedly thickened appendix (*arrow*). (*From* Katz DS, Stein LB, Mazzie JP. Recurrent non-Hodgkin's lymphoma of the appendix. AJR Am J Roentgenol 2002;179(6):1444; with permission.)

incidence of 0.015%.[41] In children, Burkitt's lymphoma is most common, and in adults, either large-cell or low-grade B cell lymphomas predominate. Symptoms may mimic acute or chronic appendicitis. The appendix may be massively enlarged but maintain its vermiform appearance (**Fig. 44**).[1] The differential diagnosis would include carcinoma, appendicitis, and mucocele.[42] Again, the tendency for uniform intermediate density without necrosis or mural stratification would argue in favor of lymphoma, but other diagnoses, even with this appearance, remain far more common.

## PERITONEAL LYMPHOMATOSIS

Omental masses with ascites may occur with intra-abdominal lymphoma, especially affecting the GI tract (see **Fig. 26**C). The appearance can be identical to that of the more common peritoneal carcinomatosis. Associated findings that may be distinctive include lymphadenopathy, aneurysmal dilatation of a gut segment with wall thickening, and splenic enlargement.[43,44]

## HODGKIN'S DISEASE

Hodgkin's disease (HD) accounts for 25% of all lymphomas. Reportedly those occurring in the GI tract account for 0.5% of all cases of HD. Among GI tract lymphomas, only 1% to 1.7% represent HD.[45,46] Extranodal HD is extremely rare. Proof of its existence in the GI tract using immunohistochemistry was lacking historically for many cases, and its incidence is likely even less than quoted

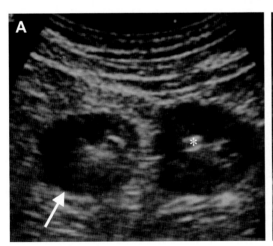
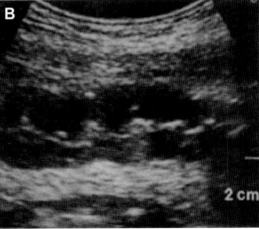

Fig. 45. Non-Hodgkin lymphoma of low-grade malignancy involving small bowel. (*A*) Transverse sonogram demonstrates two bowel loops with hypoechoic wall thickening (*arrow*) and echogenic lumen (*asterisk*) demonstrating typical target appearance because of transmural circumferential infiltration. (*B*) longitudinal sonogram of small bowel loop shows its tubular appearance. (*From* Georg C, Schwerk WB, Georg K, et al. Gastrointestinal lymphoma: sonographic findings in 54 patients. AJR Am J Roentgenol 1990;155:795–98; with permission.)

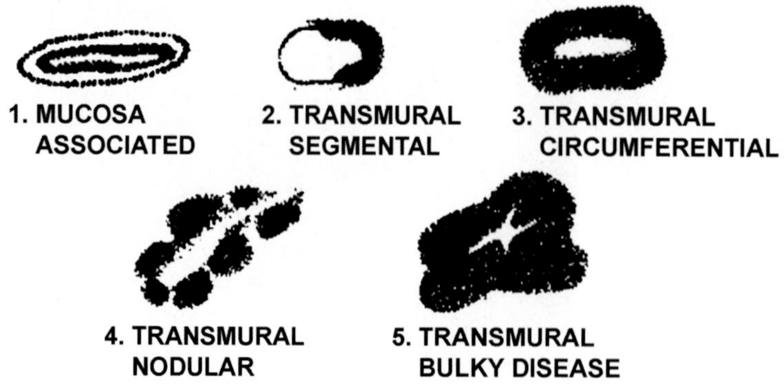

**1. MUCOSA ASSOCIATED**　　**2. TRANSMURAL SEGMENTAL**　　**3. TRANSMURAL CIRCUMFERENTIAL**

**4. TRANSMURAL NODULAR**　　**5. TRANSMURAL BULKY DISEASE**

Fig. 46. Schematic illustration of sonographic features of gastrointestinal involvement in malignant lymphoma. (*From* Georg C, Schwerk WB, Georg K, et al. Gastrointestinal lymphoma: sonographic findings in 54 patients. AJR Am J Roentgenol 1990;155: 795–98; with permission.)

previously. Most cases with GI tract involvement occur concurrent with generalized disease and symptoms. Some authors doubt the existence of primary GI tract HD.[47] Sites of involvement in descending order of frequency include the stomach, jejunum, ileum, duodenum, and colon. Patterns of involvement in the few reported cases included masses, ulcerated lesions, fold thickening, and stricturing desmoplastic disease. Lesions in the stomach will mimic carcinoma. Associations with inflammatory bowel disease and EBV virus have been reported.[46]

## OTHER MODALITIES

There are few reports of the use of US or MR imaging in the imaging work up of GI tract lymphoma. With the increased public awareness of the risk of medical radiation, especially from CT scans, these modalities could see increased use, even for disease in the GI tract. Furthermore, pathologic processes that affect the intestine generally result in decreased peristalsis and bowel wall thickening, which may lead to decrease in luminal gas content and thus facilitate US examination.[48] Goerg and colleagues[49] studied 54 patients who had proven GI tract lymphoma using transabdominal US. Most patients showed a space-occupying mass with bright central echoes and uniformly hypoechoic wall thickening of various degrees. In most of these, loss of the normally stratified appearance characteristic at US was noted. Similar to other pathologic processes in the GI tract, the sonographic appearances have been described as showing a target, halo, (**Fig. 45**A) or pseudokidney appearance (**Fig. 45**B). In this study, most patients presented with the target appearance. Less common appearances included segmental, nodular, mucosal-only, and bulky tumor spread (**Fig. 46**). Lymphadenopathy adjacent to the diseased bowel wall also may be seen.

In a small case report by Chou and colleagues[50] using MR imaging in patients who had GI tract lymphoma, the signal intensity of GI lymphoma was homogeneous and intermediate on T1 weighted images. On T2 weighted images, there was heterogeneous increased signal intensity. Enhancement after intravenous gadolinium was mild to moderate.[50] Lohan and colleagues[51] recently studied 10 patients using sequential T2 true fast imaging with steady-state free precession (True FISP) after ingestion of 1 L of polyethylene glycol (MR enterography) to elegantly demonstrate small bowel lymphoma complicating sprue. They found that tumor signal intensity was much higher than muscle and similar to spleen. A major advantage emphasized by the authors included absence of ionizing radiation, allowing multiple delayed rescans, akin to a small bowel series, to ensure luminal distension.

## SUMMARY

In summary, GI tract lymphoma most commonly affects the stomach and small intestine. It is usually of B cell origin and may have infiltrative, nodular, polypoid, ulcerating, and endoexoenteric forms. It may even present with multiple lymphomatous polyposis. Most cases are caused by systemic lymphoma with involvement of the GI tract. Primary GI tract lymphomas are less common but have a better prognosis than systemic disease with GI involvement. CT and fluoroscopy are the most useful means to stage GI tract lymphoma and detect its myriad complications such as ulceration, perforation, intussusception, and fistulization. In differentiating lymphoma from other tumors, several important imaging features to keep in mind include its bulky nature, tendency to be a soft nonobstructing neoplasm, and tendency to be a cellular, less vascular neoplasm than carcinomas. A characteristic appearance caused by this marked cellularity is its very bland, homogenous attenuation at CT with a tendency to marked wall thickening of the involved bowel segment.

# REFERENCES

1. Ghai S, Pattison J, Ghai S, et al. Primary gastrointestinal lymphoma: Spectrum of imaging findings with pathologic correlation. Radiographics 2007;27: 1371–88.

2. Dawson I, Cornes J, Morson B. Primary malignant lymphoid tumours of the intestinal tract. Report of 37 cases with a study of factors influencing prognosis. Br J Surg 1961;49:80–9.

3. Yoo CC, Levine MS, McLarney JK, et al. Value of barium studies for predicting primary versus secondary non-Hodgkin's gastrointestinal lymphoma. Abdom Imaging 2000;25:368–72.

4. Levine MS, Rubesin SE, Brown-Pantongrag L, et al. Non-Hodgkin's lymphoma of the gastrointestinal tract: radiographic findings. AJR Am J Roentgenol 1997;168:165–72.

5. Gore RM, Levine MS. Textbook of gastrointestinal radiology. 3rd edition. Philadelphia: Saunders, Elseveier; 2008.

6. Mendelson RM, Fermoyle S. Primary gastrointestinal lymphomas: a radiological–pathological review. Part 1: stomach, oesophageus, and colon. Australas Radiol 2005;49:353–64.

7. Chung JJ, Kim MJ, Kie JH, et al. Mucosa-associated lymphoid tissue lymphoma of the esophagus coexistent with bronchus-associated lymphoid tissue lymphoma of the lung. Yonsei Med J 2005;46(4): 562–6.

8. Byun JH, Ha HK, Kim AY, et al. CT findings in peripheral T cell lymphoma involving the gastrointestinal tract. Radiology 2003;227:59–67.

9. Crump M, Gospodarowicz M, Sheperd FA. Lymphoma of the gastrointestinal tract. Semin Oncol 1999;26(3):324–37.

10. Shaye OS, Levine AM. Marginal zone lymphoma. J Natl Compr Canc Netw 2006;4(3):311–8.

11. Greenstein AJ, Gennuso R, Sachar DB, et al. Extraintestinal cancers in inflammatory bowel disease. Cancer 1985;56:2914–21.

12. Tsukada T, Ohno T, Kihira H, et al. Primary esophageal non-Hodgkin's lymphoma. Intern Med 1992; 31(4):569–72.

13. Chung HH, Kim YH, Kim JH, et al. Imaging findings of mantle cell lymphoma involving gastrointestinal tract. Yonsei Med J 2003;44(1):49–57.

14. Miyazaki T, Kato H, Masuda N, et al. Mucosa-associated lymphoid tissue lymphoma of the esophagus: case report and review of the literature. Hepatogastroenterology 2004;51:750–3.

15. Leite NP, Kased N, Hanna RF, et al. Cross-sectional imaging of extranodal involvement in abdomino–pelvic lymphoproliferative malignancies. Radiographics 2007;27:1613–34.

16. Kolve ME, Fischbach W, Wilhelm M. Primary gastric non-Hodgkin's lymphoma: requirements for diagnosis and staging. Recent Results Cancer Res 2000;156:63–8.

17. Isaacson P, Wright DH. Malignant lymphoma of the mucosa-associated lymphoid tissue: a distinctive type of B cell lymphoma. Cancer 1983;52:1410–6.

18. Rodallec M, Guermazi A, Brice P, et al. Imaging of MALT lymphomas. Eur Radiol 2002;12:348–56.

19. Park MS, Kim KW, Yu JS, et al. Radiographic findings of primary B cell lymphoma of the stomach: low-grade versus high-grade malignancy in relation to the mucosa-associated lymphoid tissue concept. AJR Am J Roentgenol 2002;179:1297–304.

20. Fischbach W, Dragosics B, Kolve-Goebeler ME, et al. Primary gastric B cell lymphoma: results of a prospective multicenter study. Gastroenterology 2000;119:1191–202.

21. Choi D, Lim HK, Lee SJ, et al. Gastric mucosa-associated lymphoid tissue lymphoma: helical CT findings and pathologic correlation. AJR Am J Roentgenol 2002;178:1117–22.

22. Rohatiner A, d'Amore F, Coiffier B, et al. Report on a workshop convened to discuss the pathological and staging classifications of gastrointestinal tract lymphoma. Ann Oncol 1994;5:397–400.

23. Pavlick AC, Gerdes H, Portlock CS. Endoscopic ultrasound in the evaluation of gastric small lymphocytic mucosa-associated lymphoid tumors. J Clin Oncol 1997;15:1761–6.

24. Yahalom J, Schecter N, Portlock C. Effective treatment of MALT lymphoma of the stomach with radiation alone. Int J Radiat Oncol Biol Phys 1998;42:129 (suppl 1, abstr 10).

25. Isaacson PG, Wright DH. Classifying primary gut lymphomas. Lancet 1988;2:1148–9.

26. Boyajian DA, Margulis AR. The GI fluoroscopy suite in the early twenty-first century. Abdom Imaging 2008;33(2):200–6.

27. Levine MS, Pantongrag-Brown L, Aguilera NS, et al. Non-Hodgkin lymphoma of the stomach: a cause of linitis plastica. Radiology 1996;201:375–8.

28. Horton KM, Fishman EK. Current role of CT in imaging of the stomach. Radiographics 2003;23: 75–87.

29. Chen CY, Hsu JS, Wu DC, et al. Gastric cancer: preoperative local staging with 3D multidetector row CT—Correlation with surgical and histopathologic results. Radiology 2007;242(2):472–82.

30. Gossios K, Katsimbri P, Tsianos E. CT features of gastric lymphoma. Eur Radiol 2000;10:425–30.

31. Lecuit M, Abachin E, Martin A, et al. Immunoproliferative small intestinal disease associated with *Campylobacter jejuni*. N Engl J Med 2004;350(3):239–48.

32. Cornes JS. Multiple lymphomatous polyposis of the gastrointestinal tract. Cancer 1961;14:249–57.

33. Catassi C, Bearzi I, Holmes GKT. Association of celiac disease and intestinal lymphomas and other cancers. Gastroenterology 2005;128:S79–86.

34. Mendelson RM, Fermoyl S. Primary gastrointestinal lymphomas: a radiological–pathological review. Part 2: small intestine. Australas Radiol 2006;50:102–13.

35. Rubesin SE, Gilchrist AM, Bronner M, et al. Non-Hodgkin lymphoma of the small intestine. Radiographics 1990;10:985–98.

36. Leone N, Brunello F, Baronio M, et al. High-grade B cell lymphoma arising in mucosa-associated lymphoid tissue of the duodenum. Eur J Gastroenterol Hepatol 2002;14:893–6.

37. Bilsel Y, Balik E, Yamaner S, et al. Clinical and therapeutic considerations of rectal lymphoma: a case report and literature review. World J Gastroenterol 2005;11(3):460–1.

38. Lee HJ, Han JK, Kim TK, et al. Primary colorectal lymphoma: spectrum of imaging findings with pathologic correlation. Eur Radiol 2002;12:2242–9.

39. Breslin NP, Urbanski SJ, Shaffer EA. Mucosa-associated lymphoid tissue (MALT) lymphoma manifesting as multiple lymphomatosis polyposis of the gastrointestinal tract. Am J Gastroenterol 1999;94(9):2540–5.

40. Kim YH, Lim HK, Han JK, et al. Low-grade gastric mucosa-associated lymphoid tissue lymphoma: correlation of radiographic and pathologic findings. Radiology 1999;212:241–8.

41. Collins DC. 71,000 human appendix specimens: a final report summarizing forty years' study. Am J Proctol 1963;14:365–81.

42. Katz DS, Stein LB, Mazzie JP. Recurrent Non-Hodgkin's lymphoma of the appendix. AJR Am J Roentgenol 2002;179:1443–5.

43. Horger M, Muller-Schimpfle M, Yirkin I, et al. Extensive peritoneal and omental lymphomatosis with raised CA 125 mimicking carcinomatosis: CT and intraoperative findings. Br J Radiol 2004;77:71–3 Carpenter BW.

44. Lynch MA, Cho KV, Jeffrey RB. CT of peritoneal lymphomatosis. AJR Am J Roentgenol 1988;151:713–5.

45. Libson E, Mapp E, Dachman AH. Hodgkin's disease of the gastrointestinal tract. Clin Radiol 1994;49:166–9.

46. Kumar S, Fend F, Quintanilla-Martinez L, et al. Epstein-Barr visus-positive primary gastrointestinal Hodgkin's disease. Am J Surg Pathol 2000;24(1):66–73.

47. Venizelos I, Tamiolakis D, Bolioti S. Primary gastric Hodgkin's lymphoma: a case report and review of the literature. Leuk Lymphoma 2005;46(1):147–50.

48. O'Malley ME, Wilson SR. US of gastrointestinal tract abnormalities with CT correlation. Radiographics 2003;23:59–72.

49. Goerg C, Schwerk EB, Goerg K. Gastrointestinal lymphoma: sonographic findings in 54 patients. AJR Am J Roentgenol 1990;155:795–8.

50. Chou CK, Chen LT, Sheu RS. MRI manifestations of gastrointestinal lymphoma. Abdom Imaging 1994;19:495–500.

51. Lohan DG, Alhajeri AN, Cronin CG, et al. MR enterography of small bowel lymphoma: potential for suggestions of histologic subtype and the presence of underlying celiac disease. AJR Am J Roentgenol 2008;190:287–93.

# Imaging of Pediatric Lymphomas

Sara J. Abramson, MD, FACR*, Anita P. Price, MD, FACR

**KEYWORDS**

• Lymphoma • Children • Non-Hodgkin • Hodgkin • Burkitt

Lymphoma is the third most common malignancy in the pediatric age group following leukemia and malignant brain tumors.[1,2] Hodgkin lymphoma (HL) and non- Hodgkin lymphoma (NHL) account for 10% to 15% of all cancers in children and adolescents younger than 20, with nearly 1700 new cases per year reported in the United Sates.[1] The incidence of lymphoma increases with age, representing 3% of cancers in children younger than 5 and 24% of cancers in adolescents aged 15 to 19. Although the total number of new cases of HL per year exceeds new cases of NHL, NHL is more frequent in children younger than 10 and HL is more common in adolescents.[1] Pediatric HL and NHL each include several different histologic subtypes. Pediatric lymphomas may not be limited to a single organ system. Classic HL involves contiguous nodal groups at presentation, unlike NHL, which is more commonly extranodal.

## HODGKIN LYMPHOMA

HL was first described as a separate entity in 1832 by Thomas Hodgkin, MD, a pathologist at Guy's Hospital in London. He reported "peculiar enlargement" of cervical and other lymph nodes associated with splenic enlargement.[3] In 1856, Samuel Wilks reported similar cases. Crediting Hodgkin with the original description of this entity, Wilks named it "Hodgkin's Disease" in 1865. In 1898, Carl Sternberg provided the first histologic description of the neoplastic cell seen in HL. Four years later, Dorothy Reed described the cellular abnormalities and clinical findings in more detail. Reed-Sternberg (RS) cells are considered the hallmark of HL. RS cells are giant multinucleated lymphocytes with eosinophilic nucleoli. The term, HL, is preferred to Hodgkin's disease.

Male incidence is slightly increased under age 15 (male-to-female ratio = 1.3) and significantly increased under age 5 (male-to-female ratio = 5.3).[1] HL is more common, however, in adolescent females over age 15. The incidence is equal in African American and Caucasian children younger than 10. Above this age, the incidence is higher in Caucasians.

Age-adjusted incidence rates comparing 1975–1979 to 1990–1995 time periods reveal comparable rates of decrease in both genders, in patients younger than 15, and a greater male than female decline in the 15- to 19-year-old age group.

The overall 5-year survival for HL diagnosed in patients younger than 20 is reported to be 91%. Although the 5-year survival for both genders and all age groups is similar, the 5-year survival is slightly decreased (84%) in African Americans.[1]

Epstein-Barr virus (EBV) is associated with an increased risk for developing HL. EBV is associated with nearly 50% of HL in developed countries and up to 90% in developing countries. EBV-infected B cells may inhibit normal apoptosis of Reed Sternberg (RS) cells.[4,5] EBV in RS cells occurs more frequently in the mixed cellularity (MC) subtype, male patients, children younger than 10, and lower socioeconomic groups.[6,7] Increasing evidence links EBV-positive HL and infectious mononucleosis. Increased risk factors for developing HL in adolescents and young adults are socioeconomic status, smaller family size, and early birth order.[1] The incidence of HL is increased

Department of Radiology, Memorial Sloan-Kettering Cancer Center, New York, NY, USA
* Corresponding author.
*E-mail address:* abramsos@mskcc.org (S.J. Abramson).

Radiol Clin N Am 46 (2008) 313–338
doi:10.1016/j.rcl.2008.03.009
0033-8389/08/$ – see front matter © 2008 Elsevier Inc. All rights reserved.

in immunocompromised individuals, congenital and acquired, including HIV-infected patients. Some of these patients also are EBV positive. Such patients have a worse prognosis.[8,9]

The classification of HL is based on morphology, immunohistochemistry, and clinical behavior. The World Health Organization (WHO) classification separates the uncommon nodular lymphocyte predominant (LP) form of HL from the relatively common form, designated classical HL. WHO subtypes of classical HL are nodular sclerosis (NS), lymphocyte rich (LR) (previously LP), mixed cellularity (MC), and lymphocyte depletion (LD). Each subtype is discussed.[10]

National Cancer Institute Surveillance, Epidemiology, and End Results (SEER) statistics for the period 1975–1995 reveal the NS subtype of HL accounted for 70% of cases of HL in patients younger than 20. The incidence of NS is followed by MC (16%), LR (7%), and LD (2%). Age and gender are important factors in pediatric HL. Eighty percent of female patients and 67% of male patients aged 15 to 19 had NS subtype. MC subtype accounts for 32% of all HL cases in children younger than 10 compared with 15% in the 10- to 14-year-old age group and 13% in the 15 to 19 year olds. MC is more common in male (70%) than female patients younger than 20.[1] MC is associated with EBV.[1,6,7] LR is more common in patients younger than 10 with a male predominance.[1,11] LD is rare in the pediatric population and presents with extensive disease frequently involving bone and bone marrow and retroperitoneal lymph nodes. HIV infection and immunosuppression after solid organ transplantation are associated factors in the development of the LD subtype.[1,11,12]

Before the nearly curative current therapy protocols for HL, the ratio of lymphocytes to abnormal cells in the MC, LR, and LD subtypes was associated with prognosis. Response to therapy is in these subtypes currently is independent of histology subtype.[11]

RS cells are most abundant in the NS subtype with fewer numbers in MC and LD subtypes. NS is characterized by lymph nodes that have thickened capsules and are separated into macronodules by collagenous bands. The presence of collagen and fibrous stroma contributes to the presence of residual mediastinal soft tissue even after no viable disease remains. RS cells are rare in the LR subtype of HL often requiring evaluations of multiple tissue sections before the diagnosis can be made. The benign appearance of these lymphocytes and their characteristic cellular proliferation may result in misdiagnosis of lymphoid hyperplasia.[11]

## NON-HODGKIN LYMPHOMA

NHL comprises 10% to 15% of all childhood cancers.[13] These lymphomas arise from constituent cells of the immune system that normally circulate throughout the body, thus making NHL a systemic disease. Pediatric NHL differs in several important ways from NHL in adults:

> This group of neoplasms derives from mature and immature cells as compared with the adult population where most tumors derive from mature cells.
>
> In the pediatric age groups NHL encompasses high-grade tumors that usually are diffuse in nature.[14]
>
> Pediatric NHLs are divided more evenly between B-cell and T-cell neoplasms as opposed to adults where the majority of tumors are of B-cell origin.

In the pediatric population there are only four major subtypes of NHL as opposed to the many subtypes of NHL in adults (**Table 1**).

The World Health Organization (WHO) divides pediatric NHL into four major histologic subtypes: Burkitt lymphoma (BL), diffuse large B-cell lymphoma (DLBCL), anaplastic large cell lymphoma (ALCL), and lymphoblastic lymphoma (LBL). Each of these subtypes is discussed.

NHL is more common than HL in children younger than 10[1] but less common than HL in older children. The incidence of NHL increases with age. There is a notable male predominance for NHL in children, with 70% occurring in male children.[1] This male predominance is seen in all age groups, although it is more pronounced in those younger than 15. The incidence of NHL among Causasian children is 1.4 times higher than for African Americans younger than 15. The incidence of NHL has remained stable for those younger than 15 from 1975 to 2004. The incidence among 15 to 19 year olds, however, increased from 10.7 per million in 1979 to 16.3 per million in 1995.[1]

| Table 1 Incidence of subtypes of non-Hodgkin lymphoma in the pediatric population | |
|---|---|
| Subtype | Incidence (%) |
| Burkitt lymphoma | 40 |
| Diffuse large B-cell lymphoma | 20 |
| Anaplastic large cell lymphoma | 10 |
| Lymphoblastic lymphoma | 30 |

The 5-year survival rate for children younger than 10 is 76% versus 70% for children and adolescents 10 to 19 years old. Survival is similar for Caucasian and African American children and is similar for male and female children.[1]

## Burkitt Lymphoma

BL takes its name from Denis Burkitt,[15] a surgeon working in equatorial Africa, who identified a group of children who had jaw masses. WHO classifies BL into three clinical variants: endemic, sporadic, and immunodeficiency associated.[16] BL is a B-cell lymphoma. These mature lymphocytes are medium-sized round blue cells with a very high mitotic rate. Microscopic sections may demonstrate a "starry sky" appearance as a result of tingible bodies–laden macrophages scattered among the abnormal lymphocytes. BL is one of the fastest growing malignancies, with a tumor doubling time of 12 to 24 hours.[17] BL typically expresses certain B-cell surface antigens, including CD19,

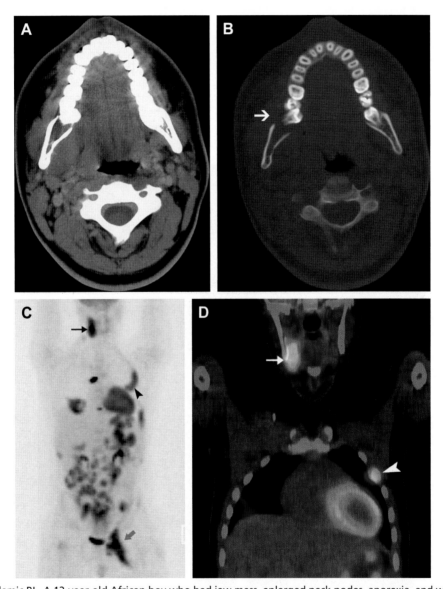

Fig. 1. Endemic BL. A 12-year-old African boy who had jaw mass, enlarged neck nodes, anorexia, and weight loss. CTs of soft tissue (A) and bone (B) reveal a destructive lesion in the right mandible with "floating teeth" (*white arrow*), soft tissue mass, and enlarged neck nodes. Maximum intensity projection (MIP) PET image (C) demonstrates the lesion in the mandible (*black arrow*) and left rib (*arrowhead*), gastrointestinal, and nodal disease. Mass involving the left obturator muscle also is seen (*gray arrow*). Fused coronal PET image (D) shows right mandibular (*arrow*) and left rib disease (*arrowhead*).

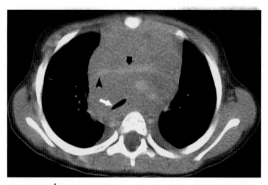

**Fig. 2.** A 3½ -year-old boy who had T-cell lymphoblastic NHL presented with shortness of breath and facial swelling. Contrast-enhanced chest CT. A large mediastinal mass encases the great vessels producing a superior vena cava syndrome. The trachea is displaced posteriorly and narrowed (*white arrow*). Superior vena cava (*black arrowhead*) and left brachiocephalic vein (*black arrow*) are compressed and displaced posteriorly.

CD20, CD22, CD10, and BCL6. A characteristic chromosomal translocation (8:14) (q24:q32) involving cMYC proto-oncogene is seen in BL.[18] The majority of children display features of classic BL.[19,20]

Endemic BL is found in young African children with a propensity for erosion of the mandible and maxilla, with characteristic involvement of the developing molar teeth (**Fig. 1**). These masses may be associated with large abdominal tumors.[21] BL, the most common pediatric malignancy in this part of the world, is considered endemic.[22] The occurrence is greater in areas of heavy rainfall and less prevalent in areas of higher altitude and cooler temperatures. The geographic and climatic associations are similar to the distribution of malaria. The exact relationship between malaria and endemic BL is unclear. It is believed, however, that in the presence of EBV, the reactive lymphoid hyperplasia occurring in patients who have malaria leads EBV to become

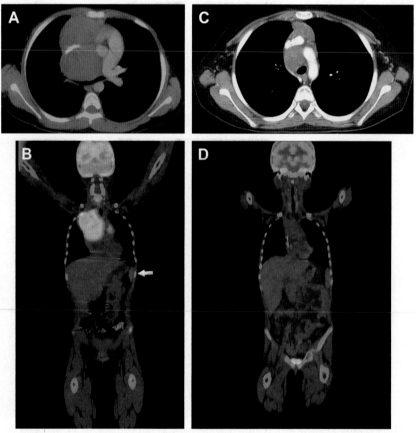

**Fig. 3.** A 9-year-old girl who had NS HL presented with cough on exertion, night sweats, weight loss, and pallor. Contrast-enhanced chest CT (*A*) and fused PET-CT images (*B*) at diagnosis. Large anterior mediastinal and precarinal masses that compress the airway (*A*) are hypermetabolic on PET (*B*). Increased FDG uptake also is seen in the spleen (*white arrow*). CT (*C*) and PET-CT (*D*) after 1 month of therapy demonstrate residual mediastinal masses on CT (*C*) with resolution of hypermetabolic activity on PET (*D*), indicating response to therapy.

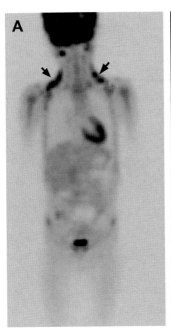
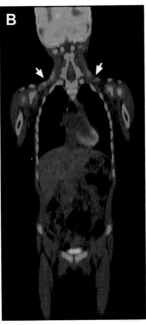

Fig. 4. A 5½-year-old boy who had BL presented with intussusception. MIP (*A*) and fused PET-CT (*B*). Physiologic activity in brown fat is present (*arrows*).

oncogenic.[15] It is now recognized that BL occurs in a worldwide distribution.[16] This form of the disease is more common in male children usually younger than 8.[19] Clonal EBV DNA is found in up to 95% of these tumors.[16,23]

Sporadic or nonendemic BL is found worldwide and makes up 40% of all NHL in children in the United States and Western Europe.[24] BL occurs throughout childhood and adolescence. The median age at diagnosis is 8, with 40% of patients between 5 and 9 years old, 24% of patients between 0 and 4 years old, 28% of patients between 10 and 14 years old, and 9% of patients between 15 and 21 years old. A 4:1 male to female ratio is seen.[23,25,26] Sporadic BL is associated with EBV in up to 20% of cases.

Immunodeficiency-associated BL refers to BL associated with HIV[27] and to BL seen in patients who are allograft recipients[28] or who have congenital immunodeficiencies. BL accounts for up to 40% of NHL in HIV-positive patients.[29] Forty percent of these HIV-associated BL are also EBV positive.[25] Most transplant patients who have BL are solid organ recipients but recipients of stem cells also may be affected. EBV is present in 30% to 40% of such cases.[28,30] A 5-year, event-free survival rate (EFS) in patients who have high-risk diseases is over 80%.[31] In patients who have low-stage disease, 5-year EFS rate is up to 98%.[32]

### Diffuse Large B-Cell Lymphoma

DLBCL makes up 20% of pediatric NHL.[13] The incidence increases with increasing age of the pediatric population. It is the most common form of NHL in 15 to 19 year olds and is uncommon in children younger than 5.[1] It is more common in male children.[1] Although DLBCL is a heterogeneous group of tumors with many subtypes identified in adults, only two subtypes are identified in children: (1) disease localized to the mediastinum,

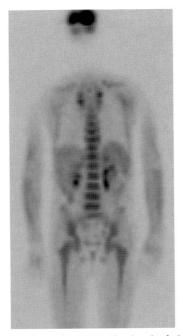

Fig. 5. Coronal PET image at the level of the spine. Diffuse increased FDG uptake in the spine represents post–GCSF treatment effects.

**Table 2**
**Normal measurements of the thymus on CT: mean values**

| Age (y) | AP Diameter in cm (SD) | Thickness of Limbs in cm (SD) | Craniocaudal Length in cm (SD) | Width in cm (SD) |
|---|---|---|---|---|
| 0–10 | 2.52 (0.82) | 1.5 (0.46) | 3.53 (0.99) | 3.13 (0.85) |
| 10–20 | 2.56 (0.88) | 1.05 (0.36) | 4.99 (1.25) | 3.05 (1.17) |

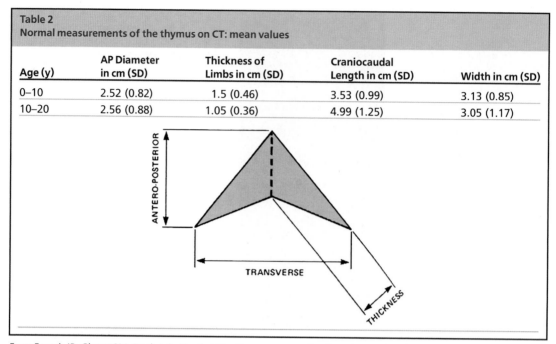

From Francis IR, Glazer GM, Bookstein FL, et al. The thymus: reexamination of age-related changes in size and shape. AJR Am J Roentgenol 1985;145:249–54; with permission.

called primary mediastinal large B lymphoma (PMBL),[33–36] and (2) disseminated disease.

PMBL occurs more commonly in adolescents and is associated with a better prognosis than the disseminated form of the disease.[33,36] PMBL is difficult to differentiate from HL on imaging studies.

Up to 75% of patients present with disseminated disease.[32] Like BL, the most common site

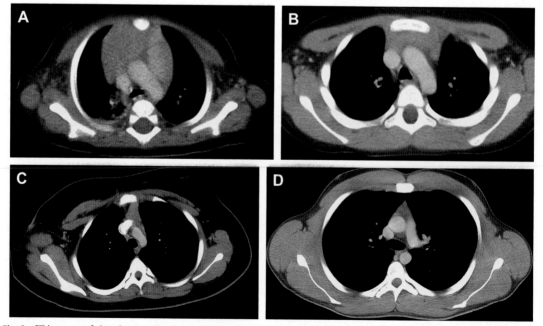

**Fig. 6.** CT images of the chest at the level of the aortic arch demonstrate the appearance of the normal thymus at representative ages. (A) 7 months, (B) 5.5 years, (C) 13 years, and (D) 20 years.

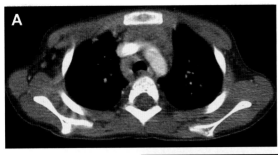
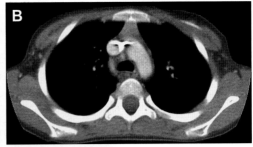
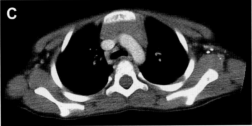

Fig. 7. Contrast-enhanced CT of the chest. A 3-year-old girl who had normal thymus at diagnosis (A). Involution of the thymus is seen after 6 months of therapy (B). Thymic rebound is noted 3 months after the completion of treatment (C).

of involvement is the gastrointestinal tract. B symptoms also frequently are present.[32]

DLBCL is associated with immunodeficiencies, inherited or acquired, and is the most common form of NHL seen in immunocompromised patients.[37-39]

All tumors contain large, mature B cells that are positive for B-cell markers CD19, CD20, CD22, and CD79a. No specific cytogenetic abnormalities are associated with DLBCL in children and adolescents.[40,41] The 5-year EFS for low-stage disease is greater than 90%.[14,31]

## Lymphoblastic Lymphoma

LBL accounts for nearly 30% of pediatric NHL although representing less than 10% of NHL in adults. Males are affected more than twice as frequently as females (male-to-female ratio = 2.5). The incidence of LBL is similar in all pediatric age groups.[1] By convention, when 25% or more of the marrow is infiltrated with lymphoblasts, the disease is termed, acute lymphoblastic leukemia (ALL).[13,42,43]

The abundance of apoptotic bodies that undergo phagocytosis by macrophages (tingible bodies–laden macrophages) and the high mitotic rate present in LBL are responsible for creating the histologic starry sky appearance akin to that seen in BL. T-cell lymphoblasts are associated with CD3, CD4, CD5, CD7, and CD8 surface markers. Translocation involving the TAL-1 gene, t(1;14), frequently is seen.[32]

Although an 80% to 90% 5-year EFS is seen in patients who have early-stage LBL, the prognosis is poor in patients who have recurrent or refractory LBL.

## Anaplastic Large Cell Lymphoma

ALCL makes up 10% of all pediatric NHL.[13,40] It is seen in older children, with a mean age of 10, and is three times more common in male children.[44,45] It is the most common mature T-cell lymphoma in the pediatric population. There is a primary cutaneous form of the disease, which is rare in children. Most pediatric patients present with advanced systemic disease.[46,47] B symptoms are common.[44,45] Morphologically, the classic features of ALCL consist of large, multinucleated tumor cells that frequently contain horseshoe-shaped nuclei with abundant cytoplasm with an area of eosinophilia near the nucleus. These are called "hallmark cells."[48,49] These findings are present in 75% of patients. Virtually all tumor cells express the CD30 (Ki-1) antigen.[50,51] ACLC cells are positive for T-cell antigens, CD2, CD3. CD4, CD5, and CD7.

## IMAGING WORK-UP

Imaging studies in lymphomas are related to emergency imaging and to studies for staging the extent of disease.

**Table 3**
**Cotswold staging classification for Hodgkin lymphoma**

| Stage | Description |
|---|---|
| Stage I | Involvement of a single lymph node region or lymphoid structure (eg, spleen, thymus, or Waldeyer's ring) or involvement of a single extralymphatic site (IE). |
| Stage II | Involvement of two or more lymph node regions on the same site of the diaphragm (II) or localized contiguous involvement of any one extranodal organ or side and its regional lymph nodes with or without other lymph node regions on the same side of the diaphragm (IIE). |
| Stage III | Involvement of lymph node regions on both sides of the diaphragm (III), which also may be accompanied by involvement of the spleen (IIIS) or by localized contiguous involvement of only one extranodal organ side (IIIE) or both (IIISE). |
| Stage IV | Disseminated (multifocal) involvement of one or more extranodal organs or tissues, with or without associated lymph node involvement or isolated extralymphatic organ involvement with distant (nonregional) nodal involvement. |
| Designations applicable to any disease stage | |
| A | No symptoms |
| B | Fever (temperature >38°C), night sweats, unexplained loss of more than 10% of body weight during the previous 6 months. |
| X | Bulky disease in pediatric patients: a contiguous nodal aggregate that measures >6 cm in the longest transverse diameter or a mediastinal mass where the tumor diameter is greater than one third of the thoracic diameter. |
| E | Involvement of a single extranodal site that is contiguous or proximal to the known nodal site. |

*Modified from* Lister TA, Crowther D, Sutcliffe SB, et al. Report of a committee convened to discuss the evaluation and staging of patients with Hodgkin disease: Cotswolds meeting. J Clin Oncol 1989;7:1630–6. Reprinted with permission of the American Society of Clinical Oncology.

## Emergency Imaging

Some emergencies that may be present at diagnosis include airway compromise or superior vena cava syndrome from large mediastinal masses (**Fig. 2**). Chest film and chest CT are necessary for evaluation of these thoracic emergencies. Patency of the airway must be assessed before anesthesia can be given. Gastrointestinal obstruction may be the result of tumor infiltration of bowel. Obstruction of the kidneys, biliary tree, or gastrointestinal tract may be secondary to mass effect of tumor on these structures. CT of the abdomen and pelvis is necessary to evaluate abdominal emergencies. Before performing intravenous contrast studies, urinary function tests (serum urea nitrogen and creatinine) must be obtained. If they are abnormal, no intravenous contrast may be administered. Abnormal renal function may be secondary to tumor lysis syndrome. If CT is unavailable, ultrasonography (US) or MR imaging may be used to evaluate mediastinal masses and intraabdominal organs. Symptoms related to cord compression must be urgently evaluated. MR imaging should be performed for central nervous system (CNS) emergencies. If MR imaging is contraindicated, myelogram should be performed.[52]

## Initial Staging by Imaging

Advances in diagnostic imaging, especially cross-sectional imaging and nuclear medicine, have replaced surgical intervention in the staging of most lymphomas. Staging studies for pediatric

| Table 4 |
| --- |
| **St. Jude staging system for childhood non-Hodgkin lymphoma** |
| **Stage I** |
| A single tumor (extranodal) or single anatomic area (nodal), with the exclusion of the mediastinum or abdomen |
| **Stage II** |
| A single tumor (extranodal) with regional node involvement |
| Two or more nodal areas on the same side of the diaphragm |
| Two single (extranodal) tumors with or without regional node involvement on the same side of the diaphragm |
| A primary gastrointestinal tract tumor, usually in the ileocecal area, with or without involvement of associated mesenteric nodes only |
| **Stage III** |
| Two single tumors (extranodal) on opposite sides of the diaphragm |
| Two or more nodal areas above and below the diaphragm |
| All primary intrathoracic tumors (mediastinal, pleural, and thymic) |
| All extensive primary intra-abdominal disease |
| All paraspinal or epidural tumors, regardless of other tumor side(s) |
| **Stage IV** |
| Any of the previous with initial CNS or bone marrow involvement |

Bone marrow involvement is defined as less than 25% of marrow replacement by tumor and the absence of circulating blast cells. If more than 25% of the marrow is involved the patient is considered to have leukemia.
*From* Murphy S. Childhood non-Hodgkin's lymphoma. N Engl J Med 1978; 299:1446–8; with permission.

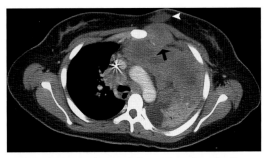

Fig. 8. Contrast-enhanced chest CT. A female 19 year old who had MC HL presented with cough and B symptoms. Anterior mediastinal and precarinal adenopathy displace the airway. A large left internal mammary lymph node (*black arrow*) is seen on the same plane as a metastatic soft tissue nodule (*white arrowhead*).

lymphomas should include a chest radiograph and CT of the chest, abdomen, and pelvis. All CT imaging in children should be guided by the As Low As Reasonably Achievable (ALARA) principle. CT of the neck is performed when there are symptoms and signs referable to the neck. When evaluating superificial lymph nodes, color Doppler US may be helpful in differentiating reactive from malignant lymphadenopathy. Distortion of intranodal vascular architecture, such as aberrant vessels, focal absence of perfusion, and amputated short subcapsular vessels and vessel displacement, are described patterns of altered intranodal angioarchitecture in malignant nodes.[53] Baseline MR imaging of the brain in the absence of symptoms usually is not performed. Bone scan or MR

imaging of the bone may be performed in patients who have focal bone disease.

Whole-body screening may be performed to detect known sites of disease and to delineate sites of disease that otherwise would remain unrecognized. This may be performed with whole-body MR,[54] which may aid in the in the detection of bone and bone marrow involvement, which frequently are spotty in nature.

Whole-body imaging also may be performed using nuclear medicine imaging with gallium 67 or with positron emission tomography (PET) using fluorodeoxyglucose (FDG). Gallium is well known to be positive in lymphoma, and gallium scanning with single photon emission CT (SPECT) enhances lesion conspicuity.[55] Recent studies have confirmed the increased sensitivity of PET compared with gallium in diagnosis and follow-up of pediatric lymphoma.[56–62] PET provides a 1-day scan with better resolution and lower radiation exposure, less intestinal activity, and semiquantitative measurement of metabolic activity.[63] PET-CT correlates anatomic abnormalities with function and is replacing gallium scanning in the diagnosis and follow-up of children who have lymphoma.[64,65]

FDG PET-CT is shown to alter staging in up to one third of pediatric patients who have lymphomas.[56,59,66–69] Image fusion has an impact on therapeutic management.[69] The combination of CT and PET scans helps determine whether or not residual mass-like opacities on CT represent disease. Areas of fibrosis may persist on CT but are not active on PET (**Fig. 3**). PET provides incremental clinically important information in 21% HL and 33% NHL and is especially useful in distinguishing scar tissue from residual disease at the end of therapy.[55,68] In HL and NHL, PET has higher sensitivity and specificity than CT/MR imaging and gallium.[69] Combining ALARA-based diagnostic CT with PET/PET-CT is important to reduce overall

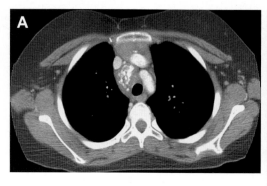

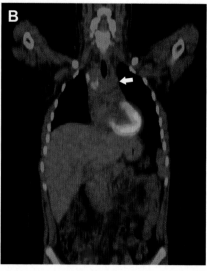

Fig. 9. Contrast-enhanced CT chest (A) and PET (B). A 10 year old after completion of treatment of NS HL Residual calcified mediastinal mass (A), which is not FDG avid. (B) Nonspecific thymic activity is seen (white arrow).

radiation exposure in children by eliminating the need to perform separate diagnostic CT scans.[59] Combined reading of PET and conventional imaging modalities is essential for accurate staging in pediatric HL.

Nonmalignant FDG activity includes reactive nodes, inflammatory lung disease, and infection.[70,71] Radiation pneumonitis also may be PET positive.

Brown adipose tissue is metabolically active in children, decreasing with age. Sites of FDG avidity include the neck, around the coronary arteries, the perinephric space, and the para-aortic and intercostal regions (Fig. 4).[72] Granulocyte colony-stimulating factor (GCSF) causes proliferation and activation of neurophil-granulocyte lines causing conversion of yellow marrow to red marrow. Increased FDG uptake is seen in spine, pelvis, long bones, and spleen and mimics lymphomatous involvement (Fig. 5).[73] False-positive PET also occurs with muscle tension.[71]

PET-CT has become extremely important in the follow-up and prognosis of pediatric lymphoma.[74] Early PET responsive disease is associated with a excellent prognosis and is used to modify therapy.[56,63,75] Likewise, persistent FDG uptake after front-line chemotherapy in patients who have lymphoma is associated with relapse.[56,76–79]

New PET-based response criteria are discussed in Chapter 2.

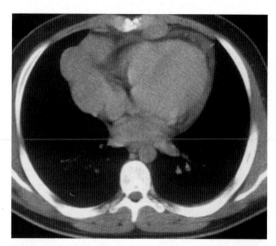

Fig. 11. Contrast-enhanced chest CT. A male 18 year old diagnosed with MC HL presented with fatigue, wheezing, and a right supraclavicular mass. Pericardial effusion, left internal mammary adenopathy, and extensive inferior mediastinal adenopathy are present.

Fig. 10. Contrast-enhanced chest CT. A 15-year-old girl who had NS HL presenting with palpable neck and supraclavicular nodes. Multiple pulmonary nodules at diagnosis (arrows).

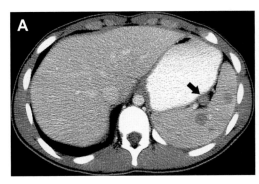
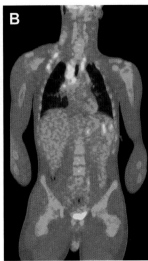

Fig. 12. A 15-year-old boy who had NS HL presented with night sweats and right cervical and supraclavicular adenopathy. Contrast-enhanced CT of the abdomen (*A*). The spleen is enlarged with multiple hypoattenuating lymphomatous lesions. A 1.5-cm gastrosplenic ligament lymph node is present (*arrow*). PET-CT coronal fused image (*B*) confirms multiple splenic lesions and adjacent lymph node involvement. Cervical and mediastinal adenopathy also is identified.

## Imaging of the Thymus in Pediatric Patients

Familiarity with the imaging spectrum of the thymus is important in differentiating disease from normal physiologic states. The normal thymus varies in size, shape, and composition with age (**Table 2**).[80,81]

The thymus, a bilobed structure, maintains a quadrilateral shape with convex borders in children younger than 5 (**Fig. 6A**). In late childhood and adolescence, the thymus becomes triangular in configuration with concave or flat margins and a more prominent left lobe (**Fig. 6**B,C).[82,83] The homogenous soft tissue attenuation of the thymus seen on CT of infants becomes heterogeneous as fatty infiltration begins after the first year of life (**Fig. 6**D).[84] Normal anatomic variants, such as a posterior mediastinal extension between the superior vena cava and trachea, extension between the right brachiocephalic vein and innominate artery, and superior mediastinal extension anteriomedial to the left brachiocephalic vein must be recognized. These variants may be confused with pathologic mediastinal masses because they may cause superior mediastinal widening on plain radiographs and increased soft tissue on cross-sectional imaging. Increased FDG activity may be seen on PET. Normal thymic tissue does not displace or compress adjacent structures.[83,85,86] When present, these findings are indicative of thymic infiltration or mass. Stress-induced thymic involution may be followed by a period of thymic rebound (**Fig. 7**). Although thymic

rebound, a form of true hyperplasia, usually appears within 6 to 12 months after the cessation of chemotherapy, it can develop in a period as short as 1 week.[63,87,88] Rebound hyperplasia can occur in ectopic thymic tissue and be misinterpreted as new disease. Thymic rebound affects 25% of pediatric patients who have HL and is self-limiting and reversible. The size and shape of the thymus on CT plus the degree of activity on PET scan help differentiate new or persistent disease from benign thymic hyperplasia. In some cases the nonmalignant enlarged thymus may be

| Table 5 | |
|---|---|
| **Normal spleen size versus age (ultrasound)** | |
| **Age** | **Spleen Length (cm)[a]** |
| 0–3 months | ≤6 |
| 3–6 months | ≤6.5 |
| 6–12 months | ≤7 |
| 1–2 years | ≤8 |
| 2–4 years | ≤9 |
| 4–6 years | ≤9.5 |
| 6–8 years | ≤10 |
| 8–10 years | ≤11 |

[a] Measurement obtained in the coronal longitudinal plane.
*Data from* Rosenberg HK, Markowitz RI, Kolbeg H, et al. Normal splenic size in infants and children: sonographic measurements. AJR 1991;157:119–21.

**Table 6**
**Sites of involvement in pediatric non-Hodgkin lymphoma**

| Feature | Burkitt | Diffuse Large B-cell | Anaplastic | T-cell Lymphoblastic |
|---|---|---|---|---|
| Peripheral adenopathy | Uncommon: sporadic Common: endemic | Common | Common | Common |
| Bone marrow | Common: sporadic Rare: endemic | Rare | Occurs | Common: if >25% involvement designated as ALL |
| Cortical bone | Common | Occurs | Common | Rare |
| CNS | Uncommon: sporadic Common: endemic | Rare | Rare | Common: receive IT MIX[a] prophylaxis |
| Mediastinum | Rare | Common | Common | Common |
| Lung: nodular or infiltrative pattern | Rare | Rare | Common | Rare |
| Gastrointestinal | Common | Common | Rare | Rare |
| Liver/spleen | Uncommon | Uncommon | Rare | Spleen common |
| Renal | Common | Occurs | Rare | Common |
| Skin and soft tissue | Rare | Rare | Common | Rare |
| B symptoms | Occurs | Common | Common | Common |

[a] Intrathecal methotrexate.

positive on nuclear imaging studies. Then, the size and shape of the thymus and degree of uptake determine the status of the disease.[59,60,68,89]

### Sequence of Imaging

CT of chest abdomen and pelvis should be performed before institution of chemotherapy and obtained after surgery and before chemotherapy begins. Burkitt tumors have such a fast doubling rate that residual tumor may grow significantly between the time of surgery and the beginning of chemotherapy.

Follow-up CT scans should be performed on a routine basis in conjunction with gallium or PET scans. They should be performed after a single cycle of chemotherapy to assess response to treatment and then at suitable intervals to detect new disease.

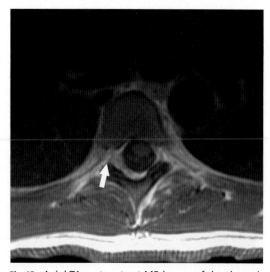

Fig. 13. Axial T1 postcontrast MR image of the thoracic spine. Endemic BL. A 12-year-old African boy who had disease extending into the right neural foramen (*arrow*).

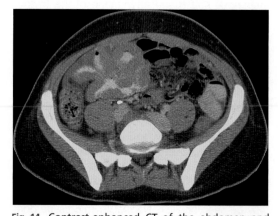

Fig. 14. Contrast-enhanced CT of the abdomen and pelvis. Sporadic BL. A 14-year-old boy who had abdominal pain, back pain, and weight loss. Extensive infiltration of small bowel with bowel wall thickening and aneurysmal dilatation of small bowel loops.

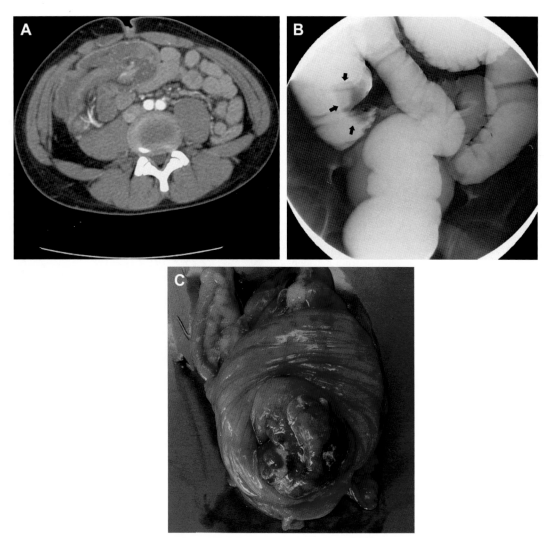

Fig.15. A 10-year-old boy who had sporadic BL who presented with abdominal pain (*A*). Contrast-enhanced CT of the abdomen demonstrates an ileocolic intussusception (*B*). Barium enema demonstrates non-reduced intussusception (*arrows*) (*C*). Pathologic specimen shows BL as lead point of intussusception.

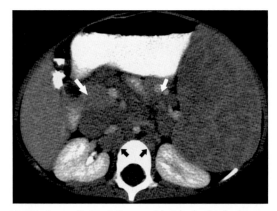

Fig.16. Sporadic BL. A 3-year-old girl who had adenopathy and splenomegaly. Contrast-enhanced CT. Enlarged, diffusely infiltrated spleen with extensive retroperitoneal adenopathy (*white and black arrows*).

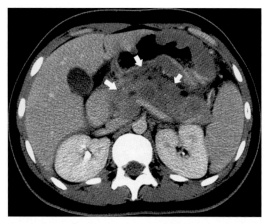

Fig. 17. Sporadic BL. An 8-year-old boy who had abdominal pain. Contrast-enhanced CT. Tumor infiltration of the pancreas and peripancreatic area (*arrows*).

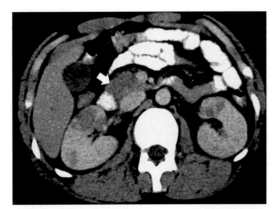

Fig. 18. Sporadic BL. A 13-year-old boy who had ab-dominal pain and weight loss. Contrast-enhanced CT. Multiple bilateral low-attenuation lesions in both kidneys. Biopsy-proved disease. Retroperitoneal aden-opathy also is present (*arrow*).

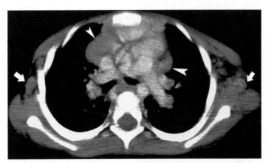

Fig. 19. Sporadic BL. A 4-year-old boy. Contrast-en-hanced CT. Mediastinal (*arrowheads*) and axillary ad-enopathy (*arrows*).

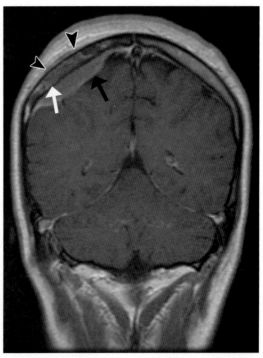

Fig. 21. Coronal T1 post–contrast-enhanced MR image of the brain. Sporadic BL. A 14-year-old boy who had known disease and diffuse bone pain and headache. Marrow abnormality along the right parietal bone (*white arrow*) with epidural disease causing mild mass effect on the underlying brain (*black arrow*). Ex-tracranial soft tissue extension into the right parietal scalp (*arrowheads*).

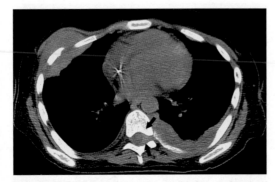

Fig. 20. Sporadic BL. A 12-year-old boy who had relapse. Noncontrast CT of chest. Lobulated left pleu-ral disease with tumor extension into the left neural canal (*arrows*). Right rib involvement and soft tissue mass.

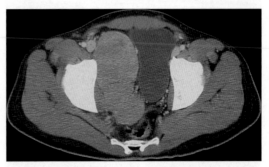

Fig. 22. DLBCL. A 16-year-old boy who had fever, night sweats, and weight loss. Contrast-enhanced CT of the pelvis. Conglomerate nodal mass in the right pelvis, displacing the bladder to the left.

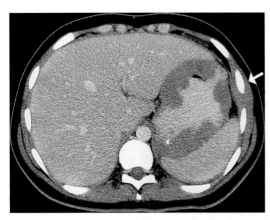

Fig. 23. DLBCL. A 12-year-old boy who had abdominal pain and distension and early satiety. Contrast-enhanced CT of the abdomen. Extensive tumor involvement of the gastric wall with decreased gastric lumen. Left rib involvement with accompanying soft tissue mass (*white arrow*).

## STAGING
### Hodgkin Lymphoma

Because classic HL involves contiguous nodal groups at presentation and early spread is to adjacent nodes, accurate staging using diagnostic imaging is critical in determining treatment and prognosis. Clinical staging has replaced surgical staging with laparotomy and splenectomy, eliminating postoperative complications and infection associated with splenectomy.

The Ann Arbor/Cotswold staging classification (**Table 3**), used to stage patients who have HL, is an anatomically based system that considers the number of sites of lymph node involvement, existence of extranodal disease, and a history of B symptoms.[90,91] For purposes of staging, the spleen is designated as a nodal group.[92] Staging is defined further with suffixes. Suffixes A and B relate to clinical symptoms at presentation. Asymptomatic patients are classified as having A disease. B disease is assigned to patients who have temperature greater than 38°C for 3 consecutive days, drenching nights sweats, or unexplained weight loss of 10% or greater during the 6-month period before diagnosis. Symptoms including B criteria are seen in 25% to 30% at diagnosis.[11] Pruritus and alcohol-induced pain are infrequent non-B symptoms that resolve with response to therapy.[11,52] The Cotswold modification of the Ann Arbor classification deals with the presence of bulky disease, something that was a weakness in the Ann Arbor system.[90]

### Non-Hodgkin Lymphomas

NHLs frequently involve multiple organ systems and generally are considered disseminated at the time of diagnosis. Staging classifications are used to reflect the tumor volume rather than the degree of spread. B symptoms do not affect the stage of the disease. These staging systems provide for a description of the extent of disease and for estimating prognosis by dividing patients into those who have "limited" (stages I and II) and those who have "extensive" (stage III and IV) disease. Bone marrow and CNS involvement reflect the most widespread forms of disease. Approximately 30% of patients present with limited-stage disease (I or II) and 70% have widespread disease (III or IV) at diagnosis. Important prognostic factors include tumor burden and staging, rapidity of response to therapy, age, gender, and histology.[52]

The St. Jude/Murphy staging system (**Table 4**) is most commonly used for staging all NHLs.[93] Because of the nature of the disease, all staging systems are problematic. The primary purpose of staging is to delineate the extent of disease, which determines the intensity of treatment.

## RADIOGRAPHIC FINDINGS IN HODGKIN LYMPHOMA

Anatomic areas of involvement vary with subtypes. Painless cervical or, less commonly, supraclavicular adenopathy is the most common presentation of NS HL in older adolescents and young adult patients.[11] Infrequently axillary adenopathy may be the initial presenting finding. Lymph nodes measuring greater than 1 cm in short axis are considered abnormal. MC HL is characterized by advanced disease and extranodal involvement and presents with upper-body peripheral adenopathy (**Fig. 8**).[52,94] LR HL presents with localized disease.

Mediastinal disease is seen in two thirds of the patients. The mediastinal mass may be demonstrated on chest radiograph.[95] On upright posteroanterior chest radiograph, tumor diameter greater than one third the thoracic diameter measured transversely at the dome of the diaphragm is diagnostic of bulk disease. Although uncommonly seen at presentation, mediastinal calcification and cysts are post-treatment findings (**Fig. 9**). Respiratory symptoms can occur if there is tracheal compression.[96,97]

Hilar and subcarinal adenopathy are indicators of microscopic lung disease.[95] Lung involvement is seen in less than 5% of children younger than 10 and 15% of adolescents and teenagers.[98] Nodules greater than 1 cm are the most common pulmonary finding in HL (**Fig. 10**).[99]

A reticular interstitial pattern and lobar or segmental consolidation are other pulmonary

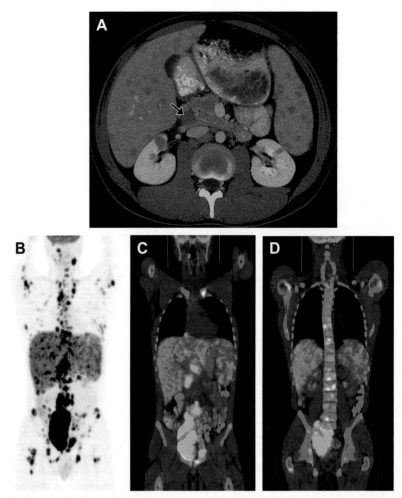

Fig. 24. DLBCL. A 16-year-old boy who had abdominal distension, fever, and vague abdominal discomfort. Contrast-enhanced CT of the abdomen. (*A*) Hepatosplenomegaly with multiple low-attenuation lesions in the liver, spleen, and kidneys representing lymphomatous infiltration. Precaval adenopathy (*black arrow*) (*B*) MIP PET. Numerous sites of nodal disease in the mediastinum, abdomen, and pelvis. FDG uptake in liver, spleen, and axial and appendicular skeleton. Coronal fused PET-CT image (*C*) shows liver, spleen, abdominal, and pelvic nodes and pericardial node. Posterior coronal fused PET-CT image (*D*) demonstrates FDG-avid disease in the spine, right ileum, proximal humeri, and proximal right femur in addition to the liver and spleen.

manifestations of HL.[82,99,100] Pleural and pericardial effusions are infrequent findings in HL (**Fig. 11**). Pleural effusions usually are negative for malignant cells.[95,101] Pericardial effusion suggests tumor involvement of the pericardium from direct extension of a mediastinal mass. MR imaging is better than CT in evaluating pericardial involvement.

Primary infradiaphragmatic disease is rare, occurring in less that 4% of HL.[82,99] Single nodes or nodal conglomerates in the retroperitoneum may be involved. US or CT may demonstrate conglomerate mesenteric nodal involvement with encasement of mesenteric vessels (sandwich sign).[102] On CT, a contiguous nodal conglomerate in any region

that measures greater than 6 cm in longest transverse diameter is considered bulk disease. Inguinal adenopathy is an uncommon presenting finding. Among patients who have HL, 35% have splenic involvement presenting as nodules or generalized splenic enlargement. When present, multiple small nodules in the spleen are more common than large lesions.[101] Adenopathy in the splenic hilum may be seen (**Fig. 12**).[103] Hepatic involvement in the absence of splenic involvement is uncommon.[82,92]

The size of the normal spleen varies with age (**Table 5**).[104]

Renal involvement is rare in pediatric HL.[95] On CT, renal disease may be manifest as diffuse infiltration or multinodular involvement.[82]

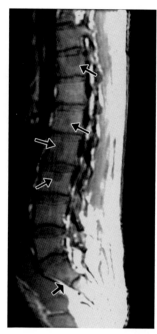

Fig. 25. Sagittal T1 MR image of lumbar spine. DLBCL. A 13-year-old boy who had weight loss, abdominal pain, and diffuse back pain. Multilevel, multifocal, low-signal osseous metastases without acute vertebral collapse (*arrows*).

Cortical bone involvement in HL is rare.[2,82] When present, bone lesions usually are lytic and may have accompanying periosteal reaction. Sclerotic bone lesions are less common and may represent reactive bone formation adjacent to involved soft tissues. Ivory vertebra describes sclerotic involvement of the spine.[95]

At diagnosis, marrow involvement is uncommon except in patients who have LD subtype, where it is present in greater than 50% of cases. Bone marrow involvement is more common in patients who have advanced disease. Although involvement may be diffuse, focal areas of marrow involvement are not uncommon.[52] MR imaging is an excellent imaging modality for evaluating diffuse and spotty marrow involvement. Marrow involvement is characterized by low signal on T1-weighted images, high signal on T2-weighted images, and enhancement after contrast administration.

Primary CNS involvement is rare with HL. CNS involvement with disseminated disease also is uncommon and can present as spinal cord compression and intramedullary cord involvement.[82]

## RADIOGRAPHIC FINDINGS IN NON-HODGKIN LYMPHOMA

Imaging findings vary with the subtype of NHL (**Table 6**).

### Burkitt Lymphoma

Endemic BL has a high propensity for the mandible and maxilla with characteristic involvement of the developing molar teeth. It also may involve the orbit. Abdominal involvement is common with masses and nodes invading the mesentery and omentum. Involvement of the right iliac fossa is uncommon. Liver, spleen, and ovary frequently

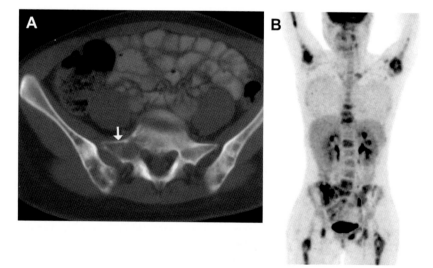

Fig. 26. DLBCL. Primary bone disease. A 12-year-old girl who had diffuse bone pain. CT of the pelvis (*A*) demonstrates multiple lytic destructive lesions in both iliac bones and in the right side of the sacrum (*white arrow*). MIP PET (*B*) shows diffuse osseous disease without evidence of soft tissue involvement.

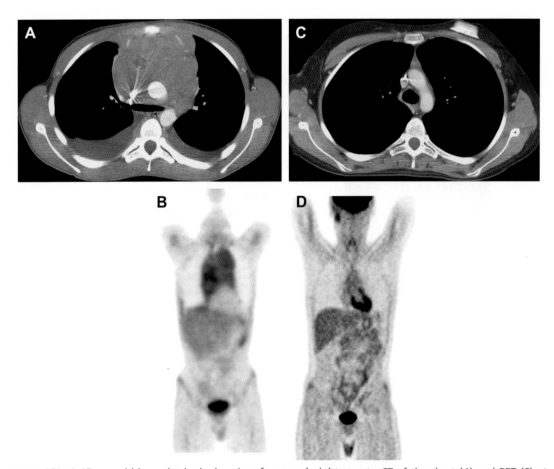

Fig. 27. LBL. A 15-year-old boy who had wheezing, fever, and night sweats. CT of the chest (A) and PET (B) at diagnosis. CT (A) demonstrates a large anterior mediastinal mass displacing the carina and bilateral pleural effusions. PET (B) demonstrates FDG uptake in the anterior mediastinal mass. Imaging after 5 months of therapy demonstrates resolution of the mediastinal mass on CT (C) and PET (D) with no evidence of FDG avid disease.

are involved. Unlike sporadic BL, 60% of these patients demonstrate peripheral adenopathy. Up to 15% of patients present with paraplegia caused by extradural masses extending into the neural canal (Fig. 13) and compressing the spinal cord. CNS disease is seen in up to 30% of patients. Bone marrow involvement is rare.[23]

Sporadic BL is an extranodal disease. The most common presentation is a right lower quadrant abdominal mass that may involve the terminal ileum, cecum, ascending colon, or appendix (Fig. 14). Intussusception is a common presentation of this disease (Fig. 15). Involvement of the liver and spleen is uncommon. Retroperitoneal and mesenteric nodal masses frequently are present (Fig. 16). Any of these masses may cause obstruction of ureters, kidneys, or biliary tree and may lead to gastrointestinal obstruction. Pancreatic involvement is rare (Fig. 17). Malignant ascites frequently

is seen.[105] In girls, ovarian involvement is common. Involvement of the kidneys and omentum also are common (Fig. 18).[106] If the abdominal disease can be completely resected, surgical intervention is indicated. This correlates with a good prognosis. Peripheral adenopathy is uncommon in BL. Mediastinal and pulmonary parenchymal involvement is rare (Fig. 19). Pharyngeal and tonsilor tumors infrequently are seen. Bone involvement is uncommon (Fig. 20). When jaw tumors are present, they do not involve the developing molar teeth, as commonly seen in endemic BL, but may be associated with diffuse bone marrow involvement. Bone marrow involvement is common (22%) (Fig. 21) but CNS involvement is infrequent (12%). Although these may be seen at diagnosis, they are more common in progressive disseminated disease. When present, they signify a poor prognosis.[52]

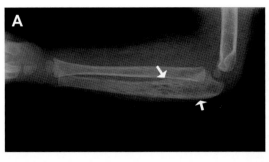

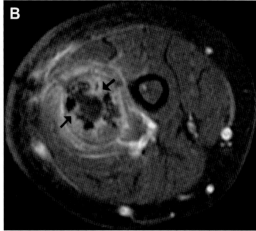

Fig. 28. A 4-year-old boy who had LBL. Left forearm (*A*) and axial T1 postcontrast fat-saturation MR images (*B*). Image of the left forearm (*A*) shows permeative changes and periosteal reaction (*white arrows*). T1 axial postcontrast MR image (*B*) demonstrates cortical destruction (*black arrows*) and enhancing soft tissue mass.

## Diffuse Large B-Cell Lymphoma

Most patients present with disseminated disease.[32] Patients may present with single or multiple masses in nodal and extranodal sites (**Fig. 22**). Patients who have DLBCL who present with disease localized to the mediastinum may be difficult to distinguish from HL. The presence of peripheral adenopathy makes DLBCL the more likely diagnosis. The gastrointestinal tract is the most common extranodal site of involvement (**Fig. 23**). Liver, spleen, and renal involvement occur. Mesenteric and retroperitoneal adenopathy also are seen (**Fig. 24**).[32] In patients who present

with gastrointestinal manifestations, distinction from BL may not be possible. Peripheral adenopathy and bone involvement make DLBCL the more likely diagnosis (**Figs. 25** and **26**).[52] Bone marrow and CNS involvement are rare.[107]

## Lymphoblastic Lymphoma

Anterior mediastinal and/or bulky cervical/supraclavicular adenopathy is characteristic of LBL. Up to 70% of patients have a mediastinal mass, which may cause dyspnea, stridor, head and neck swelling, and superior vena cava syndrome (**Fig. 27**).[32] Malignant pericardial effusion can

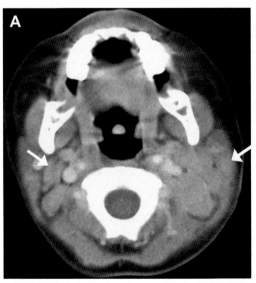

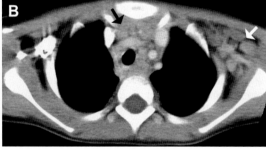

Fig. 29. ALCL. A 5-year-old girl who had fever, night sweats, and left neck pain and swelling. CT of the neck (*A*) demonstrates bilateral lymphadenopathy, left greater than right (*arrows*). CT of the upper thorax (*B*) shows extensive mediastinal (*black arrow*) and left axillary adenopathy (*white arrow*).

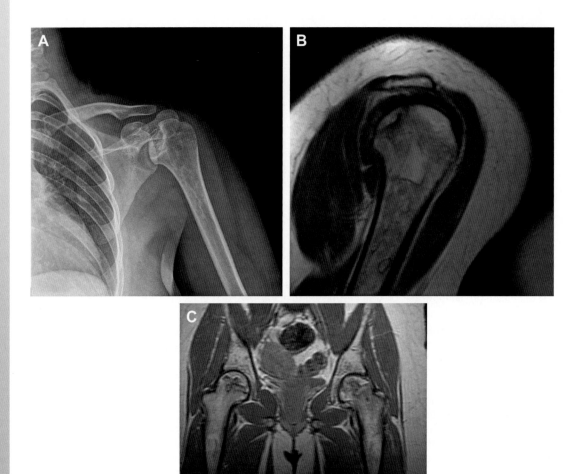

Fig. 30. A 14-year-old girl who had with avascular necrosis of the shoulder post treatment of LBL. Irregular lucency and sclerosis of the humeral head is present on radiograph (A). Signal abnormalities on T2 fast spin-echo MR image shoulder (B) and coronal PD fat-saturation MR image pelvis (C) demonstrate multiple areas of bone infarction.

result from pericardial invasion. Malignant pleural effusion also may be seen.[107] Painless adenopathy in the head and neck, axilla, and inguinal regions may occur. Hepatosplenomegaly may be present but renal involvement is more common. Cross-sectional imaging of the kidneys demonstrates renal enlargement associated with hypoattenuating cortical masses. Dissemination to CNS, bone marrow, or gonads may be present at diagnosis. Bone, soft tissue, and peripheral lymph nodes can be involved (Fig. 28).[108,109]

CNS involvement is common. CNS prophylaxis is given to all patients, even if CNS disease is not detectable at presentation.

### Anaplastic Large Cell Lymphoma

The majority of patients present with disseminated disease. Among patients who have ACLC, 90% present with peripheral adenopathy, an important clinical feature.[110] Mediastinal masses are common (Fig. 29).[111] Retroperitoneal adenopathy

also is seen.[112] The most common sites of extranodal disease include skin, soft tissues, bone, and lung.[45] Masses in the soft tissues and muscles are common. Skin nodules may be single or multiple and may be ulcerated.[113] Lung disease may be manifest as nodules or as infiltrate. Malignant effusions may be present. Bone involvement is common and the lesions may simulate primary bone tumors. Rarely, there is involvement of the pancreas, kidneys, liver, or gastrointestinal tract. CNS and bone marrow involvement are uncommon.[114,115]

### IMMUNODEFICIENCY-ASSOCIATED LYMPHOMAS

BL is the most common form of lymphoma identified in HIV-infected children unlike in adults, in whom DLBCL is more common.[116] Among children who have AIDS, 4% develop primary CNS lymphoma representing the AIDS-defining diagnosis in 0.4% of these children.[117,118] These CNS lymphomas

**Table 7**
**Summary of late effects identifiable with imaging studies**

| Late Effect | Therapy-Related Risk | Factors Associated with Risk | Disease |
|---|---|---|---|
| Breast cancer | Radiation to chest | Increasing doses, female | HL |
| Coronary disease/myocardial infarction | Radiation to chest | Increasing doses | HL |
| Pulmonary fibrosis, interstitial pneumonitis | Bleomycin, radiation to chest | Younger age at treatment Bleomycin dose >400 U/m² | |
| Secondary CNS tumors | Cranial radiation | Increasing dose, younger age at treatment | NHL |
| Hypothyroidism/thyroid cancer | Radiation to thyroid gland (neck, mantle) | Increasing dose, female, younger age at treatment | Both HL and NHL |
| Osteopenia/avascular necrosis | Corticosteroids, high-dose radiation to any bone, methotrexate | Adolescence | Both HL and NHL |
| Cardiomyopathy/congestive heart failure | Anthracyclines | Dose and age related | Both HL and NHL |

*Data from* Robison LL. The Childhood Cancer Survivor Study: a resource for research of long-term outcomes among adult survivors of childhood cancer. Minn Med 2005;88:45–9.

usually are associated with EBV.[119] On imaging studies, solitary or multiple contrast enhancing lesions are seen in the periventricular white matter, in the basal ganglia, or at the gray/white matter interface. The lesions may demonstrate ring enhancement.[117] Extranodal sites of involvement include lung, gastrointestinal tract, and bone.[118]

Congenital immune deficiency syndromes, such as Wiskott-Aldrich syndrome, are associated with an increased incidence of NHL, in particular DLBCL. The risk for malignancy increases with age. These patients develop extranodal disease, including brain involvement.[120]

## RELAPSE

HL can recur in areas original disease and in new sites. Recurrence in retroperitoneal lymph nodes and spleen can be seen, even when these areas initially were disease free.

Evaluation of lymph nodes is essential for diagnosing relapsed or progressive disease, in both HL and NHL. In NHL, evaluation with CT, MR imaging, and PET may be necessary to determine the full extent of the relapse. New PET-based criteria for evaluating response to therapy have been developed.[121]

## LATE EFFECTS

Although advances in the therapy for childhood lymphoma have resulted in improved survival, treatment-related long-term effects are seen.

Secondary neoplasms occur in all form of childhood lymphoma, more commonly in HL than in NHL.[122,123] In patients who have HL, the risk of secondary leukemia plateaus 10 to 15 years post therapy.[122] Autologous stem cell transplantation for the treatment of lymphoma is associated with secondary myelodysplastic syndrome and acute myelogenous leukemia. The incidence of NHL after HL is reported to be 4% to 8%.[92] The risk for secondary solid malignancies, including sarcoma; melanoma; and lung, thyroid, gastrointestinal, brain, and breast cancer, increases with time and is greater in patients who are younger at diagnosis and relapse. There is an increased incidence of hypothyroidism and thyroid cancer in patients receiving mantle radiation.[92,117,124]

Lymphoma survivors exposed to anthracycline or thoracic radiation are at risk for long-term cardiac toxicity, including delayed pericarditis, pancarditis, pericardial and myocardial fibrosis, functional valve injury, conduction defects, and coronary artery disease.[52,125] Anthracycline is particularly associated with cardiomyopathy. Younger age at diagnosis and female gender are risk factors for developing cardiomyopathy.[126]

Pulmonary fibrosis is an uncommon sequela of childhood lymphoma. It is more common in patients who have received radiation therapy than in those who have received pulmonary toxic chemotherapy, such as bleomycin.[127]

Radiation effects on the ovary are age and dose dependent, increasing with age.

Avascular necrosis is a not infrequent complication of steroid therapy and radiation therapy in children who have lymphoma (**Fig. 30**).[52]

**Table 7** describes the more common treatment-related complications in childhood lymphoma that are identifiable on imaging.

## SUMMARY

HL and NHL represent 10% to 15% of all malignancies occurring in children younger than 20. Advances in cross-sectional imaging and the increasing availability of PET and PET-CT have had a major impact on the imaging and management of pediatric patients. This article reviews the clinical features of lymphoma and focuses on the spectrum of imaging findings seen in the diagnosis, staging, and follow-up of pediatric patients who have HL and NHL. Pediatric NHL is divided into four major histologic subtypes: BL, DLBCL, ALCL, and LBL. The most important subtype of HL is NS.

## ACKNOWLEDGMENTS

The authors wish to thank Ms. Evelyn Tolliver-Lopez and Ms. Rachel Kronman for their help in the preparation of this manuscript.

## REFERENCES

1. Percy CL, Smith M, Linet M, et al. Lymphomas and reticuloendothelial neoplasms. In: Ries LAG, S M, Gurney JG, et al, editors. Cancer incidence and survival among children and adolescents: United States SEER Program. Bethesda (MD): NIH; 1999. p. 35–50.
2. Parker BR, Castellino RA. Hodgkin's disease. St. Louis (MO): CV Mosby; 1977.
3. Jackson H Jr, Parker FJ. Hodgkin's disease and allied disorders. New York: Oxford University Press; 1947.
4. Portis T, Dyck P, Longnecker R. Epstein-Barr Virus (EBV) LMP2A induces alterations in gene transcription similar to those observed in Reed-Sternberg cells of Hodgkin lymphoma. Blood 2003;102: 4166–78.
5. Fingeroth JD, W J, Tedder TF, et al. Epstein-Barr virus receptor of human B lymphocytes is the C3d receptor CR2. Proc Natl Acad Sci U S A 1984;81: 4510–4.
6. Jarrett RF. Risk factors for Hodgkin's lymphoma by EBV status and significance of detection of EBV genomes in serum of patients with EBV-associated Hodgkin's lymphoma. Leuk Lymphoma 2003; 44(Suppl 3):S27–32.
7. Gandhi MK, Tellam JT, Khanna R. Epstein-Barr virus-associated Hodgkin's lymphoma. Br J Haematol 2004;125:267–81.
8. Massarweh S, Udden MM, Shahab I, et al. HIV-related Hodgkin's disease with central nervous system involvement and association with Epstein-Barr virus. Am J Hematol 2003;72:216–9.
9. Glaser SL, Clarke CA, Gulley ML, et al. Population-based patterns of human immunodeficiency virus-related Hodgkin lymphoma in the Greater San Francisco Bay Area, 1988–1998. Cancer 2003;98: 300–9.
10. Lukes RJ, Butler JJ. The pathology and nomenclature of Hodgkin's disease. Cancer Res 1966;26: 1063–83.
11. Hudson MM, Donaldson SS. Hodgkin's disease. Pediatr Clin North Am 1997;44:891–906.
12. Hutchinson RE, Uner A. Biology and pathology of Hodgkin's disease. In: Weinstein HJ, Hudson MM, Link MP, editors. Pediatric lymphomas. Berlin: Springer-Verlag; 2007. p. 7–27.
13. Cairo MS, Raetz E, Perkins SL, et al. Non-Hodgkin's lymphomas in children. London: B.C. Decker Inc.; 2003.
14. Sandlund JT, Downing JR, et al. Non-Hodgkin's lymphoma in childhood. N Engl J Med 1996;334: 1238–48.
15. Burkitt DP. The discovery of Burkitt's lymphoma. Cancer 1983;51:1777–86.
16. Ferry JA. Burkitt's Lymphoma: clinicopathologic features and differential diagnosis. Oncologist 2006;11:375–83.
17. Iverson O, Iverson U, et al. Cell kinetics in Burkitt's lymphoma. Eur J Cancer 1974;10:1507–12.
18. Sanger W. Primary (8q24) and secondary chromosome abnormalities (1q, 6q, 13q, 17p) are similar in pediatric Burkitt lymphoma/Burkitt leukemia & Burkitt-like lymphoma: a report of the international pediatric B-cell non-Hodgkin lymphoma study. Blood 2003;102:845a.
19. Diebold J. Burkitt lymphoma. In: Jaffe E, Harris N, Stein H, et al, editors. Pathology and genetics of tumours of haematopoietic and lymphoid tissues. Washington, DC: IARC Press; 2001. p. 181–4.
20. The Non-Hodgkin's Lymphoma Classification Project. National Cancer Institute sponsored study of classifications of non-Hodgkin's lymmphomas: summary and description of a working formulation for clinical usage. Cancer 1982;49:2112.
21. Burkitt D. A sarcoma involving the jaws in African children. Br J Surg 1958;46:218–23.
22. van den Bosch CA. Is endemic Burkitt's lymphoma an alliance between three infections and a tumour promoter? Lancet Oncol 2004;5:738–46.
23. Magrath IT. African Burkitt's lymphoma. History, biology, clinical features, and treatment. Am J Pediatr Hematol Oncol 1991;13:222–46.

24. Blum KA, Lozanski G, Byrd JC. Adult Burkitt leukemia and lymphoma. Blood 2004;104:3009–20.

25. Hecht JL, Aster JC. Molecular biology of Burkitt's lymphoma. J Clin Oncol 2000;18:3707–21.

26. Young L, Alfieri C, Hennessy K, et al. Expression of Epstein-Barr virus transformation-associated genes in tissues of patients with EBV lymphoproliferative disease. N Engl J Med 1989;321(16): 1080–5.

27. McClain KL, Joshi VV, Murphy SB. Cancers in children with HIV infection. Hematol Oncol Clin North Am 1996;10:1189–201.

28. Gong JZ, Stenzel TT, Bennett ER, et al. Burkitt lymphoma arising in organ transplant recipients: a clinicopathologic study of five cases. Am J Surg Pathol 2003;27:818–27.

29. Knowles DM. Etiology and pathogenesis of AIDS-related non-Hodgkin's lymphoma. Hematol Oncol Clin North Am 2003;17:785–820.

30. Carbone A, Gloghini A. AIDS-related lymphomas: from pathogenesis to pathology. Br J Haematol 2005;130:662–70.

31. Patte C, Auperin A, Michon J, et al. The Societe Francaise d'Oncologie Pediatrique LMB89 protocol: highly effective multiagent chemotherapy tailored to the tumor burden and initial reponse in 561 unselected children with B-cell lymphomas and L3 leukemia. Blood 2001;97:3370–9.

32. Shukla NN, Trippett TM. Non-Hodgkin's lymphoma in children and adolescents. Curr Oncol Rep 2006;8:387–94.

33. Seidemann K, Tiemann M, Lauterbach J, et al. Primary mediastinal large B-cell lymphoma with sclerosis in pediatric and adolescent patients: treatment and results from three therapeutic studies of the Berlin-Frankfurt-Munster Group. J Clin Oncol 2003;21(9):1782–9.

34. Rosenwald A, Wright G, Leroy K, et al. Molecular diagnosis of primary mediastinal B-cell lymphoma identifies a clinically favorable subgroup of diffuse large B-cell lymphoma related to Hodgkin lymphoma. J Exp Med 2003;198:851–62.

35. Savage KJ, Monti S, Kutok JL, et al. The molecular signature of mediastinal large B-cell lymphomas and shares features with classical Hodgkin lymphoma. Blood 2003;102:3871–9.

36. Lones MA, Perkins SL, Sposto R, et al. Large-cell lymphoma arising in the mediastinum in children and adolescents is associated with an excellent outcome: a Children's Cancer Group report. J Clin Oncol 2000;18:3845–53.

37. Cotelingham J, Witesby E, et al. Malignant lymphoma in patients with the Wiscott-Aldrich syndrome. Cancer Investigation 1985;3:515–22.

38. Preciado MV, Fallo A, Chabay P, et al. Epstein Barr virus-associated lymphoma in HIV-infected children. Pathol Res Pract 2002;198(5):327–32.

39. van Krieken JH. Lymphoproliferative disease associated with immune deficiency in children. Am J Clin Pathol 2004;122:S122–7.

40. Perkins SL, Morris SW. Biology and pathology of pediatric non-hodgkin lymphoma. In: Weinstein HJ, Hudson MM, Link MP, editors. Pediatric lymphomas. Berlin: Springer Verlag; 2007. p. 91–127.

41. Heerema N, Poirel H, Swansbury J, et al. Chromosomal abnormalities of pediatric (ped) and adult diffuse large B-cell lymphoma (DLBCL) differ and may reflect potential differences in oncogenesis. An international pediatric mature B-cell non-Hodgkin lymphoma study (FAB/LMB96). Blood 2003;102:3139.

42. Perkins SL. Work-up and diagnosis of pediatric non-Hodgkin's lymphomas. Pediatr Dev Pathol 2000;3:374–90.

43. Reddy KS, Perkins SL. Advances in the diagnostic approach to childhood lymphoblastic malignant neoplasms. Am J Clin Pathol 2004;122:S3–18.

44. Reiter A. Anaplastic large-cell lymphoma. In: Weinstein HJ, Hudson MM, Link MP, editors. Pediatric lymphomas. Berlin: Springer Verlag; 2007. p. 175–92.

45. Brugieres L, Deley MC, Pacquement H, et al. CD30(+) anaplastic large-cell lymphoma in chidlren: analysis of 82 patients enrolled in two consecutive studies of the French Society of Pediatric Oncology. Blood 1998;92:3591–8.

46. Alessandri AJ, Pritchard SL. A population-based study of pediatric anaplastic large cell lymphoma. Cancer 2002;94:1830–5.

47. Massimino M, Gasparini M, Giardini R. Ki-1 (CD30) anaplastic large-cell lymphoma in children. Ann Oncol 1995;6(9):915–20.

48. Kinney M, Collins R, Greer JP, et al. A small-cell predominant variant of primary Ki-1 (CD30)+ T-cell lymphoma. Am J Surg Pathol 1993;17(9): 859–68.

49. Kinney MC, Kadin ME. The pathologic and clinical spectrum of anaplastic large cell lymphoma and correlation with ALK gene dysregulation. Am J Clin Pathol 1999;111:S56–67.

50. Goldsby RE, Carroll WL. The molecular biology of pediatric lymphmas. J Pediatr Hematol Oncol 1998;20:282–96.

51. Oertel J, Huhn D. Immunocytochemical methods in haematology and oncology. J Cancer Res Clin Oncol 2000;126:425–40.

52. Weinstein HJ, Hudson MD, Ling MP. Pediatric lymphomas. Berlin: Springer; 2007.

53. Tschammler A, Ott G, Schang T, et al. Lymphadenopathy: differentiation of benign from malignant disease–color Doppler US assessment of intranodal angioarchitecture. Radiology 1998;208: 117–23.

54. Kellenberger CJ, Miller SF, Khan M, et al. Initial experience with FSE STIR whole-body MR imaging for staging lymphoma in children. Eur Radiol 2004;14:1829–41.

55. Bar-Shalom R, Mor M, Yefremov N, et al. The value of Ga-67 scintigraphy and F-18 fluorodeoxyglucose positron emission tomography in staging and monitoring the response of lymphoma to treatment. Semin Nucl Med 2001;31:177–90.

56. Kaste SC, Shulkin BL. 18F-Fluorodeoxyglucose PET/CT in childhood lymphomas. PET Clinics 2006;1:265–73.

57. Rini JN, Leonidas JC, Tomas MB, et al. 18F-FDG PET versus CT for evaluating the spleen during initial staging of lymphoma. J Nucl Med 2003;44:1072–4.

58. Depas G, De Barsy C, Jerusalem G, et al. 18F-FDG PET in children with lymphomas. Eur J Nucl Med Mol Imaging 2005;32:31–8.

59. Miller E, Metser U, Avrahami G, et al. Role of 18F-FDG PET/CT in staging and follow-up of lymphoma in pediatric and young adult patients. J Comput Assist Tomogr 2006;30:689–94.

60. Edeline V, Bonardel G, Brisse H, et al. Prospective study of 18F-FDG PET in pediatric mediastinal lymphoma: a single center experience. Leuk Lymphoma 2007;48:823–6.

61. Montravers F, McNamara D, Landman-Parker J, et al. [(18)F]FDG in childhood lymphoma: clinical utility and impact on management. Eur J Nucl Med Mol Imaging 2002;29:1155–65.

62. Yamamoto F, Tsukamoto E, Nakada K, et al. 18F-FDG PET is superior to 67Ga SPECT in the staging of non-Hodgkin's lymphoma. Ann Nucl Med 2004;18:519–26.

63. Hudson MM, Krasin MJ, Kaste SC. PET imaging in pediatric Hodgkin's lymphoma. Pediatr Radiol 2004;34:190–8.

64. Jerusalem G, Beguin Y, Fassotte MF, et al. Whole-body positron emission tomography using 18F-fluorodeoxyglucose for posttreatment evaluation in Hodgkin's disease and non-Hodgkin's lymphoma has higher diagnostic and prognostic value than classical computed tomography scan imaging. Blood 1999;94:429–33.

65. Spaepen K, Stroobants S, Dupont PL, et al. Prognostic value of positron emission tomography (PET) with fluorine-18 fluorodeoxyglucose ([18F]FDG) after first-line chemotherapy in non-Hodgkin's lymphoma: is [18F]FDG-PET a valid alternative to conventional diagnostic methods? J Clin Oncol 2001;19:414–9.

66. Bar-Sever Z, Keidar Z, Ben-Barak A, et al. The incremental value of 18F-FDG PET/CT in pediatric malignancies. Eur J Nucl Med Mol Imaging 2007;34(5):630–7.

67. Hernandez-Pampaloni M, Takalkar A, Yu JQ, et al. F-18 FDG-PET imaging and correlation with CT in staging and follow-up of pediatric lymphomas. Pediatr Radiol 2006;36:524–31.

68. Mody RJ, Bui C, Hutchinson RJ, et al. Comparison of (18)F Flurodeoxyglucose PET with Ga-67 scintigraphy and conventional imaging modalities in pediatric lymphoma. Leuk Lymphoma 2007;48:699–707.

69. Furth C, Denecke T, Steffen I, et al. Correlative imaging strategies implementing CT, MRI, and PET for staging of childhood Hodgkin disease. J Pediatr Hematol Oncol 2006;28:501–12.

70. Weinblatt ME, Zanzi I, Belakhlef A, et al. False-positive FDG-PET imaging of the thymus of a child with Hodgkin's disease. J Nucl Med 1997;38:888–90.

71. Meany HJ, Gidvani VK, Minniti CP. Utility of PET scans to predict disease relapse in pediatric patients with Hodgkin lymphoma. Pediatr Blood Cancer 2007;48:399–402.

72. Kaste SC, Howard SC, McCarville EB, et al. 18F-FDG-avid sites mimicking active disease in pediatric Hodgkin's. Pediatr Radiol 2005;35:141–54.

73. Hollingshead LM, Goa KL. Recombinant granulocyte colony-stimulating factor (rG-CSF). A review of its pharmacological properties and prospective role in neutropenic conditions. Drugs 1991;42:300–30.

74. Jadvar H, Connolly LP, Fahey FH, et al. PET and PET/CT in pediatric oncology. Semin Nucl Med 2007;37:316–31.

75. Jerusalem G, Hustinx R, Beguin Y, et al. Evaluation of therapy for lymphoma. Semin Nucl Med 2005;35:186–96.

76. Spaepen K, Stroobants S, Dupont P, et al. Early restaging positron emission tomography with (18)F-fluorodeoxyglucose predicts outcome in patients with aggressive non-Hodgkin's lymphoma. Ann Oncol 2002;13:1356–63.

77. Spaepen K, Stroobants S, Verhoef G, et al. Positron emission tomography with [(18)F] FDG for therapy response monitoring in lymphoma patients. Eur J Nucl Med Mol Imaging 2003;30:S97–105.

78. Zinzani PL, Chierichetti F, Zompatori M, et al. Advantages of positron emission tomography (PET) with respect to computed tomography in the follow-up of lymphoma patients with abdominal presentation. Leuk Lymphoma 2002;43:1239–43.

79. Zinzani PL. Lymphoma: diagnosis, staging, natural history, and treatment strategies. Semin Oncol 2005;32:S4–10.

80. Frush DP. Imaging evaluation of the thymus and thymic disorders in children. In: Lucaya J, Strife JL, editors. Pediatric chest imaging: chest imaging in infants and children. New York: Springer Verlag; 2002. p. 187–208.

81. Francis IR, Glazer GM, Bookstein FL, et al. The thymus: reexamination of age-related changes in size and shape. AJR Am J Roentgenol 1985;145:249–54.

82. Toma P, Granata C, Rossi A, et al. Multimodality imaging of Hodgkin disease and non-Hodgkin lymphomas in children. Radiographics 2007;27:1335–54.

83. Siegel MJ, Glazer HS, Wiener JI, et al. Normal and abnormal thymus in childhood: MR imaging. Radiology 1989;172:367–71.

84. Sklair-Levy M, Agid R, Sella T, et al. Age-related changes in CT attenuation of the thymus in children. Pediatr Radiol 2000;30:566–9.

85. Swischuk LE, John SD. Normal thymus extending between the right brachiocephalic vein and the innominate artery. AJR Am J Roentgenol 1996;166:1462–4.

86. Smith CS, Schoder H, Yeung HW. Thymic extension in the superior mediastinum in patients with thymic hyperplasia: potential cause of false-positive findings on 18F-FDG PET/CT. AJR Am J Roentgenol 2007;188:1716–21.

87. Bogot NR, Quint LE. Imaging of thymic disorders. Cancer Imaging 2005;5:139–49.

88. Michel F, Gilbeau JP, Six C, et al. Progressive mediastinal widening after therapy for Hodgkin's disease. Acta Clin Belg 1995;50:282–7.

89. Levine JM, Weiner M, Kelly KM. Routine use of PET scans after completion of therapy in pediatric Hodgkin disease results in a high false positive rate. J Pediatr Hematol Oncol 2006;28:711–4.

90. Lister TA, Crowther D, Sutcliffe SB, et al. Report of a committee convened to discuss the evaluation and staging of patients with Hodgkin's disease: Cotswolds meeting. J Clin Oncol 1989;7:1630–6.

91. Rademaker J. Hodgkin's and Non Hodgkin's lymphomas. In: Hricak H, Panicek DM, editors. Radiologic clinics of North America: update on radiologic evaluation of common malignancies. Philadelphia: Elsevier/Saunders; 2007. p. 69–83.

92. Sullivan MP. Hodgkin's disease in children. Hematol Oncol Clin North Am 1987;1:603–20.

93. Murphy S. Childhood non-Hodgkin's lymphoma. N Engl J Med 1978;299:1446–8.

94. Donaldson SS, Link MP. Childhood lymphomas: Hodgkin's disease and non-Hodgkin's lymphoma. Baltimore (MD): Williams and Wilkins; 1986.

95. Parker BR. Leukemia and lymphoma in childhood. Radiol Clin North Am 1997;35:1495–516.

96. Mandell GA, Lantieri R, Goodman LR. Tracheobronchial compression in Hodgkin lymphoma in children. AJR Am J Roentgenol 1982;139:1167–70.

97. Jeffrey GM, Mead GM, Whitehouse JMA. Life-threatening airway obstruction at the presentation of Hodgkin's disease. Cancer 1991;67:506–10.

98. Blinova GA, Kolygin BA. Clinical and morphological correlation of Hodgkin's disease in children. Tumori 1973;59:409–18.

99. Krikorian JG, Portlock CS, Mauch PM. Hodgkin's disease presenting below the diaphragm: a review. J Clin Oncol 1986;4:1551–62.

100. Au V, Leung AN. Radiologic manifestations of lymphoma in the thorax. AJR Am J Roentgenol 1997;168:93–8.

101. White KS. Thoracic imaging of pediatric lymphomas. J Thorac Imaging 2001;16:224–37.

102. Mueller PR, Ferrucci JT Jr, Harbin WP, et al. Appearance of lymphomatous involvement of the mesentery by ultrasonography and body computed tomography: the "sandwich sign". Radiology 1980;134:467–73.

103. Neumann CH, Parker BR, Castellino RA. Hodgkin's disease and the non-Hodgkin's lymphoma. New York: Pergamon; 1985.

104. Rosenberg HK, Markowitz RI, Kolbeg H, et al. Normal splenic size in infants and children: sonographic measurements. AJR Am J Roentgenol 1991;157:119–21.

105. Boerma EG, van Imhoff GW, Appel IM, et al. Gender and age-related differences in Burkitt lymphoma–epidemiological and clinical data from The Netherlands. Eur J Cancer 2004;40:2781–7.

106. Magrath I. Small noncleaved cell lymphomas (Burkitt and Burkitt-like lymphomas). In: Magrath I, editor. The non Hodgkin's lymphomas. 2nd edition. New York: Arnold; 1997. p. 781–811.

107. Magrath IT. Malignant Non-Hodgkin's lymphomas and practice of pediatric oncology. In: Pizzo PA, Poplack DG, editors. Principles and practices of pediatric oncology. Philadelphia: Lippincott/Williams and Wilkins; 2002. p. 661–705.

108. Lin P, Jones D, Dorfman DM, et al. Precursor B-cell lymphoblastic lymphoma: a predominantly extranodal tumor with low propensity for leukemic involvement. Am J Surg Pathol 2000;24:1480–90.

109. Neth O, Seidemann K, Jansen P, et al. Precursor B-cell lymphoblastic lymphoma in childhood and adolescence: clinical features, treatment, and results in trials NHL-BFM 86 and 90. Med Pediatr Oncol 2000;35:20–7.

110. Reiter A, Schrappe M, Tiemann M, et al. Successful treatment strategy for Ki-1 anaplastic large-cell lymphoma of childhood: a prospective analysis of 62 patients enrolled in three consecutive Berlin-Frankfurt-Munster Group Studies. J Clin Oncol 1994;12:899–908.

111. Williams DM, Hobson R, Imeson J, et al. Anaplastic large-cell lymphoma in childhood: analysis of 72 patients treated on The United Kingdom Children's Cancer Study Group chemotherapy regimens. Br J Haematol 2002;117:812–20.

112. Mori T, Kiyokawa T, Shimada H, et al. Anaplastic large-cell lymphoma in Japanese children: retrospective analysis of 34 patients diagnosed at the National Research Institute for Child Health and Development. Br J Haematol 2003;121:94–6.

113. Kadin ME, Sako D, Berliner N, et al. Childhood Ki-1 lymphoma presenting with skin lesions and peripheral lymphadenopathy. Blood 1986;68: 1042–9.

114. Sandlund JT, Pui CH, Roberts WM, et al. Clincopathologic features and treatment outcome of children with large-cell lymphoma and the t(2;5)(p23;q35). Blood 1994;84:2467–71.

115. Sandlund JT, Pui CH, Santana VM, et al. Clinical features and treatment outcome for children with CD30+ large-cell non-Hodgkin's lymphoma. J Clin Oncol 1994;12:895–8.

116. McClain KL, Leach CT, Jenson HB, et al. Molecular and virologic characteristics of lymphoid malignancies in children with AIDS. J Acquir Immune Defic Syndr 2000;23:152–9.

117. Jeanes AC, Owens CM. Imaging of HIV disease in children. Imaging 2002;14:8–23.

118. Mueller BU. Cancers in human immunodeficiency virus-infected children. J Natl Cancer Inst Monogr 1998;23:31–5.

119. Fallo A, De Matteo E, Preciado MV, et al. Epstein-Barr virus associated with primary CNS lymphoma and disseminated BCG infection in a child with AIDS. Int J Infect Dis 2005;9:96–103.

120. Gilson D, Taylor RE. Long-term survival following non-Hodgkin's lymphoma arising in Wiskott-Aldrich syndrome. Clin Oncol (R Coll Radiol) 1999;11: 283–5.

121. Cheson BD, Pfistner B, Juweid ME, et al. Revised response criteria for malignant lymphoma. J Clin Oncol 2007;25:579–86.

122. Bhatia S, Yasui Y, Robison LL, et al. High risk of subsequent neoplasms continues with extended follow-up of childhood Hodgkin's disease: report from the late effects study group. J Clin Oncol 2003;21:4386–94.

123. Inskip PD. Thyroid cancer after radiotherapy for childhood cancer. Med Pediatr Oncol 2001;36: 568–73.

124. Acharya S, Sarafoglou K, LaQuaglia M, et al. Thyroid neoplasms after therapeutic radiation for malignancies during childhood or adolescence. Cancer 2003;97:2397–403.

125. Adams MJ, Lipsitz SR, Colan SD, et al. Cardiovascular status in long-term survivors of Hodgkin's disease treated with chest radiotherapy. J Clin Oncol 2004;22:3139–48.

126. Kremer LC, Caron HN. Anthracycline cardiotoxicity in children. N Engl J Med 2004;351:120–1.

127. Mertens AC, Yasui Y, Liu Y, et al. Pulmonary complications in survivors of childhood and adolescent cancer. A report from the Childhood Cancer Survivor Study. Cancer 2002;95:2431–41.

# Imaging of Lymphoma of the Central Nervous System, Spine, and Orbit

Sofia Haque, MD[a,b,*], Meng Law, MD[c],
Lauren E. Abrey, MD[d,e], Robert J. Young, MD[a,b]

**KEYWORDS**
- Lymphoma • Primary CNS lymphoma (PCNSL)
- Non-Hodgkin lymphoma • Magnetic resonance (MR)
- Computed tomography (CT) • Spectroscopy • Perfusion
- Diffusion tensor

Both systemic lymphoma and primary central nervous system (CNS) lymphoma (PCNSL) may directly involve the neuraxis. These non-Hodgkin lymphomas (NHL) are usually caused by the malignant transformation of B lymphocytes, although some systemic T-cell lymphomas can also have high rates of CNS involvement. A total of 10% to 15% of patients with systemic lymphoma have CNS disease caused by disseminated disease. This number may vary depending on the definition of CNS involvement by imaging, clinical, or cerebrospinal fluid (CSF) criteria, with most disseminated disease manifesting in the CSF.

PCNSL represents 1% of all lymphomas, less than 5% of all NHLs, and only 3% to 5% of all primary brain tumors.[1] The increased incidence that has occurred since the 1990s cannot be explained simply by increased imaging.[2] Most PCNSL are aggressive malignancies of the diffuse large B-cell lymphoma type. Patients with PCNSL should have disease that is restricted entirely to the brain, eye, and spinal cord; careful extent of disease evaluation in patients with presumed PCNSL discovers a reservoir of systemic disease in 4% to 8% of the patients.[3,4]

Lymphomas are aggressive malignancies that require rapid diagnosis. Imaging findings that are suggestive for lymphoma should preclude corticosteroid therapy and facilitate stereotactic biopsy rather than resection. Evidence of CSF or ocular involvement or vitrectomy may be used to provide the tissue diagnosis if present without brain biopsy.

## PART I: INTRACRANIAL LYMPHOMA
### Clinical Features

The clinical prodrome is relatively short, as most cases are diagnosed within 1 to 2 months after the onset of symptoms. The presentation is determined by the location and size of the tumor, and may include nonspecific focal neurologic deficits, behavioral and personality changes, headaches, hydrocephalus, or seizures. Although systemic lymphoma can present with focal enhancing mass lesions like PCNSL, systemic lymphoma

a Department of Radiology, Memorial Sloan-Kettering Cancer Center, 1275 York Avenue, MRI-1159, New York, NY 10065, USA
b Department of Radiology, New York Presbyterian Hospital/Weill Cornell Medical College, New York, NY, USA
c Departments of Radiology and Neurosurgery, Mount Sinai Medical Center, One Gustave L. Levy Place, New York, NY 10029, USA
d Department of Neurology, Memorial Sloan-Kettering Cancer Center, 1275 York Avenue, New York, NY 10065, USA
e Department of Neurology, New York Presbyterian Hospital/Weill Cornell Medical College, New York, NY, USA
* Corresponding author. Department of Radiology, Memorial Sloan-Kettering Cancer Center, 1275 York Avenue, MRI-1159, New York, NY 10065.
E-mail address: haques@mskcc.org (S. Haque).

Radiol Clin N Am 46 (2008) 339–361
doi:10.1016/j.rcl.2008.04.003

more typically manifests with disseminated leptomeningeal disease.

## Prognosis

The overall survival of patients with PCNSL is significantly worse than that in patients with similar types of extranodal NHL. The most widely accepted prognostic factors are age and performance status at time of diagnosis.[5] Poor prognostic factors include disease in deep brain structures, decreased performance status, increased patient age, increased serum lactate dehydrogenase, and increased CSF protein.[6] With an increased number of risk factors, the 2-year survival falls from 80% to 48% to 15%.[6]

## Imaging Evaluation

The initial study for most patients with new neurologic signs or symptoms is a noncontrast CT scan, particularly for patients with acute findings or who present to the emergency department. This noncontrast CT is then followed by a contrast study. PCNSL involves the supratentorial brain in 87% of cases.[7] Typical locations include the cerebral hemispheres, periventricular white matter, deep gray matter, corpus callosum, subependymal region, and adjacent to other CSF spaces (**Fig. 1**). Lymphomas of the corpus callosum are nearly double the size of lymphomas at other locations.[8] Atypical locations for PCNSL include the brainstem, cranial nerves, cavernous sinuses, pineal gland, and pituitary gland (**Fig. 2**). The tendency to abut the ependymal surface in 28% to 38% or meningeal surface in 8% to 13% may reflect the PCNSL origin from the periadventitial cells of arterioles penetrating through the Virchow-Robin spaces in these regions (**Fig. 3**).[9,10,11,12] The imaging differences between immunocompetent and immunocompromised patients are summarized in **Table 1**.

## Immunocompetent Patients

Lymphoma is usually hyperdense on noncontrast CT scans because of its high cellularity and nucleus-to-cytoplasm ratio. On MR imaging, this high cellularity results in tumors that are isointense to hypointense relative to gray matter on T1-weighted images, and isointense to hypointense on T2-weighted images.[9] With iodinated (CT) or gadolinium (MR imaging) contrast agent, more than two thirds of tumors reveal moderate to intense homogeneous enhancement and mild to absent peritumoral edema.[9,12] Focal tumors that are hyperintense on T2-weighted images and have moderate heterogeneous to absent enhancement may represent low-grade lymphomas.[13]

Lymphoma may also uncommonly present as diffusely infiltrative or nonenhancing lesions.

## Immunocompromised Patients

Disruption of the normal immune system from any cause (eg, HIV and AIDS; posttransplant pharmacologic immunosuppression; congenital diseases, such as IgA deficiency, severe combined immunodeficiency, and ataxia-telangiectasia) is an important risk factor for PCNSL.

The immunocompromised patient is more likely to have lymphoma occur in an atypical location. Intratumoral calcifications and blood products are uncommon but may be seen (**Figs. 4** and **5**). Nearly one half of immunocompromised patients have heterogeneous, often peripheral rim-enhancing tumors with cystic or necrotic components and marked peritumoral edema,[9] whereas some may have no enhancement at all. The presence of necrosis and heterogeneous enhancement are important differences between the imaging appearance of lymphoma in immunocompromised versus immunocompetent patients.

## Differential Diagnosis

The typical imaging features of lymphoma can be used to narrow the differential diagnosis, initiate stereotactic biopsy, and prompt chemotherapy and radiation therapy. The different diagnostic clues are discussed next.

### Signal intensity

Lymphoma shows prominent CT hyperdensity and MR imaging T2 shortening (hypointense signal) because of its high nucleus-to-cytoplasm ratio and relatively low intratumoral water content. This hypointense T2 signal distinguishes lymphoma from other lesions that usually demonstrate hyperintense T2 signal, such as gliomas, metastases, and demyelinating disease. Some highly cellular gliomas may also show hypointense T2 signal, but these are much more likely to contain blood products, have infiltrative margins, and reveal heterogeneous enhancement. Blood products are more typical for metastatic disease from melanoma, renal cell, breast, and lung carcinomas. These metastases are usually located at the gray-white junctions and often incite marked peritumoral edema, unlike the little peritumoral edema of lymphoma.

### Corpus callosum

The main differential possibility for lymphoma centered at the corpus callosum is a glioblastoma multiforme. These high-grade gliomas show hemorrhagic and cystic-necrotic changes with heterogeneous enhancement in 95%, compared with lymphomas that are usually homogeneous with

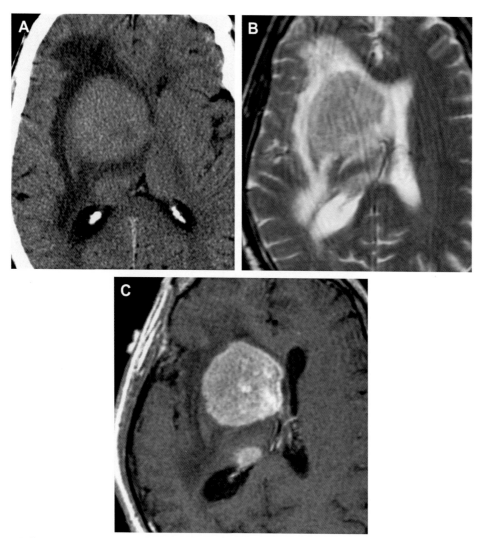

**Fig. 1.** Multifocal PCNSL in the right basal ganglia and thalamus. The tumors are hyperdense on axial noncontrast CT (*A*), hypointense to isointense (relative to gray matter) on T2-weighted image (*B*), and homogeneously enhancing on contrast T1-weighted image (*C*). Mass effect compresses the right lateral ventricle and causes mild contralateral midline shift.

solid enhancement (unless the patient is immunocompromised) (**Fig. 6**). Subependymal disease may occur in both lymphoma and high-grade glioma. Involvement of the corpus callosum by metastatic or demyelinating disease is much less common than callosal involvement by lymphoma, although the incidence of lymphoma is overall much lower than these two diseases.

### Extra-axial disease

Leptomeningeal lymphoma is a common manifestation of systemic lymphoma. PCNSL usually causes focal enhancing masses in the brain parenchyma and spares the extra-axial spaces. Leptomeningeal disease portends a worse prognosis for patients with systemic lymphoma. More than

two thirds of the patients do not have any symptoms, whereas some may present with cranial nerve palsies.[14] Contrast T1-weighted and fluid-attenuated inversion recovery images are the most sensitive ways to detect subarachnoid space disease, although the leptomeningeal disease can occasionally be visible on CT as hyperdense masses even without contrast (**Fig. 7**). Leptomeningeal disease is nonspecific and may alternatively occur after invasion by other primary and systemic malignancies into the subarachnoid spaces.

Dural disease usually reflects involvement by systemic lymphomas. Dural lymphoma may also represent a low-grade marginal zone subtype. These present as hyperdense dural-based enhancing tumors that may be mistaken for

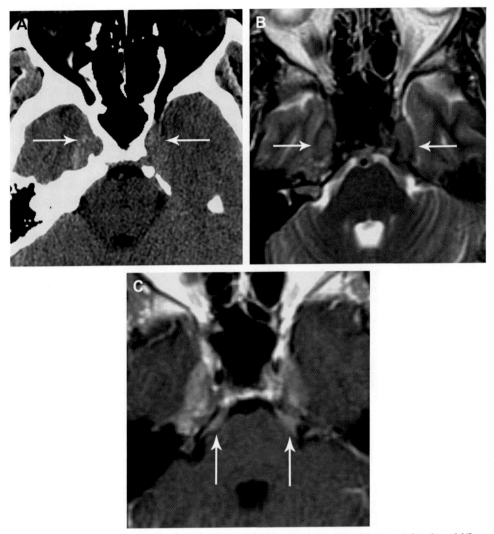

**Fig. 2.** Cavernous sinus and perineural PCNSL in AIDS. (*A*) Axial noncontrast CT, (*B*) T2-weighted, and (*C*) contrast T1-weighted images reveal tumor filling the cavernous sinuses (*arrows, A*), Meckel's caves (*arrows, B*), and perineural disease along the cisternal trigeminal nerves (*arrows, C*). The tumor is hyperdense on CT and nearly isointense on T2-weighted images.

meningiomas. Most patients have complete responses and excellent local control, although the risk for systemic relapse is high, possibly related to the dura mater lying outside the normal blood-brain barrier.[15]

### Immunocompromised patients

In the immunocompromised patient, a heterogeneous, peripherally enhancing lymphoma with cystic-necrotic areas may mimic a brain abscess. Careful inspection of the T2-weighted images may reveal a thin hypointense peripheral rim around the brain abscess that represents free radicals released by the inflammatory process.[16] Deep gray matter and periventricular lymphoma may be mistaken for infections, such as toxoplasmosis.

Lymphoma and toxoplasmosis may both present as single, multiple, or coexisting collision (containing both tumor and infection) lesions. Despite these overlapping features, lymphoma is favored if a solitary hyperdense mass lesion is found or if subependymal extension or ventricular encasement is present (**Fig. 8**).[17] Accurate distinction is important because prompt, appropriate therapy for lymphoma can more than triple life expectancy in the immunocompromised patient.[18] Diffuse periventricular enhancement without a focal mass lesion in an immunocompromised patient with lymphoma may also mimic infectious ventriculitis, most commonly from cytomegalovirus infection. Posttransplant lymphoproliferative disorder may present with similar peripherally

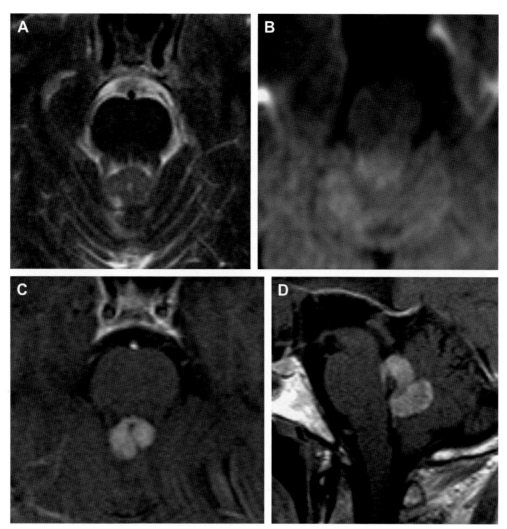

**Fig. 3.** Intraventricular PCNSL. (*A*) Axial T2-weighted, (*B*) diffusion-weighted, and (*C*) axial and (*D*) sagittal contrast T1-weighted images demonstrate a lobulated tumor in the fourth ventricle, which was initially thought to represent an ependymoma or medulloblastoma. Both lymphoma and medulloblastoma may show diffusion restriction; medulloblastoma is usually round and arises from the roof of the fourth ventricle.

enhancing mass lesions and surrounding edema. Correlation with the patient's clinical history is important, because the primary treatment in these cases is reduced immunosuppression and antiviral therapy for Epstein-Barr infection.[19]

## INTRAVASCULAR LYMPHOMA

Intravascular lymphoma is an extremely rare type of systemic large B-cell lymphoma that deserves mention because of its strong CNS predilection. The disease is limited to the lumens of medium to small blood vessels including the capillary beds. The diagnosis is often difficult because of nonspecific imaging features that are similar to other vasculitides and ischemic diseases.[20] Patients may present with multiple small

fluctuating T2 hyperintense, diffusion restricted, and enhancing lesions.[21] Intravascular lymphoma may follow a relapsing-remitting or relapsing-progressive clinical course caused by fluctuating ischemic damage by the small vascular occlusions. The spinal cord is often involved, although the sensitivity of MR imaging is poor.[21] These cases require a strong index of suspicion, an aggressive work-up, and low threshold for biopsy.[22] If skin nodules are present, sampling these often reveals the diagnosis.

## OCULAR AND ORBITAL LYMPHOMA

Primary intraocular lymphomas are an uncommon form of NHL that can be considered a subtype of PCNSL. Up to 80% of patients with primary ocular

**Table 1**
**Differences in brain lymphoma between immunocompetent and immunocompromised patients**

|  | Immunocompetent | Immunocompromised |
|---|---|---|
| Age (mean) | 60 (years) | 30 |
| Multiple lesions | 30%–50% | 63%–81% |
| Necrotic change | Rare | Common |
| *CT* |  |  |
| Density | Hyperdense | Hyperdense |
| Enhancement | Homogeneous | Heterogeneous |
| *MR imaging* |  |  |
| T1 signal | Iso- to hypo- | Iso- to hypo- |
| T2 signal | Iso- to hypo- | Iso- to hypo- |
| Enhancement | Homogeneous | Heterogeneous |

*Data from* Refs. [8,9,17,18,60].

lymphoma go on to develop PCNSL in the brain, whereas only 10% to 20% of patients with PCNSL have ocular involvement.[23,24] The median age is 65 years in immunocompetent patients and younger in immunocompromised patients.[25] CT and MR imaging are usually normal, although occasionally enhancing soft tissue mass lesions may be seen involving the vitreous, choroid, iris, ciliary body, retina, or optic nerve.[26] Tumor cells in the vitreous may cause decreased or blurry vision. Near half of the patients with primary ocular lymphoma have bilateral disease, which along with a corticosteroid refractory course is helpful in distinguishing lymphoma from chronic intermediate or posterior uveitis.

Lymphomas of the orbit usually reflect orbital spread of systemic NHL, although only 1.3% of patients with systemic lymphoma have orbital involvement.[27] Mucosa-associated lymphoid tissue lymphoma is the most common primary NHL of the orbit. The median age is 63 years.[28] Proptosis, visual disturbances, diplopia, and restricted motion are common symptoms, but unlike orbital pseudotumor patients do not complain of pain. The tumors are hyperdense on CT, hypointense on T1-weighted images, and hypointense to hyperintense on T2-weighted images with homogeneous enhancement. These are typically soft tumors that mold to rather than destroy the confining bony rim; bone erosion is rare unless the tumor

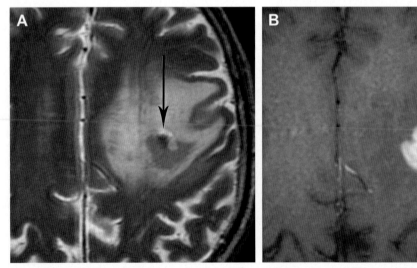

**Fig. 4.** Hemorrhagic PCNSL in the left centrum semiovale. (*A*) Axial T2-weighted image demonstrates focal hypointense blood products (*arrow*) at the anterior margin of the enhancing tumor seen on the (*B*) contrast T1-weighted image.

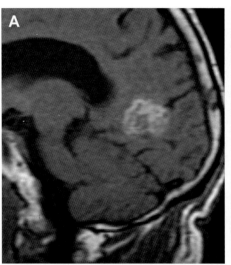
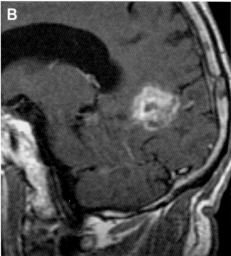

Fig. 5. Parietal occipital T-cell lymphoma. Sagittal (A) precontrast and (B) postcontrast T1-weighted images show abundant hyperintense blood products and mild heterogeneous enhancement.

has high-grade histology. Any portion of the orbit may be affected in a focal or diffuse manner (**Figs. 9** and **10**). The imaging features are not specific and often mimic other tumors, such as metastatic disease from systemic tumors and primary lacrimal gland tumors.

## SPINAL LYMPHOMA

Lymphoma of the spine may occur, in decreasing order of frequency, in the bony, extradural-epidural, intradural extramedullary, or intradural intramedullary compartments.

Spinal epidural lymphoma is usually caused by local invasion of the epidural space from systemic lymphoma of the adjacent vertebral or paravertebral disease. Epidural lymphoma presents as an isointense, homogeneous tumor that spans multiple segments and may extend through the neural foramina.

Leptomeningeal lymphoma in the intradural extramedullary space usually reflects hematogenous dissemination or perineural extension of systemic lymphoma. Primary leptomeningeal lymphoma in the absence of any parenchymal lesions is uncommon. The leptomeningeal tumor can manifest with enhancing nodular mass lesions along the surface of the cord or with nerve root thickening and enhancement (**Fig. 11**). The nodules are usually isointense relative to the cord on T1- and T2-weighted images.

Intramedullary lymphoma is the least common form of PCNSL. Most cases of spinal cord lymphoma are not isolated disease but instead represent secondary invasion of the spinal cord by disseminated leptomeningeal disease (**Fig. 12**).[29] These are poorly circumscribed T1 isointense, T2 hyperintense intramedullary mass lesions with variable enhancement that may be patchy, confluent, infiltrating, or discrete.

### Differential Diagnosis

A spinal epidural or subdural hematoma may show signal characteristics similar to lymphoma, but these often contain hyperintense blood products and the patients should have more acute clinical presentations. An epidural abscess typically shows peripheral rather than solid enhancement and has associated diskitis-osteomyelitis inflammatory changes in the adjacent bone. Epidural metastases from carcinomas and sarcomas are usually associated with adjacent expansile bone disease and reveal hyperintense T2 signal that is greater than that of epidural lymphoma and adjacent fat.

It is often not possible to distinguish leptomeningeal lymphoma from other neoplastic, granulomatous, and infectious causes of leptomeningeal disease. In these cases, the patient's clinical history, CSF analysis, and imaging of the brain and total spine are important.

Intramedullary lymphomas are distinctly less common than other spinal cord tumors. Lymphoma usually does not have an associated cystic or hemorrhagic component, as opposed to other tumors, such as astrocytomas and ependymomas. Transverse myelitis may have a very similar appearance. Of the other poorly circumscribed, isointense to slightly hyperintense T2 signal lesions in the spinal cord, posttraumatic contusion

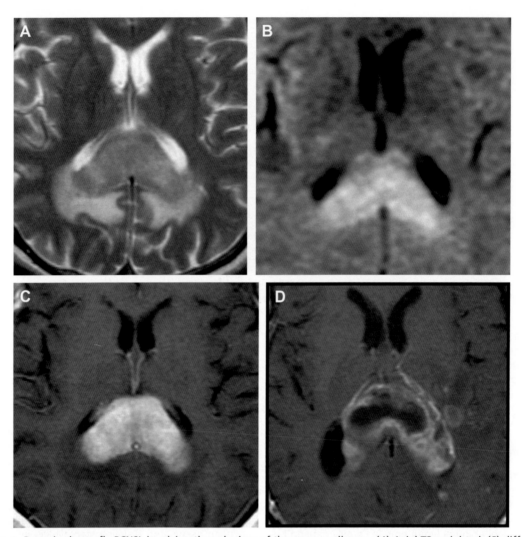

**Fig. 6.** Posterior butterfly PCNSL involving the splenium of the corpus callosum. (*A*) Axial T2-weighted, (*B*) diffusion-weighted, and (*C*) contrast T1-weighted images demonstrate a homogeneously enhancing tumor with diffusion restriction at the splenium of the corpus callosum. The companion case glioblastoma (*D*) also located in the corpus callosum is heterogeneously enhancing and has marked cystic-necrotic changes that could mimic lymphoma in an immunocompromised patient; these features are less common in an immunocompetent patient.

can be excluded by history, spondylotic myelopathy by the lack of abnormal enhancement, and demyelinating disease by finding typical lesions in the brain.

## NEUROLYMPHOMATOSIS

Neurolymphomatosis is a rare form of NHL that manifests by lymphoma infiltration of cranial and peripheral nerves, plexii, and roots. Nearly three fourths of patients later develop systemic lymphoma and one fourth reveal evidence of PCNSL.[30] Patients may present with painful mononeuropathy or polyneuropathy. If isolated, a nerve biopsy is necessary for diagnosis. The prognosis is similar to that of PCNSL. CT has poor sensitivity for neurolymphomatosis but may

show fusiform or nodular thickening of the affected nerve or plexus. With MR imaging, the lymphomatous nerve shows hypointense to isointense T1 signal and hyperintense T2 and short tau inversion recovery signal. The enhancement is variable with both modalities. Fluorine-18 fluoro-2-deoxyglucose positron emission tomography (PET) can reveal hypermetabolic activity localized to the nerve and can be very useful for disease diagnosis and management (**Fig. 13**).

## TREATMENT AND MANAGEMENT

Lymphoma is highly sensitive to both radiation therapy and chemotherapy, including corticosteroids. Corticosteroids induce cytolysis or

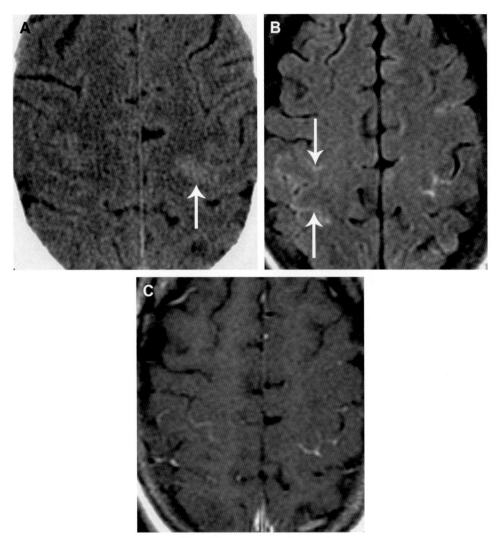

Fig. 7. PCNSL in an AIDS patient. (*A*) Axial noncontrast CT shows a hyperdense mass lesion in the left central sulcus (*arrow*). In addition to the left central sulcus disease, fluid-attenuated inversion recovery image (*B*) also demonstrates T2 hyperintense subarachnoid space disease in the right paracentral sulci (*arrows*), and contrast T1-weighted image (*C*) confirms the bilateral enhancing leptomeningeal disease.

apoptosis and can cause significant tumor regression and clinical improvement. Although useful for symptomatic treatment, steroids can interfere with biopsy results and definitive pathologic diagnosis. Use of steroids can cause complete disappearance of contrast-enhancing abnormalities on CT and MR imaging. Most of these responses are transient, however, and almost all patients develop resistance after long-term treatment with steroids. In addition, other intracranial processes, such as multiple sclerosis, sarcoidosis, and occasionally gliomas, can respond similarly to steroid treatment. For these reasons, steroids should be avoided in suspected but undiagnosed PCNSL, with the exception of patients who show evidence of overt or impending brain herniation. Similarly,

debulking surgery is only useful for relief of symptoms from herniation and does not improve patient survival. Stereotactic needle biopsy for histopathologic examination is preferred, followed by chemotherapy and radiation therapy. During and after therapy, multiplanar contrast MR imaging is the imaging modality of choice, but some patients may undergo precontrast and postcontrast CT scans at the same time as whole-body CT or PET-CT imaging.

High-dose methotrexate-based regimens given before radiation therapy have improved response rates and patient survival. Therapy-related neurotoxicity is a problem that affects nearly all patients greater than 60 years. Newer regimens aim to minimize such toxicity while maintaining the survival

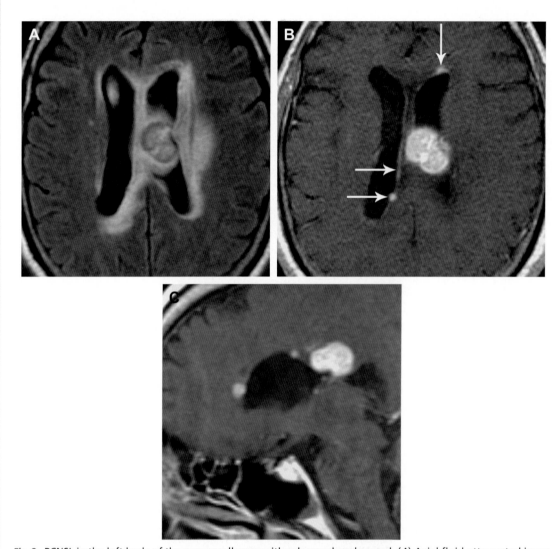

**Fig. 8.** PCNSL in the left body of the corpus callosum with subependymal spread. (*A*) Axial fluid-attenuated inversion recovery image shows the lobulated T2 hypointense tumor and moderate periventricular T2 hyperintense changes. (*B*) Contrast axial and (*C*) sagittal T1-weighted images reveal nodular enhancement of the dominant callosal tumor and additional linear and nodular enhancement along the ventricular margins (*arrows*).

benefit of combined modality treatment. The standard dose of whole-brain radiation therapy is 40 to 50 Gy, although induction chemotherapy may allow a reduction in the whole-brain radiation therapy dose to 23.4 Gy and avoid neurocognitive decline.[31] No benefit is noted with the addition of a radiation boost to the tumor bed.[1] Doses of radiation can be adjusted to account for age and response to chemotherapy, but targeted or image-guided radiation is not useful because patients treated with focal radiation therapy suffer unacceptably high recurrence rates outside of the radiation field and in treated ports.[1] This is because PCNSL is a diffusely infiltrative malignancy that is often underestimated by imaging, despite the appearance of well-circumscribed

enhancing tumors on CT and MR imaging. Although available chemotherapy and radiation therapy protocols induce complete remission in approximately 80%, nearly all patients remain at high risk for recurrence at any location including sites distant from the original disease, such as the brain, eyes, spine, CSF, or systemic (**Figs. 14 and 15**). The risk for relapse is 50% to 60%, with most (80%) occurring within 2 years of the diagnosis.

## RESPONSE CRITERIA

The International Primary CNS Lymphoma Collaborative Group developed standardized baseline evaluation, response criteria, and outcome measures for immunocompetent patients with PCNSL

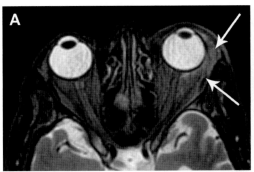
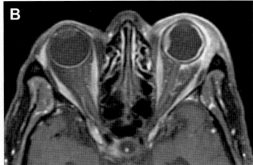

Fig. 9. Systemic lymphoma involving the orbit. Axial (A) fat-saturated T2-weighted image and (B) contrast axial T1-weighted image show enhancing tumor in the anterior left orbit centered at the lacrimal fossa (arrows) with circumferential involvement of the globe, which reveals abnormal scleral, choroid, and retinal enhancement. There is also infiltration of the conjunctiva and eyelids.

enrolled in clinical trials.[32] Patients can be stratified into complete response (CR), unconfirmed complete response (CRu), partial response (PR), and progressive disease (PD) categories (Table 2). These guidelines are based on changes in the contrast-enhancing mass lesions, with size measured using the single largest dimension or two perpendicular dimensions. For example, an enhancing lesion with a greater than 50% decrease in size from 2 × 2 cm to 0.5 × 0.5 cm is considered a PR.

Complete ophthalmologic including slit-lamp examination is required for patients with ocular disease at baseline; CSF analysis is required for patients with abnormal CSF cytology at baseline.

Patients must be corticosteroid free for a minimum of 2 weeks to be considered CR; otherwise, they are categorized as CRu. Corticosteroids are irrelevant for the PR and PD categories. PET has not been incorporated into the standardized criteria for PCNSL because only limited data regarding its use are currently available. The clinically determined primary end points of event-free survival, progression-free survival, and overall survival should be complemented by routine MR imaging monitoring for at least 10 years to detect recurrent disease and late treatment-related neurotoxicity. No standardized criteria have been developed for immunocompromised patients.

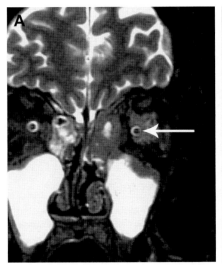
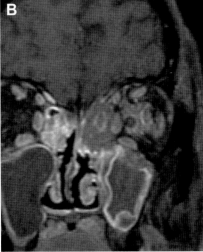

Fig. 10. Human T-cell lymphotropic type 1–associated cutaneous T-cell lymphoma. Coronal (A) T2-weighted and (B) contrast T1-weighted images demonstrate hypointense enhancing tumor infiltrating from the paranasal sinus into the left orbit with encasement of the optic nerve (arrow). Tumor is also present in the left maxillary sinus roof. The more marked T2 hyperintense and peripherally enhancing inflammatory changes in the remaining maxillary sinuses and right ethmoid sinus are readily distinguished from tumor.

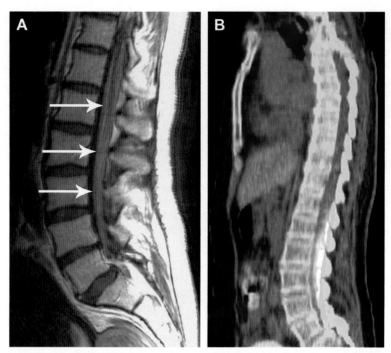

**Fig.11.** Leptomeningeal PCNSL. (*A*) Sagittal contrast T1-weighted image shows enhancing leptomeningeal disease in the lumbar spine coating the distal spinal cord, conus, and cauda equina (*arrows*). (*B*) Sagittal fused PET-CT reveals corresponding hypermetabolic activity.

## PART II: FUNCTIONAL IMAGING OF BRAIN LYMPHOMA

Functional imaging of brain lymphoma provides information about tumor biology that goes beyond the gross anatomic changes seen with standard contrast CT and MR imaging studies. Biophysiologic data can be obtained about tumor metabolism, metabolite formation, water diffusion, microvascularity, and blood-brain barrier permeability. This information can be used to improve diagnostic accuracy for lymphoma (**Table 3**).[33,34,35]

## NUCLEAR MEDICINE

PET and PET-CT are useful to stage systemic lymphoma and to predict and monitor treatment responses.[4] The most common radiopharmaceutical is the glucose analogue fluorine-18 fluoro-2-deoxyglucose, which has a reported sensitivity of 87% for brain disease, 80% sensitivity for spinal disease, but only 20% sensitivity for orbital disease.[3] The disproportionate accumulation by viable tumor cells and tumor-associated macrophages means that many lymphomas show increased activity at PET (**Fig. 16**). The normal high background brain activity makes it difficult to assess lymphomas that have lower uptake at initial presentation and lymphomas with lower residual uptake after treatment, although PET is commonly used to make clinical management decisions.

The older single-photon emission CT studies retain usefulness when PET is not readily available. The most common single-photon emission CT tracer is thallium-201. Thallium single-photon emission CT is particularly useful in the immunocompromised patient to diagnosis hypermetabolic lymphoma rather than hypometabolic toxoplasmosis with 55% to 100% sensitivity and 85% to 100% specificity.[36,37,38] The sensitivity and specificity are improved if the contrast-enhancing lesions are greater than a critical size of 2 cm.[39] Both PET-CT and thallium single-photon emission CT can distinguish recurrent lymphoma (increased activity) from treatment necrosis (decreased to absent activity) after chemotherapy and radiation therapy.

## DIFFUSION IMAGING

Diffusion-weighted imaging reflects the macromolecular motion of extracellular water, and is very helpful in distinguishing lymphoma from other tumors and tumor-mimicking lesions. The high cellularity of lymphoma decreases the extracellular space and restricts the normal random or brownian motion of water molecules. This is readily apparent as tumor hyperintensity on diffusion-weighted imaging and hypointensity on apparent

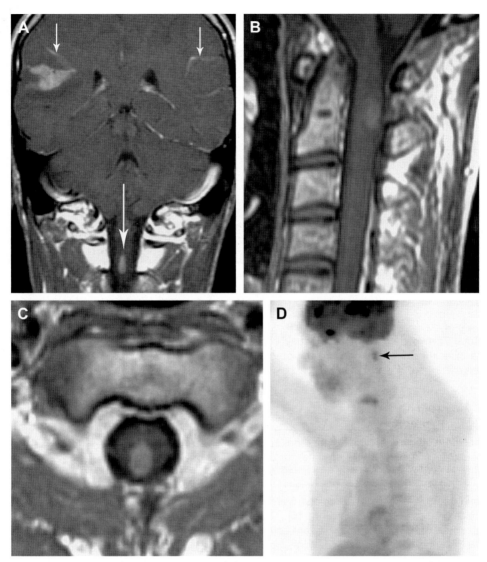

Fig. 12. Meningeal lymphoma from a systemic NHL. (A) Coronal contrast T1-weighted image of the brain reveals bilateral perisylvian leptomeningeal disease with right brain invasion and edema (*short arrows*), and intramedullary lymphoma of the cervical cord (*long arrow*). (B) Sagittal and (C) axial contrast T1-weighted images reveal a focal T2 hyperintense, homogeneously enhancing tumor in the dorsal midline cervical cord. (D) Oblique sagittal FDG-PET shows the hypermetabolic cord (*arrow*) and multiple brain tumors, which are poorly seen against the normal high background brain FDG activity.

diffusion coefficient (ADC) maps. Decreased ADC is suggestive for increased cellularity.[40] A lesion with restricted diffusion with an ADC threshold value of $1.1 \times 10^{-3}$ mm$^2$/s has been recommended to help differentiate lymphoma from other intracranial masses lesions.[34] During treatment, increasing ADC values suggest positive response to therapy, whereas decreasing ADC values suggest tumor progression.[41]

Diffusion tensor imaging takes advantage of the highly ordered directionality of white matter (WM) fibers caused by preferential water diffusion along the longitudinal axes of axons and myelin sheaths.[42,43,44] The two most common metrics are fractional anisotropy (FA) that measures diffusion directionality, and mean diffusivity (MD) as derived from the ADC maps that measures diffusion magnitude. Increasing tumor cellularity has been correlated with decreasing fractional anisotropy (FA) and increasing mean diffusivity (MD).[45] Corticosteroids can be problematic if given to reduce edema and mass effect before the diagnosis of lymphoma is definitely established; reductions in tumor enhancement, diffusion restriction, and

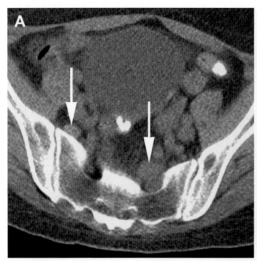
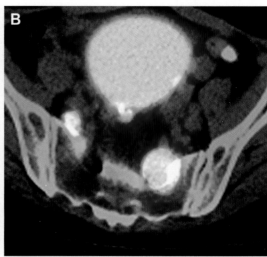

Fig. 13. Neurolymphomatosis in a patient with progressive foot pain and weakness. Axial noncontrast CT (*A*) and fused FDG–PET and CT (*B*) show thickening of the bilateral sacral nerves (*arrows*) and corresponding hypermetabolic activity.

peritumoral T2 hyperintensity and MD may confuse the clinical picture and obscure the correct diagnosis.[46]

### Differential Diagnosis

The diffusion restriction of lymphoma is not specific because diffusion bright lesions include other tumors, such as high-grade gliomas and cystic-necrotic metastases, and nonmalignancies, such as acute stroke and cerebritis or cerebral abscess (see **Figs. 3, 6,** and **16**). The minimal ADC values of lymphoma are lower than the minimal ADC values for high-grade gliomas, although there is some overlap with metastases.[47] Expressed as a ratio relative to normal-appearing brain, the ADC ratio of lymphoma is also lower than that of high-grade gliomas; this correlates with histologic estimates of greater cellularity and nuclear-to-cytoplasm ratios in lymphoma than in high-grade gliomas (1.45 versus 0.24).[40] Similarly, the ADC of lymphoma is lower than that of toxoplasmosis in the immunocompromised patient.[48] Acute infarcts also demonstrate diffusion restriction but should be located within a vascular distribution, have classic clinical signs and symptoms, and show reduced or delayed perfusion.

Lymphoma demonstrates a more marked decrease in FA and in ADC than glioblastoma multiforme, which is the most common differential consideration (**Fig. 17**).[49] Most other tumors also show less marked decreases in FA than lymphoma. Brain abscesses may cause increased

FA because of up-regulated adhesive molecules and aggregated leukocytes.[50]

### PERFUSION IMAGING

MR perfusion imaging allows estimation of tumoral angiogenesis and permeability at the capillary level. MR perfusion imaging can be used to help establish the diagnosis of lymphoma before histopathologic confirmation, and can be used to assist management and treatment issues. Dynamic susceptibility contrast imaging uses the signal decrease that occurs with injection of gadolinium contrast to calculate perfusion measures. Lymphoma has a characteristic angiocentric growth pattern at histopathology with perivascular tumor infiltration that surrounds blood vessels with multiple cell layers and late vascular invasion (**Fig. 18**). Only mild increases in relative cerebral blood volume (rCBV) are observed. In some settings, particularly when the lymphoma is very cellular or there is considerable perivascular or intravascular tumor infiltration, the rCBV may actually be decreased.[51] Lymphoma also shows a typical increase in the intensity-time curve above baseline because of marked leakage of contrast into the interstitial space, in contrast to most other tumors.[52]

### Differential Diagnosis

A large, avidly enhancing mass lesion with marked mass effect and surrounding edema-type changes is usually thought to represent a high-grade glioma until proved otherwise. High-grade gliomas induce

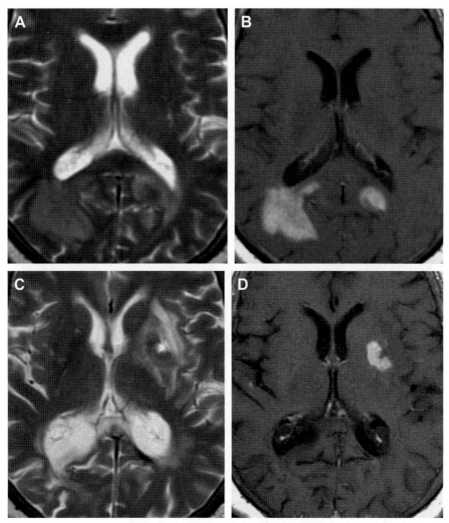

**Fig. 14.** Remote PCNSL lymphoma recurrence. (*A*) Axial T2-weighted and (*B*) contrast T1-weighted images reveal enhancing tumors in the bilateral parietal occipital lobes and splenium of the corpus callosum. (*C*) Axial T2-weighted and (*D*) contrast T1-weighted images obtained 3 years later reveal lymphoma recurrence in the left basal ganglia. Note mild gliotic posttherapeutic changes at the original disease sites.

abundant endothelial proliferation and neovascularity that manifest with markedly increased perfusion and increased permeability, features that are absent in lymphomas. These gliomas display marked increases in rCBV that are double to triple the increased rCBV of lymphoma.[47,52,53] Gliomas also show increased peritumoral rCBV and increased choline of high-grade gliomas because of infiltrating tumor cells in the T2 hyperintense nonenhancing abnormality,[54] features that are absent in the bland peritumoral edema of lymphoma and metastases. The peripherally enhancing portion of a brain abscess, such as toxoplasmosis, shows decreased perfusion with rCBV slightly less than normal white matter.[55] Lymphoma may be thought of as having mildly increased or occasionally decreased perfusion that is less

than that of high-grade gliomas but more than that of infections.

## SPECTROSCOPIC IMAGING

Proton MR spectroscopy provides for the semi-quantitative evaluation of metabolites, such as N-acetylaspartate (NAA), choline, creatine, lactate, and lipids. Lymphoma typically shows decreased NAA, decreased creatine, increased choline, and present lipid-lactate peaks (**Fig. 19**).[56] The NAA decrease reflects decreased neuronal density and variability in the tumor, the creatine decrease suggests higher tumor metabolism and energy consumption, and the choline increase indicates phosphorylcholine and glycerophosphorylcholine release by cell membrane

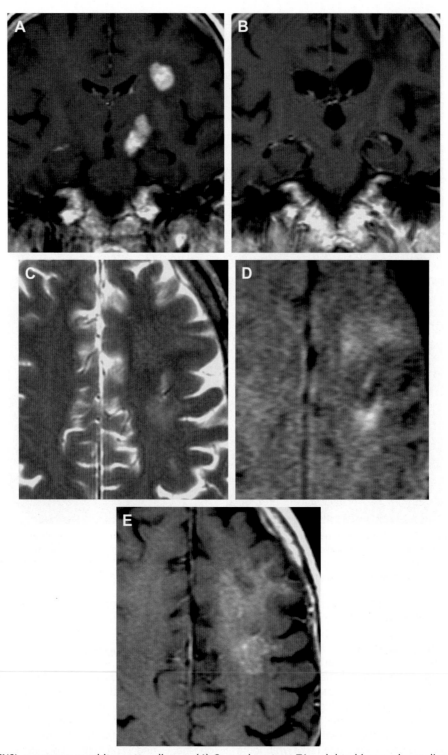

**Fig. 15.** PCNSL recurrence as white matter disease. (*A*) Coronal contrast T1-weighted image shows discontinuous lobulated enhancing tumors in the left centrum semiovale and midbrain along the region of the corticospinal tract. Two years later, (*B*) coronal contrast T1-weighted image shows resolution of the original tumors. At that time, (*C*) axial T2-weighted and (*D*) diffusion-weighted images reveal new confluent lesions in the frontal subcortical and deep white matter. (*E*) Contrast T1-weighted image demonstrates abnormal enhancement consistent with recurrent tumoral disease rather than posttherapeutic or microvascular change.

**Table 2**
**Response for primary central nervous system lymphoma**

| Response | Brain Imaging | Corticosteroid Dose | Eye Examination | CSF Cytology |
|---|---|---|---|---|
| CR | No contrast enhancement | None | Normal | Negative |
| CRu | No contrast enhancement | Any | Normal | Negative |
| | Minimal abnormality | Any | Minor RPE abnormality | Negative |
| PR | 50% decrease in enhancing tumor[a] | Irrelevant | Minor RPE abnormality or normal | Negative |
| | No contrast enhancement | Irrelevant | Decrease in vitreous cells or retinal infiltrate | Persistent or suspicious |
| PD | 25% increase in esion | Irrelevant | Recurrent or new ocular disease | Recurrent or positive |
| | Any new site of disease: central nervous system or systemic | | | |

*Abbreviations:* CR, complete response; CRu, unconfirmed complete response; CSF, cerebrospinal fluid; PD, progressive disease; PR, partial response; RPE, retinal pigment epithelium.
[a] Lesion size may be determined using a single or two perpendicular measurements.
*Data from* Abrey LE, Batchelor TT, Ferreri AJ. Report of an international workshop to standardize baseline evaluation and response criteria for primary CNS lymphoma. J Clin Oncol 2005;23(22):5034–43.

**Table 3**
**Advanced imaging characteristics of masslike lymphoma lesions of the brain versus other lesions**

| | Lymphoma | High-Grade Gliomas | Metastasis | Infection |
|---|---|---|---|---|
| *MR imaging* | | | | |
| DWI | Hyper- | Hypo- > hyper- | | Hyper- |
| ADC minimum | Hypo- | Hyper- > hypo- | Hyper- | Hypo- |
| ADC (x10-3 mm²/s) | 0.51–0.63 | 0.75–0.96 | 0.68–2.2 | 0.7 |
| ADC ratio (tumor/normal) | 0.83–1.15 | 1.26–1.68 | | |
| *DTI* | | | | |
| FA | 0.14 | 0.16–0.23 | 0.14 | 0.13–0.44 |
| *Perfusion* | | | | |
| rCBV | 1.0–2.3 | 3.7–6.3 | 3.1–5.2 | 0.7–0.9 |
| *Spectroscopy* | | | | |
| Cho | Increased | Increased | Increased | Increased |
| Cho/Cr | 2.05–3.12 | 3.92–4.12[a] | 1.84–4.56 | 1.48 |
| NAA | Decreased | Decreased | Decreased | Decreased |
| Lipid/lactate | Present | Present | Present | Present[b] |
| *FDG-PET* | | | | |
| Uptake | Increased | Increased | Increased | Decreased |

*Abbreviations:* ADC, apparent diffusion coefficient; Cho, choline; Cr, creatine; DWI, diffusion-weighted imaging; DTI, diffusion tensor imaging; FA, fractional anisotropy; FDG, fluorodeoxyglucose; NAA, *N*-acetylaspartate; PET, positron emission tomography; rCBV, relative cerebral blood volume.
[a] Peritumoral Cho/Cr also increased (>2.3) because of infiltrating tumor cells.
[b] Short TE (30 ms) preferred to show minor metabolites, such leucine, isoleucine, valine, alanine, acetate, succinate, glycine rather than usual long TE (144 ms).
*Data from* Refs. [34,35,47,49,50,54,57,61,62].

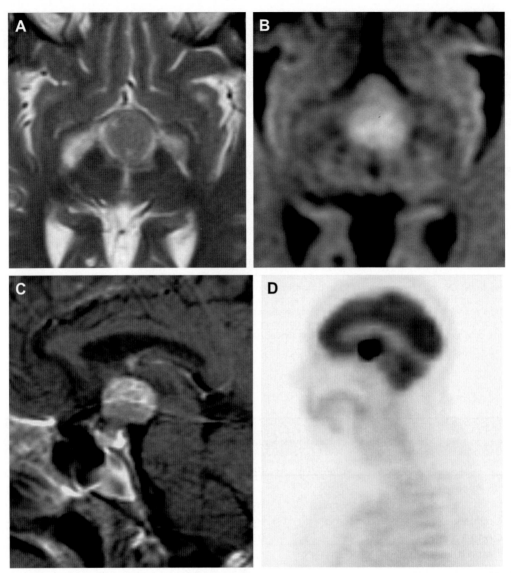

**Fig. 16.** PCNSL of the infundibulum. (*A*) Axial T2-weighted image demonstrates a rounded tumor and mild adjacent basal ganglia edema. (*B*) Axial diffusion-weighted image reveals corresponding diffusion restriction that helps to distinguish hyperintense lymphoma from hypointense nongranulomatous diseases, such as sarcoidosis. Highly cellular germinomas that may also have diffusion restriction are often separable on clinical grounds. (*C*) Sagittal contrast T1-weighted image shows homogeneous enhancement, whereas (*D*) sagittal FDG-PET demonstrates marked hypermetabolic activity.

destruction or synthesis. Increasing Cho/NAA and Cho/Cr ratios indicate tumor progression and perhaps increased aggressiveness but do not correlate with increased tumor grade. Often because of the very high cellularity of lymphoma, the Cho concentration can be very high, even greater than in high-grade gliomas. The lactate represents anaerobic glycolysis after failed aerobic oxidation in areas of ischemia, or accumulation similar to lipid because of poor washout in cystic-necrotic regions. The presence of lactate or lipid at baseline is associated with poor progression-free and

overall survival.[57] Lactate and lipid as necrosis signatures have also been demonstrated in immunocompromised patients with lymphoma.[35]

## Differential Diagnosis

The spectral pattern of lymphoma is not specific, because similar spectra may be seen with metastases and high-grade gliomas. NAA should be absent in metastases, because metastases reflect the primary systemic tumor and lack neuroglial elements.[58] In practical terms, however, the

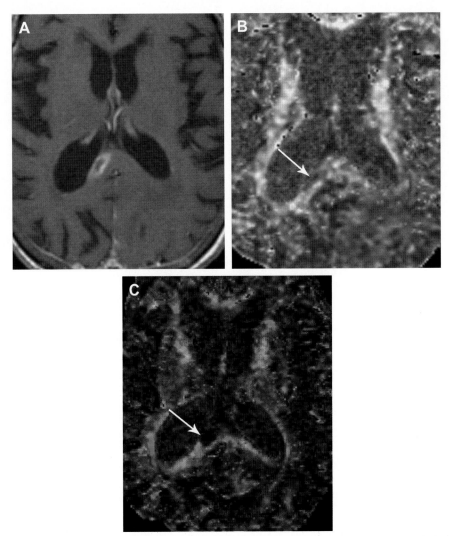

**Fig. 17.** PCNSL of the right splenium of the corpus callosum. (*A*) Axial contrast T1-weighted image shows a heterogeneously enhancing tumor. The direct axial (*B*) FA and (*C*) color FA maps (with slight differences in slice angulation) reveal focal decreased anisotropy or disruption of the highly organized white matter in the corpus callosum (*arrow*). The color FA map is directionally encoded with blue fibers oriented in the craniocaudal direction, red in the transverse direction, and green in the anteroposterior direction.

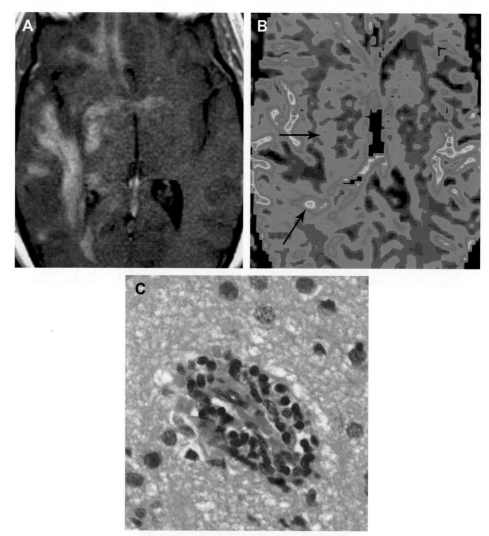

**Fig. 18.** Diffuse enhancing PCNSL. (*A*) Axial contrast T1-weighted image demonstrates diffuse enhancing tumor in the right cerebral hemisphere and corpus callosum that extends through the anterior commissure into the contralateral hemisphere. (*B*) Axial rCBV map reveals corresponding areas of mild hyperperfusion with rCBV increased to 1.8 times the contralateral normal white matter, which are most conspicuous in the right basal ganglia and periatrial region (*arrows*). (*C*) A 400× hematoxylin-eosin stain shows typical angiocentric growth with perivascular cuffing by the neoplastic lymphocytes before they spill into the brain parenchyma. The tumor and the angiocentric growth are responsible for only modest hyperperfusion, compared with high-grade gliomas with marked hyperperfusion caused by neovascularity (*Courtesy of* Diane L. Carlson, MD, New York, NY.)

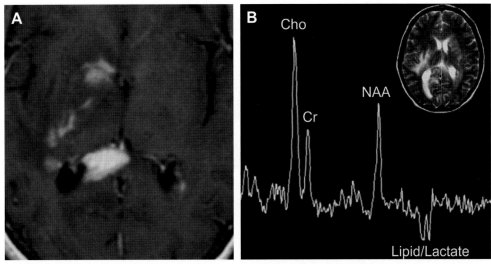

Fig.19. (A) Axial contrast T1-weighted image shows PCNSL of the right basal ganglia, right splenium of the corpus callosum, and left periatrial region. (B) Spectroscopy (TE =136) of the dominant callosal lesion shows elevated choline, decreased NAA, and inverted lipid-lactate peaks. This spectrum is not specific, and may be seen with a variety of high-grade malignancies. Cho, choline; Cr, creatine; NAA, N-acetylaspartate.

presence of NAA is often unreliable because of partial volume effects with normal brain in the same voxel. The peritumoral choline is decreased for lymphomas and metastases, whereas the peritumoral choline is increased for high-grade gliomas because of infiltrating tumor cells.[54] In the immunocompromised patient, both toxoplasmosis and lymphoma may display increased lactate and lipid, although there may sometimes be greater levels of lactate and lipid in toxoplasmosis than that seen in lymphoma, and decreased to absent other metabolites.[33,59] A thallium scan or PET-CT is useful in this setting to differentiate between toxoplasmosis and lymphoma.

## SUMMARY

Diagnostic imaging has a central role in the diagnosis, prognosis, and management of systemic and primary lymphomas of the neuraxis. This is a heterogeneous group of lymphomas that vary in epidemiology, presentation, and distribution, particularly between immunocompetent and immunocompromised patients. Functional imaging techniques using PET and advanced MR imaging can help improve the understanding of tumor biology, and may lead to further refinements of the response criteria that are currently based on changes in lesion contrast enhancement.

## REFERENCES

1. Mohile NA, Abrey LE. Primary central nervous system lymphoma. Neurol Clin 2007;25:1193–207.

2. Olson JE, Janney CA, Rao RD, et al. The continuing increase in the incidence of primary central nervous system non-Hodgkin lymphoma: a surveillance, epidemiology, and end results analysis. Cancer 2002; 95:1504–10.

3. Karantanis D, O'Neill BP, Subramaniam RM, et al. 18F-FDG PET/CT in primary central nervous system lymphoma in HIV-negative patients. Nucl Med Commun 2007;28:834–41.

4. Mohile NA, Deangelis LM, Abrey LE. The utility of body FDG PET in staging primary central nervous system lymphoma. Neurol Oncol 2008;10:223–8.

5. Abrey LE, Ben-Porat L, Panageas KS, et al. Primary central nervous system lymphoma: the Memorial Sloan-Kettering Cancer Center prognostic model. J Clin Oncol 2006;24:5711–5.

6. Ferreri AJ, Blay JY, Reni M, et al. Prognostic scoring system for primary CNS lymphomas: the International Extranodal Lymphoma Study Group experience. J Clin Oncol 2003;21:266–72.

7. Bataille B, Delwail V, Menet E, et al. Primary intracerebral malignant lymphoma: report of 248 cases. J Neurosurg 2000;92:261–6.

8. Kuker W, Nagele T, Korfel A, et al. Primary central nervous system lymphomas (PCNSL): MRI features at presentation in 100 patients. J Neurooncol 2005; 72:169–77.

9. Johnson BA, Fram EK, Johnson PC, et al. The variable MR appearance of primary lymphoma of the central nervous system: comparison with histopathologic features. AJNR Am J Neuroradiol 1997;18:563–72.

10. Helle TL, Britt RH, Colby TV. Primary lymphoma of the central nervous system: clinicopathological

study of experience at Stanford. J Neurosurg 1984; 60:94–103.

11. Jack CR Jr, O'Neill BP, Banks PM, et al. Central nervous system lymphoma: histologic types and CT appearance. Radiology 1988;167:211–5.

12. Roman-Goldstein SM, Goldman DL, Howieson J, et al. MR of primary CNS lymphoma in immunologically normal patients. AJNR Am J Neuroradiol 1992; 13:1207–13.

13. Jahnke K, Schilling A, Heidenreich J, et al. Radiologic morphology of low-grade primary central nervous system lymphoma in immunocompetent patients. AJNR Am J Neuroradiol 2005;26:2446–54.

14. Balmaceda C, Gaynor JJ, Sun M, et al. Leptomeningeal tumor in primary central nervous system lymphoma: recognition, significance, and implications. Ann Neurol 1995;38:202–9.

15. Iwamoto FM, Abrey LE. Primary dural lymphomas: a review. Neurosurg Focus 2006;21:1–5.

16. Smirniotopoulos JG, Murphy FM, Rushing EJ, et al. Patterns of contrast enhancement in the brain and meninges. Radiographics 2007;27:525–51.

17. Dina TS. Primary central nervous system lymphoma versus toxoplasmosis in AIDS. Radiology 1991;179: 823–8.

18. Baumgartner JE, Rachlin JR, Beckstead JH, et al. Primary central nervous system lymphomas: natural history and response to radiation therapy in 55 patients with acquired immunodeficiency syndrome. J Neurosurg 1990;73:206–11.

19. Brennan KC, Lowe LH, Yeaney GA. Pediatric central nervous system posttransplant lymphoproliferative disorder. AJNR Am J Neuroradiol 2005;26: 1695–7.

20. Song DK, Boulis NM, McKeever PE, et al. Angiotropic large cell lymphoma with imaging characteristics of CNS vasculitis. AJNR Am J Neuroradiol 2002; 23:239–42.

21. Baehring JM, Henchcliffe C, Ledezma CJ, et al. Intravascular lymphoma: magnetic resonance imaging correlates of disease dynamics within the central nervous system. J Neurol Neurosurg Psychiatry 2005;76:540–4.

22. Beristain X, Azzarelli B. The neurological masquerade of intravascular lymphomatosis. Arch Neurol 2002;59:439–43.

23. Ferreri AJ, Blay JY, Reni M, et al. Relevance of intraocular involvement in the management of primary central nervous system lymphomas. Ann Oncol 2002;13:531–8.

24. Peterson K, Gordon KB, Heinemann MH, et al. The clinical spectrum of ocular lymphoma. Cancer 1993;72:843–9.

25. Grimm SA, Pulido JS, Jahnke K, et al. Primary intraocular lymphoma: an International Primary Central Nervous System Lymphoma Collaborative Group report. Ann Oncol 2007;18:1851–5.

26. Gill MK, Jampol LM. Variations in the presentation of primary intraocular lymphoma case reports and a review. Surv Ophthalmol 2001;45:463–71.

27. Rosenberg SA, Diamond HD, Jaslowitz B, et al. Lymphosarcoma: a review of 1269 cases. Medicine (Baltimore) 1961;40:31–84.

28. Martinet S, Ozsahin M, Belkacemi Y, et al. Outcome and prognostic factors in orbital lymphoma: a rare cancer network study on 90 consecutive patients treated with radiotherapy. Int J Radiat Oncol Biol Phys 2003;55:892–8.

29. Schild SE, Wharen RE Jr, Menke DM, et al. Primary lymphoma of the spinal cord. Mayo Clin Proc 1995;70:256–60.

30. Baehring JM, Damek D, Martin EC, et al. Neurolymphomatosis. Neuro Oncol 2003;5:104–15.

31. Shah GD, Yahalom J, Correa DD, et al. Combined immunochemotherapy with reduced whole-brain radiotherapy for newly diagnosed primary CNS lymphoma. J Clin Oncol 2007;25:4730–5.

32. Abrey LE, Batchelor TT, Ferreri AJ, et al. Report of an international workshop to standardize baseline evaluation and response criteria for primary CNS lymphoma. J Clin Oncol 2005;23:5034–43.

33. Al-Okaili RN, Krejza J, Wang S, et al. Advanced MR imaging techniques in the diagnosis of intraaxial brain tumors in adults. Radiographics 2006; 26(Suppl 1):S173–89.

34. Al-Okaili RN, Krejza J, Woo JH, et al. Intraaxial brain masses: MR imaging-based diagnostic strategy–initial experience. Radiology 2007;243:539–50.

35. Zacharia T, Law M, Naidich T, et al. Central nervous system lymphoma characterized by diffusion weighted imaging and MR spectroscopy. J Neuroimaging, in press.

36. Miller RF, Hall-Craggs MA, Costa DC, et al. Magnetic resonance imaging, thallium-201 SPET scanning, and laboratory analyses for discrimination of cerebral lymphoma and toxoplasmosis in AIDS. Sex Transm Infect 1998;74:258–64.

37. O'Malley JP, Ziessman HA, Kumar PN, et al. Diagnosis of intracranial lymphoma in patients with AIDS: value of 201Tl single-photon emission computed tomography. AJR Am J Roentgenol 1994; 163:417–21.

38. Ruiz A, Ganz WI, Post MJ, et al. Use of thallium-201 brain SPECT to differentiate cerebral lymphoma from toxoplasma encephalitis in AIDS patients. AJNR Am J Neuroradiol 1994;15:1885–94.

39. Young RJ, Ghesani MV, Kagetsu NJ, et al. Lesion size determines accuracy of thallium-201 brain single-photon emission tomography in differentiating between intracranial malignancy and infection in AIDS patients. AJNR Am J Neuroradiol 2005;26: 1973–9.

40. Guo AC, Cummings TJ, Dash RC, et al. Lymphomas and high-grade astrocytomas: comparison of water

diffusibility and histologic characteristics. Radiology 2002;224:177–83.

41. Dong Q, Welsh RC, Chenevert TL, et al. Clinical applications of diffusion tensor imaging. J Magn Reson Imaging 2004;19:6–18.

42. Conturo TE, Lori NF, Cull TS, et al. Tracking neuronal fiber pathways in the living human brain. Proc Natl Acad Sci U S A 1999;96:10422–7.

43. Golay X, Jiang H, Van Zijl PC, et al. High-resolution isotropic 3D diffusion tensor imaging of the human brain. Magn Reson Med 2002;47:837–43.

44. Shimony JS, McKinstry RC, Akbudak E, et al. Quantitative diffusion-tensor anisotropy brain MR imaging: normative human data and anatomic analysis. Radiology 1999;212:770–84.

45. Stadlbauer A, Ganslandt O, Buslei R, et al. Gliomas: histopathologic evaluation of changes in directionality and magnitude of water diffusion at diffusion-tensor MR imaging. Radiology 2006;240:803–10.

46. Bastin ME, Carpenter TK, Armitage PA, et al. Effects of dexamethasone on cerebral perfusion and water diffusion in patients with high-grade glioma. AJNR Am J Neuroradiol 2006;27:402–8.

47. Calli C, Kitis O, Yunten N, et al. Perfusion and diffusion MR imaging in enhancing malignant cerebral tumors. Eur J Radiol 2006;58:394–403.

48. Camacho DL, Smith JK, Castillo M. Differentiation of toxoplasmosis and lymphoma in AIDS patients by using apparent diffusion coefficients. AJNR Am J Neuroradiol 2003;24:633–7.

49. Toh CH, Castillo M, Wong AM, et al. Primary cerebral lymphoma and glioblastoma multiforme: differences in diffusion characteristics evaluated with diffusion tensor imaging. AJNR Am J Neuroradiol 2008;29:471–5.

50. Gupta RK, Hasan KM, Mishra AM, et al. High fractional anisotropy in brain abscesses versus other cystic intracranial lesions. AJNR Am J Neuroradiol 2005;26:1107–14.

51. Law M, Teicher N, Zagzag D, et al. Dynamic contrast enhanced perfusion MRI in mycosis fungoides. J Magn Reson Imaging 2003;18:364–7.

52. Hartmann M, Heiland S, Harting I, et al. Distinguishing of primary cerebral lymphoma from high-grade glioma with perfusion-weighted magnetic resonance imaging. Neurosci Lett 2003;338:119–22.

53. Cha S, Knopp EA, Johnson G, et al. Intracranial mass lesions: dynamic contrast-enhanced susceptibility-weighted echo-planar perfusion MR imaging. Radiology 2002;223:11–29.

54. Law M, Cha S, Knopp EA, et al. High-grade gliomas and solitary metastases: differentiation by using perfusion and proton spectroscopic MR imaging. Radiology 2002;222:715–21.

55. Young RJ, Knopp EA. Brain MRI: tumor evaluation. J Magn Reson Imaging 2006;24:709–24.

56. Chang L, Miller BL, McBride D, et al. Brain lesions in patients with AIDS: H-1 MR spectroscopy. Radiology 1995;197:525–31.

57. Raizer JJ, Koutcher JA, Abrey LE, et al. Proton magnetic resonance spectroscopy in immunocompetent patients with primary central nervous system lymphoma. J Neurooncol 2005;71:173–80.

58. Kwock L, Smith JK, Castillo M, et al. Clinical applications of proton MR spectroscopy in oncology. Technol Cancer Res Treat 2002;1:17–28.

59. Chinn RJ, Wilkinson ID, Hall-Craggs MA, et al. Toxoplasmosis and primary central nervous system lymphoma in HIV infection: diagnosis with MR spectroscopy. Radiology 1995;197:649–54.

60. Braus DF, Schwechheimer K, Muller-Hermelink HK, et al. Primary cerebral malignant non-Hodgkin's lymphomas: a retrospective clinical study. J Neurol 1992;239:117–24.

61. Erdogan C, Hakyemez B, Yildirim N, et al. Brain abscess and cystic brain tumor: discrimination with dynamic susceptibility contrast perfusion-weighted MRI. J Comput Assist Tomogr 2005;29:663–7.

62. Kimura T, Sako K, Gotoh T, et al. In vivo single-voxel proton MR spectroscopy in brain lesions with ring-like enhancement. NMR Biomed 2001;14:339–49.

# Imaging Hodgkin and Non-Hodgkin Lymphoma in the Head and Neck

Ashley H. Aiken, MD[a],*, Christine Glastonbury, MBBS[b]

**KEYWORDS**
- Lymphoma • Head and neck • Hodgkin lymphoma
- Non-Hodgkin lymphoma

Hodgkin lymphoma (HL) and non-Hodgkin lymphoma (NHL) are common neoplasms that frequently involve the head and neck. Lymphoma is the second most common neoplasm in the head and neck and the most common diagnosis for a unilateral neck mass in patients aged 21 to 40 years.[1] The imaging manifestations of these disease processes are protean, ranging from cervical lymphadenopathy to nonnodal lymphatic disease with pathologic enlargement of pharyngeal tonsillar tissue to nonnodal extralymphatic masses in the head and neck, such as in the orbit, cavernous sinuses, and deep face. Because of its many pathologic and clinical expressions, the radiologic appearances of lymphoma overlap with many other pathologic entities, including infectious, inflammatory, and neoplastic processes.

HL most commonly presents as cervical lymphadenopathy alone. Extranodal involvement is rare, with an incidence of approximately 4% to 5%. Conversely, NHL presents as cervical lymphadenopathy with extranodal sites of disease in as many as 23% to 30% of patients.[2–4] The only body site with more frequent extranodal lymphoma than the head and neck is the gastrointestinal tract. The most common extranodal site of lymphoma in the head and neck is Waldeyer's ring, with more than half of cases occurring here. The remaining nonlymphatic extranodal sites are the paranasal sinuses, the nasal cavity, the larynx, oral cavity, salivary glands, thyroid, and orbit. The imaging patterns of lymphomatous involvement in the head and neck have been previously described and are outlined in **Box 1**.[2,5] Essentially, a type 1 imaging pattern is purely nodal disease, type 2 purely extranodal lymphoma, type 3 both nodal and extranodal disease, and type 4 multifocal extranodal lymphoma.

Imaging with CT, MR imaging, and, more recently, positron emission tomography (PET)/CT has an important role in accurate staging, which is crucial for treatment decisions. Involved field radiation plus chemotherapy is commonly used for lower stages and chemotherapy alone for higher stages.

## CLINICAL AND RADIOGRAPHIC STAGING

Clinical staging is based on a combination of clinical, radiologic, and surgical findings, including a medical history and physical examination. The Ann Arbor staging system is now used to clinically stage HL and NHL, although it was initially designed to stage HL.[6] Conventional staging includes a complete blood count, serum liver biochemistries, and erythrocyte sedimentation rate. Bone marrow biopsy from the iliac crest is crucial because approximately 18% of NHL patients have bone marrow involvement.[4] A lumbar puncture is usually performed if there is suspected intracranial or intraspinous involvement.

Contrast-enhanced CT is routinely performed for evaluation of cervical lymph nodes, and CT of the chest, abdomen, and pelvis is also obtained. In the head and neck, CT not only evaluates for

[a] Department of Radiology, San Francisco General Hospital, University of California San Francisco, 1001 Potrero Avenue, Room 1x55, San Francisco, CA 94110, USA
[b] Department of Radiology, University of California San Francisco, Box 0628, Room-358, 505 Parnassus Avenue, San Francisco, CA 94143-0628, USA
* Corresponding author.
*E-mail address:* ashley.aiken@radiology.ucsf.edu (A.H. Aiken).

Radiol Clin N Am 46 (2008) 363–378
doi:10.1016/j.rcl.2008.03.001

nodal and nonnodal lymphatic masses but is also useful for detection of bone destruction involving the skull base, the paranasal sinuses, and the mandible or maxilla. If there is evidence of, or concern for, extension of lymphoma to multiple fascial spaces (parapharyngeal, masticator, infratemporal fossa, tongue, and nasopharynx) or concern for intracranial or intraspinal extension, MR imaging is the preferred modality owing to its greater soft tissue detail. At most institutions, 18F-FDG PET has replaced 67Ga-citrate single-photon imaging and is frequently used for the initial staging and for follow-up of many types of lymphoma. Nevertheless, it has limited sensitivity for some low-grade lymphomas, such as peripheral T-cell, marginal zone B-cell, and grade 1 cutaneous follicular lymphoma, and for early stage MALT lymphoma.

## Hodgkin Lymphoma

Classic HL has a bimodal age distribution, with an early peak at 20 to 24 years and a later peak at 80 to 84 years. The median age at diagnosis for patients with HL is around 28 years as compared with 67.2 years for patients with NHL.[2,3,7] In distinction to NHL, HL primarily affects lymph nodes (>90%) and only rarely presents in extranodal sites. In 70% to 80% of cases, HL presents with enlarging neck adenopathy, and there is frequently also disease in the mediastinum along contiguous nodal groups. Most patients with neck HL have a type 1 imaging pattern, with the internal jugular chain most frequently involved.[1]

All HLs are characterized by the presence of a small number of distinctive large neoplastic cells known as Reed-Sternberg cells that reside on a background of nonneoplastic cells and, in some cases, fibrosis. Four histologic subtypes of HL are defined by Rye's modification. The nodular sclerosing type is the most common in North America and Western Europe, usually presenting as a mediastinal mass in a young woman. The mixed cellularity type is the second most common in North America and more frequent in indigent populations. It is more often associated with subdiaphragmatic disease, extranodal sites, "B" symptoms, and an overall worse prognosis than nodular sclerosis. Lymphocyte-predominant disease classically has a favorable prognosis. Lymphocyte-depleted disease has the worst prognosis and is associated with advanced age, systemic symptoms, retroperitoneal lymphadenopathy, and extranodal sites.

## Non-Hodgkin Lymphoma

NHL comprises a diverse group of lymphoreticular neoplasia varying in prognosis based on the histologic subtype and clinical features and tending to occur in an older age group than HL. NHL has a wide spectrum of presentations and may exhibit imaging patterns 1 through to 4.[1] Also in distinction to HL, NHL frequently presents with extranodal disease (23%–30%) in the head and neck.

Various schemes have been devised over the years to classify lymphoma. The one currently used by most pathologists and oncologists is the World Health Organization system, which is based on the Revised European-American Classification of Lymphoid Tumors.[8,9] The Working Formulation, developed by the National Cancer Institute in 1982, is still used by otolaryngologists and other head and neck surgeons. This classification is based on Rappaport's clinically based system and divides NHL into low-, intermediate-, and high-grade categories.[10]

Extranodal lymphoma in the head and neck typically occurs in patients between 50 and 60 years of age and generally occurs with a slight male predominance, except for salivary gland, orbit, and thyroid lymphomas which are more common in women. The most common NHL subtypes to present in the head and neck are B-cell lymphoblastic, small lymphocytic, follicular, mantle cell, MALT, diffuse large B-cell, Burkitt's, and extranodal NK/T-cell nasal type. Diffuse large B-cell lymphoma, the most common type of NHL in the head and neck, is often encountered in the paranasal sinuses, jaw, or Waldeyer's ring. Marginal zone lymphoma (MALT type) has an affinity for the ocular adnexae, salivary glands, larynx, and the thyroid gland. NK/T-cell lymphoma has a predilection for the nasal cavity. Burkitt's lymphoma is a high-grade, B-cell NHL associated with the Epstein-Barr virus. The endemic African variant of Burkitt's lymphoma, which is more common in children, usually involves the maxilla and facial bones. Clinically aggressive lymphomas such as Burkitt's lymphoma and diffuse large B-cell lymphoma and NK/T-cell lymphoma are characterized by destruction of the facial and paranasal sinus bones, which is indistinguishable from bony destruction in other malignant tumors, such as squamous cell carcinoma, which is the most common sinus paranasal malignancy.[4]

Risk factors for NHL include congenital or acquired immunodeficiency, autoimmune disorders, and immunosuppressive regimens used for organ transplantation. Several chronic infectious or inflammatory diseases also predispose to the development of lymphoma. Chronic HIV infection poses a 100 times increased risk of lymphoma, Hashimoto's thyroiditis is found in half of all patients with thyroid lymphoma, Sjogren's syndrome increases the risk of salivary gland lymphoma, and Epstein-Barr virus is often associated with nasal lymphoma.

## IMAGING FEATURES AT DIAGNOSIS
### Nodal Disease, Non-Hodgkin Lymphoma, and Hodgkin Lymphoma

Imaging cannot reliably distinguish HL and NHL lymphadenopathy. The classic head and neck presentation of lymphoma is enlarging or persistent painless lymphadenopathy, with or without associated constitutional symptoms.[11] Both HL and NHL typically have multiple homogeneous nodes ranging in size from 2 to 10 cm that may show variable enhancement. The recommendation for the upper limit of cervical lymph node size (short axis) at CT is 10 mm. More heterogeneous nodes with necrosis before and after treatment or calcification after treatment may also be seen (**Fig. 1**). Nodal necrosis preceding treatment is more frequently seen in high-grade lymphoma.

In the head and neck, NHL or HL can be suspected with multiple large lymph nodes.[5] Classically, HL involves a single node or nodal chain and spreads contiguously, whereas NHL typically involves noncontiguous disease and more commonly has extranodal involvement. When retropharyngeal, occipital, parotid, posterior triangle, or submandibular nodes are involved, NHL should be strongly considered. HL has an affinity for the internal jugular chain lymph nodes of the neck and mediastinum. Associated mediastinal

adenopathy is more common with HL and abdominal adenopathy with NHL. Extranodal disease is much more commonly found with NHL.[3,5] Necrosis and extranodal spread suggest aggressive lymphoma and are often found with AIDS.

### Extranodal Lymphatic Disease, Non-Hodgkin Lymphoma

#### Waldeyer's ring
The pharyngeal mucosal space is rich in lymphatic tissue and not surprisingly is the most common head and neck extranodal site of NHL. Waldeyer's ring comprises the palatine tonsils, the nasopharyngeal tonsil (or adenoids), and the lingual tonsils, which are common sites of NHL in descending order of frequency. More than half of extranodal head and neck NHL occurs in this location, and 5% to 10% of patients with NHL have Waldeyer's ring as the primary site.[12] Ten percent of patients with primary Waldeyer's ring NHL have gastrointestinal involvement; therefore, their staging work-up frequently includes barium studies. As many as one third of patients with neck nodal NHL have occult involvement of Waldeyer's ring on careful inspection. Most Waldeyer's ring lymphomas are of B-cell origin and more than half occur in the palatine tonsil.[11,12] Clinical symptoms are similar to those of squamous cell carcinoma in these locations. When lymphoma involves the tonsils, it frequently presents with tonsillar swelling and a sore throat; when arising in the nasopharyngeal tonsil, patients typically present with a cervical mass, nasal obstruction, and decreased hearing from obstruction of the Eustachian tube. Lingual tonsillar lymphoma typically presents with a foreign body sensation. On clinical inspection in these cases, lymphomas appear mostly submucosal as opposed to the ulcerated mucosal masses seen in squamous cell carcinoma.

Most patients with lymphoma involving Waldeyer's ring present with intermediate-grade disease and are treated with doxorubicin-based chemotherapy (CHOP) and radiation.[12] One notable characteristic of Waldeyer's ring lymphomas is the propensity for associated gastric disease, with one large randomized study showing gastrointestinal relapse in 30% to 35% patients.[13]

Imaging of primary palatine tonsillar NHL most frequently shows a large homogeneous tumor mass of similar intensity to normal tonsillar tissue without deep invasion (**Fig. 2**). Associated ipsilateral adenopathy is typically nonnecrotic.[9] Nasopharyngeal lymphoma is also usually homogeneous, with relatively well-defined contours and mild enhancement, and frequently involves

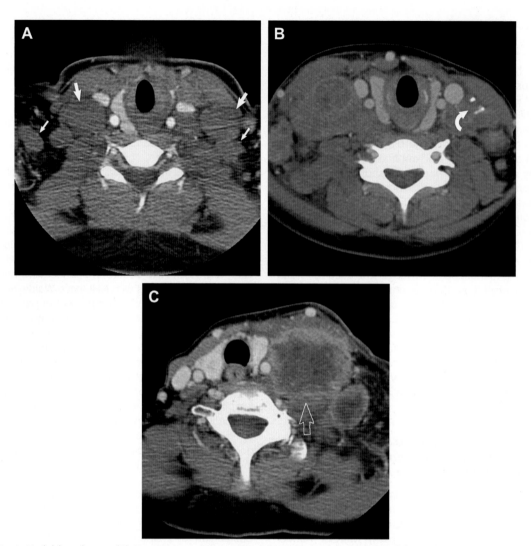

Fig. 1. Nodal lymphoma. (*A*) Homogenous bilateral lymph nodes in NHL (*arrows*). (*B*) Calcified lymph nodes in nodular sclerosing HL (*curved arrow*). (*C*) Necrotic lymph nodes in NHL (*open arrow*).

all walls of the nasopharynx, mimicking nasopharyngeal carcinoma (**Fig. 3**). Unlike in nasopharyngeal carcinoma, skull base bony erosion is rare, with nasopharyngeal lymphoma tending to grow in an exophytic fashion to fill the airway or spreading superficially to involve the nasal cavity or oropharynx rather than infiltrating into the deep tissues.[14] Deep tumor infiltration, when it occurs, is found in patients with primary NHL and is usually limited in extent and of small volume. Lymphadenopathy is frequent and extensive with nasopharyngeal lymphoma, and the nodes may show necrosis and matting. Primary lingual tonsillar lymphoma may mimic oropharyngeal squamous cell carcinoma, presenting as a large mass at the tongue base, but tends to be more homogeneous and is less likely to be necrotic (**Fig. 4**).

## Extranodal, Nonlymphatic Disease, Non-Hodgkin Lymphoma

### Sinonasal

Sinonasal lymphomas are relatively rare, representing less than 1% of all head and neck malignancies. Two distinct subgroups are recognized—B-cell lymphomas and NK/T-cell lymphoma. B-cell lymphomas are the most frequent sinonasal lymphoma and are less aggressive with a more favorable prognosis. They are more common in men, occurring at a median age of 50 years. The more uncommon NK/T-cell lymphomas present at a younger age and are mostly found in the nasal cavity. Although it is more common in Asia and South America, NK/T-cell sinonasal lymphoma has a strong association with Epstein-Barr virus infection in both Western and Asian regions.

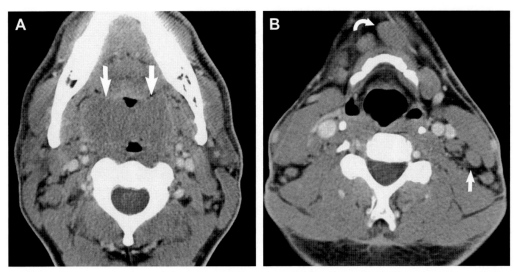

Fig. 2. NHL of the palatine tonsils. (*A*) Post contrast CT shows bilateral symmetric, homogeneous enlargement of the palatine tonsils (*solid arrows*). (*B*) With associated level I (*curved arrow*) and II (*straight arrow*) lymphadenopathy.

Low-grade sinonasal lymphomas present with obstructive symptoms, whereas high-grade lymphomas are more likely to present with symptoms suggestive of an aggressive or invasive nature, including a nonhealing ulcer, cranial nerve palsies, epistaxis, or pain. High-grade, diffuse, large B-cell lymphomas tend to present with soft tissue or osseous destruction, particularly of the orbit with proptosis. T-cell lymphomas are associated with nasal septal perforation or destruction.[15] Overall, most patients with sinonasal lymphoma tend to present with stage I or II disease.

Patients with localized sinonasal lymphoma have a favorable prognosis when treated with combined radiotherapy and chemotherapy, which is usually doxorubicin based. Some patients with paranasal sinus lymphoma may benefit from prophylactic treatment of the central nervous system with intrathecal methotrexate.[16]

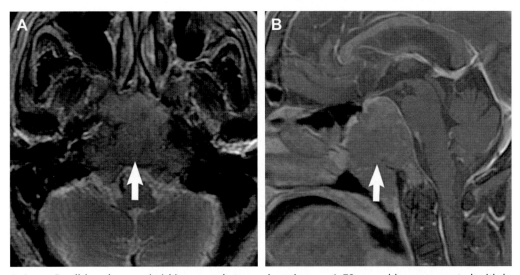

Fig. 3. Large B-cell lymphoma mimicking nasopharyngeal carcinoma. A 78-year-old man presented with headache. (*A*) Axial T2-weighted MR image shows a homogeneous mass, isointense to brain, replacing and expanding the clivus (*arrow*). (*B*) Sagittal post gadolinium T1-weighted MR image with fat saturation shows the tumor to be homogeneous but with little enhancement (*arrow*). The mass appears centered in the nasopharynx with upward extension to expand the clivus and infiltrate the sella. The well-defined borders, T2 hypointensity, homogeneous but minimal enhancement, and clival expansion favor lymphoma over nasopharyngeal carcinoma.

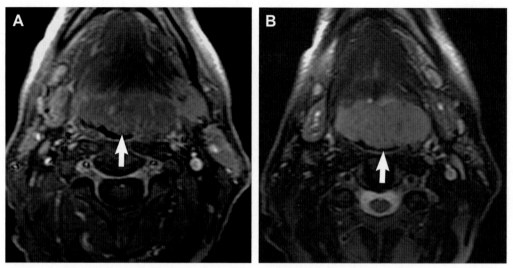

**Fig. 4.** Lingual tonsil lymphoma mimicking a base of tongue squamous cell carcinoma. A 58-year-old veteran presented with a large mass at the base of tongue. (*A*) Axial T1-weighted post gadolinium MR image with fat saturation shows a homogeneously enhancing mass at the tongue base with a low level of enhancement (*arrow*). (*B*) Axial T2-weighted MR image with fat saturation shows the mass to be relatively well defined with little infiltration of adjacent soft tissues and homogeneous (*arrow*). T2 homogeneity is not typical for a large primary squamous cell carcinoma, raising the possibility of an alternative diagnosis such as adenocarcinoma or lymphoma.

On imaging, sinonasal NHL may present as a destructive soft tissue mass and may mimic a variety of sinonasal pathologies, such as Wegener's granulomatosis and tumors such as squamous cell carcinoma and esthesioneuroblastoma. Lymphoma more frequently arises in the nasal cavity, whereas carcinoma more often arises in the paranasal sinuses. Lymphoma tends to be more homogeneous on T2 imaging, with less intense enhancement than carcinomas (**Fig. 5**). Sinonasal lymphomas are typically bulky masses with intermediate signal intensity on MR imaging and show moderate contrast enhancement. The lesions remodel and may erode adjacent bone. Most frequently, sinonasal lymphoma arises within the nasal fossa, then the maxillary sinus, less commonly in the ethmoids, and rarely in the sphenoid or frontal sinuses.[17]

### Salivary gland/parotid lymphoma

Primary lymphoma of the salivary gland is rare, comprising 2% to 5% of all salivary neoplasms. It is most common in the parotid gland (70%) and least common in the submandibular gland.[18] Histopathologically, the most common subtypes are marginal zone B cell of the MALT type, follicular lymphomas, and diffuse large B-cell lymphomas. Three criteria have been suggested to define salivary lymphoma as primary to the gland: (1) involvement of gland is the first disease manifestation; (2) histologically, disease involves gland

parenchyma and not adjacent nodes; and (3) lymphoid infiltrate is malignant.[19]

Most patients with parotid lymphoma have widespread disease at other sites and extensive adenopathy. Parotid NHL in disseminated disease is frequently bilateral. It can present as a solitary mass or unilateral or bilateral multifocal masses mimicking metastatic intraparotid nodes or a small primary parotid tumor (**Fig. 6**).

Primary parotid lymphoma is significantly less common and most often of the MALT variety with unilateral diffuse invasion of ductal and acinar tissue. There is a higher incidence of primary parotid NHL in patients with Sjogren's disease, Mikulicz's disease, and Warthin's tumors. Some series of Sjogren's disease show nearly a 40 times higher risk than in women of similar age. Primary parotid lymphoma often presents as diffuse parotid infiltration mimicking a high-grade parotid carcinoma (**Fig. 7**).[20] Primary salivary lymphoma has a favorable prognosis when compared with NHL elsewhere, especially when there is no sicca syndrome. Usually, stage I disease is treated with radiotherapy alone, whereas chemotherapy is performed for stages II to IV.[21]

### Thyroid lymphoma

Primary thyroid lymphoma is a rare disease that can be confused with anaplastic thyroid carcinoma radiographically and, in the past, even pathologically, although new immunohistochemical stains make the pathologic diagnosis easier. The

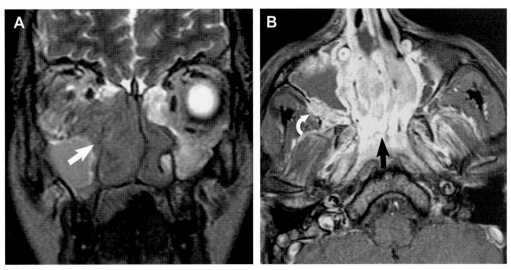

**Fig. 5.** Sinonasal NK T-cell lymphoma. A 19-year-old man was referred from an outside hospital with a presumptive diagnosis of juvenile angiofibroma after presenting with epistaxis. (*A*) Coronal T2-weighted MR image with fat saturation shows a T2 hypointense mass centered in the nasal cavity obstructing and infiltrating the right maxillary sinus and invading the inferomedial orbital floor (*arrow*). Note that there are no flow voids within this mass. (*B*) Axial T1-weighted post gadolinium MR image with fat saturation shows homogeneous intense enhancement (*black arrow*). Infiltration without significant expansion of the right pterygopalatine fossa is noted (*curved white arrow*). Although the age of the patient, location of the tumor, and presentation were in keeping with the diagnosis of juvenile angiofibroma, these imaging characteristics favored a sinonasal malignancy, with lymphoma the leading differential.

clinical presentations include an enlarging neck mass, but patients may also present with symptoms of dysphagia, hoarseness and choking, or a cold thyroid nodule. Thyroid lymphoma is more common in women, typically occurring between 70 and 80 years of age. Nearly 80% of thyroid lymphoma cases are associated with chronic lymphocytic thyroiditis (Hashimoto's).[19]

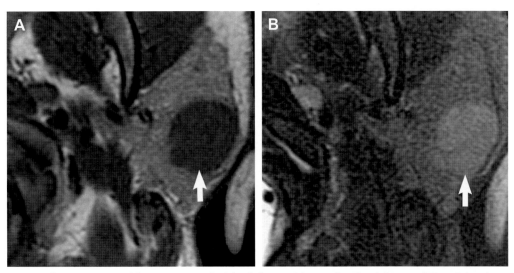

**Fig. 6.** Parotid HL. A 21-year-old man presented with a left parotid mass. (*A, B*) Axial T1- and T2-weighted precontrast MR images demonstrate a T2 isointense to slightly hyperintense, well-circumscribed mass in the left parotid (*arrows*). Post gadolinium sequences (not shown) demonstrated homogeneous enhancement. These imaging characteristics mimic a primary low-grade parotid carcinoma. Biopsy revealed nodular lymphocyte-predominant HL. Such well-defined parotid masses are usually disseminated lymphoma rather than the rare primary parotid lymphoma.

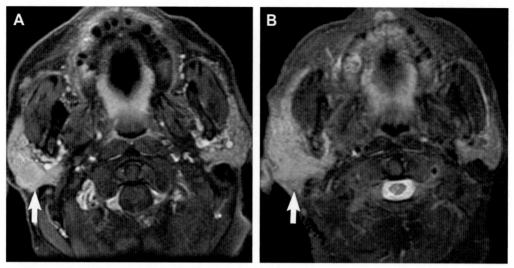

Fig. 7. Primary parotid MALT lymphoma mimicking a salivary malignancy. A 72-year-old man presented with right neck swelling and was imaged over 1 year. (A) The initial axial T1-weighted post gadolinium MR image with fat saturation shows subtle fullness and increased enhancement of the right parotid (arrow). Fine-needle aspiration was negative, and the patient elected to be followed up clinically. (B) Twelve months later, axial T2-weighted MR image with fat saturation shows a diffusely enlarged right parotid with the appearance of an infiltrative, enhancing mass (arrow). Open biopsy revealed extranodal marginal zone lymphoma (MALT). This rare primary parotid lymphoma mimics a high-grade parotid carcinoma; however, clinically, these patients usually do not have pain or facial nerve involvement and usually present with lymphadenopathy.

Most thyroid lymphomas are of B-cell origin, but there appears to be two distinct clinical and prognostic subtypes of these rare tumors. The more indolent lymphomas are the subgroup of mucosa-associated lymphoid tissue (MALT) lymphomas, comprising 6% to 27% of thyroid lymphomas. Localized disease in this subgroup (IE) responds well to total thyroidectomy or radiation, with a complete response rate of more than 90%, leading some authorities to recommend

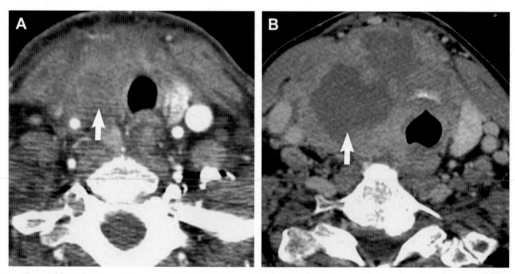

Fig. 8. Thyroid lymphoma versus anaplastic thyroid carcinoma. (A) A 60-year-old woman with a rapidly enlarging right neck mass. Axial contrast-enhanced CT shows a relatively homogeneous, noncalcified mass in the right lobe of the thyroid that infiltrates the adjacent soft tissues (arrow). Biopsy showed B-cell lymphoma. (B) A 61-year-old man with a rapidly enlarging right neck mass. Axial contrast-enhanced CT shows a similar appearance with a heterogeneous and necrotic mass replacing the right thyroid lobe and infiltrating the adjacent soft tissues (arrow). Biopsy showed anaplastic thyroid carcinoma.

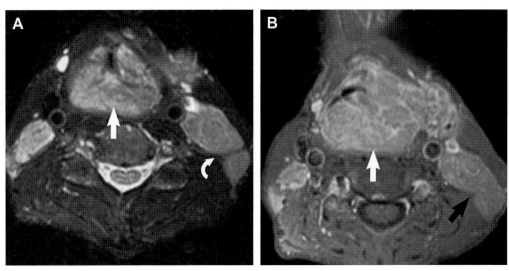

**Fig. 9.** NHL of the larynx. (*A*) Axial T2-weighted images demonstrate diffuse, circumferential involvement of the larynx (*straight arrow*) and bilateral adenopathy (*curved arrow*). (*B*) Post gadolinium images show a homogeneous T2 hyperintense mass extending exophytically into the hypopharynx (*white arrow*) and bilateral cervical lymphadenopathy (*black arrow*).

surgery as primary therapy in the treatment of localized MALT lymphomas. Because that scenario is rarely seen, surgery is not a mainstay of treatment in thyroid lymphoma. The management of low-grade lymphoproliferative disorders of MALT type may include radiotherapy, oral chlorambucil, or intravenous chemotherapy (cyclophosphamide, vincristine, and prednisone).

Diffuse large B-cell lymphoma is the more common subtype, representing 70% of thyroid lymphomas, and in some cases may arise from MALT lymphomas. This subtype appears to have the most aggressive clinical course, with almost 60% of these tumors diagnosed with disseminated disease. The management of diffuse large B-cell lymphoma is combined modality therapy with radiation and cyclophosphamide, doxorubicin, vincristine, and prednisone (CHOP) chemotherapy. The overall 5-year survival rate for this aggressive group is less then 50%.

On imaging, primary thyroid NHL most commonly presents as a solitary, rapidly enlarging

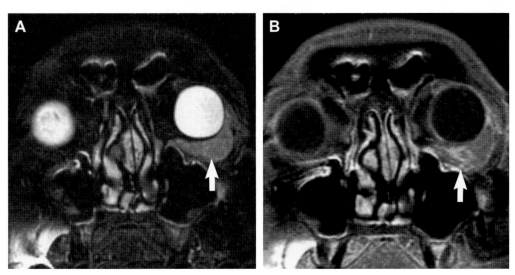

**Fig. 10.** Ocular lymphoma. (*A*) Coronal T2-weighted images show a homogeneous, T2 hyperintense mass inferior to the left globe. Biopsy revealed MALT lymphoma (*arrow*). (*B*) Coronal post gadolinium image shows mild, homogeneous enhancement (*arrow*).

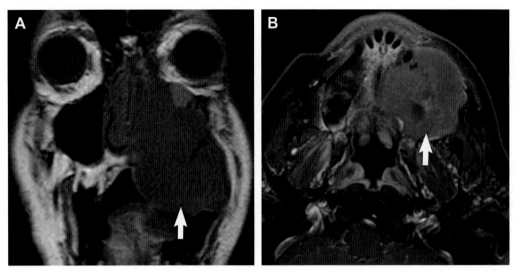

**Fig. 11.** Burkitt's lymphoma involving the maxilla. (*A*) Coronal precontrast T1-weighted image shows a large mass replacing most of the maxilla and extending superiorly into the maxillary sinus (*arrow*). (*B*) Axial postcontrast T1-weighted image shows mild, homogeneous enhancement and an exophytic soft tissue component (*arrow*).

mass mimicking anaplastic thyroid carcinoma or other aggressive carcinoma. Thyroid lymphoma may also present as multiple nodules mimicking goiter. On cross-sectional imaging, thyroid lymphoma tends to be more homogeneous than thyroid carcinoma, and calcification or cystic degeneration or necrosis is rare, distinguishing it from goiter (**Fig. 8**).[22] Although tracheal invasion is not uncommon in thyroid carcinomas, lymphoma

is rarely associated with tracheal invasion, although significant narrowing of the airway can occur.

Fine-needle aspiration has become the procedure of choice for evaluating thyroid masses at many institutions; however, this modality has yielded inconsistent results in the diagnosis of lymphoma. It can often be difficult to distinguish the lymphoid infiltrate in Hashimoto's thyroiditis from low-grade lymphomas of MALT type.[23,24]

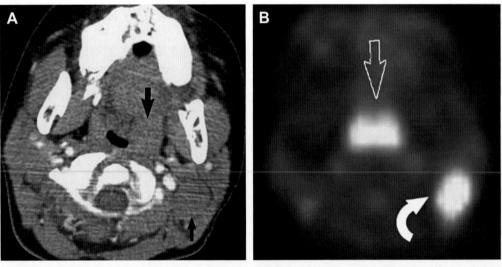

**Fig. 12.** A 35-year-old with a history of renal transplant presented with fever and a sore throat. (*A*) Axial contrast-enhanced CT shows left cervical adenopathy (*thin arrow*) and an enlarged left tonsil (*thick arrow*). The most common clinical presentation of PTLD is fever and lymphadenopathy; therefore, the history and timing of solid organ transplantation are crucial to distinguish this diagnosis from infection. Furthermore, PTLD can present with central low attenuation mimicking abscess. (*B*) PET shows increased FDG uptake in the palatine tonsils (*open arrow*) and left greater than right cervical lymphadenopathy (*curved arrow*).

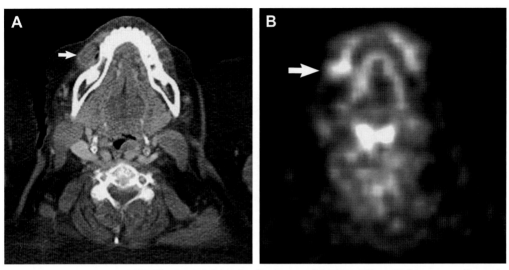

**Fig.13.** A 64-year-old woman with slow onset of a right cheek mass. (*A*) Postcontrast CT shows a small mass in the right buccal space (*arrow*). (*B*) PET at the same axial level shows increased FDG uptake (*arrow*). No other increased FDG uptake was seen on this PET study. Biopsy of this buccal mass showed low-grade NHL.

## Larynx

Primary hematologic laryngeal tumors are rare, accounting for less than 1% of laryngeal tumors. Fewer than 100 cases of primary NHL have been reported in the literature. Laryngeal lymphoma is most often marginal zone lymphoma of the MALT type and occurs in a similar age group as laryngeal squamous cell carcinoma, with a median age of 58 years. Laryngeal NHL is typically a submucosal mass centered in the supraglottis and may spread to involve the glottis and less frequently the subglottis. It tends to be homogeneous at MR imaging with moderate enhancement. Deep tumor invasion into cartilage or muscle may occur, as well as cervical lymphadenopathy. In nearly all cases, there is involvement of the hypopharynx, and superior extension to the oropharynx or even nasopharynx may occur (**Fig. 9**). The finding of submucosal tumor centered in the supraglottis should raise the possibility of NHL.[25]

## Ocular adenexa

Lymphoma of the ocular adenexa is the most common orbital malignancy in adults aged more than 60 years. Orbital lymphoma can involve the lacrimal gland, extraocular muscles, orbital fat, eyelids, and conjunctiva. The most common location is the anterior extraconal space centered in the superotemporal quadrant. Primary ocular lymphoma is most often marginal zone lymphoma of the MALT type, followed by follicular B-cell and diffuse systemic large B-cell lymphoma. Orbital involvement is seen in as much as 5% of all systemic NHL. Clinically, patients present with an enlarging painless mass and proptosis without signs of inflammation. Because lymphomas tend to mold to surrounding structures rather than invade tissues, vision loss is usually not present.

Imaging of orbital lymphoma usually demonstrates a T1- and T2-intermediate intensity, homogeneous globular mass with moderate enhancement encasing orbital structures (**Fig. 10**). Bony erosion on CT is rare; when present, this finding suggests a high-grade lymphoma.

## Mandible/maxilla

African variant Burkitt's lymphoma is a high-grade, B-cell lymphoma that involves the mandible in over 50% cases and less commonly the maxilla. It is one of the fastest growing malignancies. Before the development of aggressive therapies, children died quickly. This tumor is the most common childhood malignancy in Africa and is strongly associated with Epstein-Barr virus. CT most commonly demonstrates a large osteolytic lesion near the angle of the mandible, less commonly in the maxilla, with an associated soft tissue mass without osteoid or cartilaginous matrix (**Fig. 11**). The non-African variant of Burkitt's lymphoma involves abdominal organs.

## Posttransplant lymphoproliferative disorder

Posttransplant lymphoproliferative disorder (PTLD) represents a unique disease occurring in immunosuppressed patients after organ transplantation. It is associated with Epstein-Barr virus from infected donor lymphocytes. PTLD has an

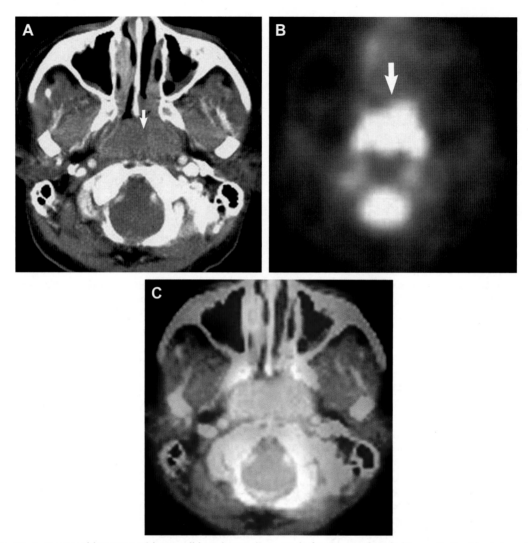

**Fig. 14.** A 44-year-old woman with NK cell lymphoma diagnosed after inguinal node biopsy. Patient had stage IV disease with marrow involvement treated with chemotherapy and was in remission. She then developed nasal stuffiness and was reimaged with CT and then PET. (*A*) CT shows prominent nasopharyngeal/adenoidal soft tissue (*arrow*) suspicious for recurrent disease. (*B, C*) PET and PET/CT fused images demonstrate abnormal FDG uptake in this prominent nasopharyngeal soft tissue (*arrow*). Biopsy confirmed relapse. No other evidence of recurrent disease was seen on the whole body PET.

overall prevalence of 2% to 3% in solid organ transplant patients, with higher rates occurring in younger patients, liver transplants, high doses of immunosuppression, and transplant recipients who are seronegative for Epstein-Barr virus. Treatment for PTLD begins with reducing immunosuppression, but rituximab and even chemotherapy and radiation may be added.

In the head and neck, it most commonly involves Waldeyer's ring and may mimic tonsillitis or pharyngitis (**Fig. 12**). PTLD is more common in patients following lung (4%–10%) and small bowel (20%) transplantation, which is thought

to be related to the type of immune suppressive agents.[26,27]

## AIDS-Related Lymphoma

Nearly 15% of patients with AIDS present with lymphoma, and B-cell NHL has become a Centers for Disease Control and Prevention criterion for presumptive HIV diagnosis.[3] NHL is the second most common malignancy of HIV-positive patients.[28] In the head and neck, oral cavity lymphoma has a predilection for HIV patients. HIV-associated lymphomas include (1) lymphomas

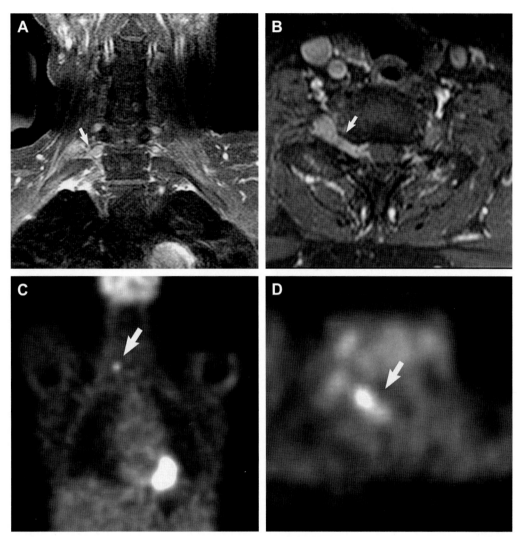

**Fig. 15.** A 71-year-old woman with a prior history of systemic NHL treated with chemotherapy and in remission. She presented with new right arm pain and underwent an MR neurogram and then PET. (*A, B*) Coronal and axial MR postgadolinium neurogram images demonstrate abnormal enlargement and enhancement of the right C8 nerve root (*white arrows*). (*C, D*) The corresponding coronal and axial PET images demonstrate abnormal FDG uptake along the C8 nerve root (*white arrows*). Subsequent MR brain images showed an additional site of relapse involving the third ventricle and infundibulum.

also occurring in the absence of HIV infection, which are mostly high-grade, B-cell lymphomas (Burkitt's lymphoma, diffuse large B-cell lymphoma with centroblastic features, and diffuse large B-cell lymphoma with immunoblastic features); and (2) unusual lymphomas occurring more specifically in HIV-positive patients, including two rare entities (ie, primary effusion lymphoma and plasmablastic lymphoma of the oral cavity).[29] Lymphomas in HIV patients are associated with a poorer prognosis—a 5-month survival for HIV-positive patients versus a 24-month survival for HIV-negative patients.[30]

## IMAGING SURVEILLANCE
### Positron Emission Tomography

Although CT has been the gold standard for staging lymphomas, it offers only structural information. The primary pitfalls of CT evaluation of lymphoma include lymph node assessment by size criteria alone and the inability to distinguish posttreatment fibrosis from residual active tumor. Although CT and MR imaging can provide high-resolution anatomic imaging, PET complements these studies by adding useful information about the metabolic activity through standardized uptake values. 18F-FDG PET has replaced 67Ga-citrate as the nuclear medicine imaging for lymphoma. The increasing role of PET/CT has added sensitivity and specificity, combining anatomic and functional information.

Early studies have demonstrated the efficacy of PET in initial staging of lymphoma and have shown the increased sensitivity when compared with CT alone (**Fig. 13**). A retrospective study by Schoder and colleagues demonstrated that PET affected clinical management in 44% patients and up-staged the disease in 21%.[31,32] PET surveillance after treatment is key to finding residual or recurrent disease that can be nonspecific on anatomic imaging (**Figs. 14 and 15**). Specifically, FDG-PET can help to distinguish posttreatment fibrosis from active residual tumor. 18F-FDG PET has a higher specificity (92% versus 17%), accuracy (96% versus 63%), and positive predictive value (94% versus 60%) than CT.[33]

PET may also be useful for early prediction of treatment response. One study evaluated 30 patients with NHL and HL before and after one cycle of chemotherapy. Fifteen patients had residual FDG-avid disease, and 87% experienced early relapse or never achieved remission. Fifteen patients had no residual FDG activity, and 87% of these patients had complete remission with a median of 19 months of follow-up.[34] At the University of California at San Francisco, patients with pathology primary to the head and neck undergo PET/CT scans with post contrast images of the chest, abdomen, and pelvis and diagnostic quality post contrast CT of the neck.

## SUMMARY

HL and NHL involving the head and neck have many overlapping imaging features, and definitive diagnosis depends on histology; however, both have imaging trends that may help distinguish them from other common pathologic entities in the head and neck. HL is predominately nodal (>90%) and frequently presents with supraclavicular and mediastinal lymphadenopathy with spread along contiguous nodal groups. NHL can be extranodal in as many as 30% of patients. Waldeyer's ring is the most common site, with more than half of head and neck extranodal NHL occurring here (**Table 1**). Specific NHL subtypes have predilections for certain locations in the head and neck. MALT lymphomas commonly involve the ocular adnexa, salivary glands, and thyroid; diffuse large B-cell lymphomas involve Waldeyer's ring and paranasal sinuses; NK cell lymphomas involve the nasal cavity; and Burkitt's lymphomas involve the maxilla and mandible (**Table 2**). Aggressive NHL subtypes such as NK cell and Burkitt's lymphoma can have permeative bone destruction, closely mimicking their squamous cell carcinoma counterparts. Other low-grade NHL subtypes such as MALT lymphoma and B-cell lymphoma are more well circumscribed and exhibit exophytic rather than infiltrative growth and lack bone destruction. Many NHL subtypes are also specifically associated with certain predisposing clinical factors, such as Sjogren's syndrome and MALT lymphoma of the parotid, HIV infection and diffuse large B-cell NHL of the oral cavity, and Hashimoto's thyroiditis and MALT lymphoma of the thyroid.

Nodal lymphoma has a myriad of imaging appearances. Nodes are most often homogeneous, ranging in size from 2 to 10 cm; however, necrosis and calcification can be seen before treatment, more commonly with NHL than HL.

MR imaging, CT, and PET are currently used for staging and surveillance imaging. A staging neck, chest, abdomen, and pelvis CT is routinely performed for evaluation of lymphadenopathy. CT is also useful for bony involvement. In the head and neck, MR imaging is performed for further soft tissue detail in extranodal disease, especially when there is transpatial disease or intracranial or intraspinal extension. Extranodal lymphoma typically has T1 hypointensity, T2 mild hyperintensity, and homogeneous mild enhancement. PET has become the mainstay of staging and

| Table 1 |
|---|
| Common imaging features of lymphoma in the head and neck: features of Hodgkin lymphoma and non-Hodgkin lymphoma |

| Type of Lymphoma | Location | Feature |
|---|---|---|
| Hodgkin | Contiguous spread, internal jugular chain and mediastinum | Lymphadenopathy |
| Non-Hodgkin | –Noncontinguous and unusual nodal chains (ie, occipital, parotid, [posterior triangle) <br> –Extranodal and extralymphatic involvement | Lymphadenopathy, mass |

**Table 2**
Common imaging features of lymphoma in the head and neck: features of the most common non-Hodgkin lymphomas

| Type of non-Hodgkin Lymphoma | Location | Feature |
|---|---|---|
| MALT | Ocular adnexa (common) | Homogenous mass encasing orbital structure |
| | Parotid | Solitary or multifocal bilateral masses[a] |
| | Thyroid | Solitary homogeneous mass or multiple nodules |
| | Larynx | Homogenous submucosal mass in supraglottis.[b] |
| Follicular | Waldeyer's ring | >50% in palatine tonsil |
| | Parotid | Solitary or multifocal bilateral masses.[a] |
| Diffuse B cell | Thyroid | Solitary homogeneous mass or multiple nodules |
| | Waldeyer's ring | >50% in palatine tonsil |
| | Larynx | Homogenous submucosal mass in supraglottis.[b] |
| | Ocular adnexa (rare) | Homogenous mass encasing orbital structure |
| NK/T cell | Sinonasal | Destructive mass most commonly arising in nasal cavity[c] |
| Burkitt | Mandible/maxilla | Large osteolytic mass, commonly near angle of mandible |

[a] Primary parotid lymphoma, often unilateral diffuse parotid infiltration.
[b] Extends to hypopharynx or glottis, less commonly to subglottis.
[c] Unlike carcinoma, more commonly arises in paranasal sinuses.

surveillance imaging and is particularly useful to distinguish posttreatment fibrosis and residual tumor.

## REFERENCES

1. DePena CA, Van Tassel P, Lee YY. Lymphoma of the head and neck. Radiol Clin North Am 1990;28(4): 723–43.
2. Lee YY, Van Tassel P, Nauert C, et al. Lymphomas of the head and neck: CT findings at initial presentation. AJR Am J Roentgenol 1987;149(3):575–81.
3. Urquhart A, Berg R. Hodgkin's and non-Hodgkin's lymphoma of the head and neck. Laryngoscope 2001;111(9):1565–9.
4. Weber AL, Rahemtullah A, Ferry JA. Hodgkin and non-Hodgkin lymphoma of the head and neck: clinical, pathologic, and imaging evaluation. Neuroimaging Clin N Am 2003;13(3):371–92.
5. Harnsberger HR, Bragg DG, Osborn AG, et al. Non-Hodgkin's lymphoma of the head and neck: CT evaluation of nodal and extranodal sites. AJR Am J Roentgenol 1987;149(4):785–91.
6. Carbone PP, Kaplan HS, Musshoff K, et al. Report of the committee on Hodgkin's disease staging classification. Cancer Res 1971;31(11):1860–1.
7. Rademaker J. Hodgkin's and non-Hodgkin's lymphomas. Radiol Clin North Am 2007;45(1):69–83.
8. Greenlee RT, Murray T, Bolden S, et al. Cancer statistics, 2000. CA Cancer J Clin 2000;50(1):7–33.
9. Harris NL, Jaffe ES, Stein H, et al. A revised European-American classification of lymphoid neoplasms: a proposal from the International Lymphoma Study Group. Blood 1994;84(5):1361–92.
10. National Cancer Institute sponsored study of classifications of non-Hodgkin's lymphomas: summary and description of a working formulation for clinical usage. The Non-Hodgkin's Lymphoma Pathologic Classification Project. Cancer 1982;49(10): 2112–35.
11. Nayak LM, Deschler DG. Lymphomas. Otolaryngol Clin North Am 2003;36(4):625–46.
12. Yuen A, Jacobs C. Lymphomas of the head and neck. Semin Oncol 1999;26(3):338–45.
13. Aviles A, Delgado S, Ruiz H, et al. Treatment of non-Hodgkin's lymphoma of Waldeyer's ring: radiotherapy versus chemotherapy versus combined therapy. Eur J Cancer B Oral Oncol 1996;32B(1):19–23.
14. King AD, Lei KI, Richards PS, et al. Non-Hodgkin's lymphoma of the nasopharynx: CT and MR imaging. Clin Radiol 2003;58(8):621–5.
15. Abbondanzo SL, Wenig BM. Non-Hodgkin's lymphoma of the sinonasal tract: a clinicopathologic

and immunophenotypic study of 120 cases. Cancer 1995;75(6):1281–91.

16. Cheung MM, Chan JK, Lau WH, et al. Primary non-Hodgkin's lymphoma of the nose and nasopharynx: clinical features, tumor immunophenotype, and treatment outcome in 113 patients. J Clin Oncol 1998;16(1):70–7.

17. Das S, Kirsch CF. Imaging of lumps and bumps in the nose: a review of sinonasal tumours. Cancer Imaging 2005;5:167–77.

18. Wolvius EB, van der Valk P, van der Wal JE, et al. Primary non-Hodgkin's lymphoma of the salivary glands: an analysis of 22 cases. J Oral Pathol Med 1996;25(4):177–81.

19. Hyman GA, Wolff M. Malignant lymphomas of the salivary glands: review of the literature and report of 33 new cases, including four cases associated with the lymphoepithelial lesion. Am J Clin Pathol 1976;65(4):421–38.

20. Stafford ND, Wilde A. Parotid cancer. Surg Oncol 1997;6(4):209–13.

21. Mehle ME, Kraus DH, Wood BG, et al. Lymphoma of the parotid gland. Laryngoscope 1993;103(1 Pt 1): 17–21.

22. Widder S, Pasieka JL. Primary thyroid lymphomas. Curr Treat Options Oncol 2004;5(4):307–13.

23. Ansell SM, Grant CS, Habermann TM. Primary thyroid lymphoma. Semin Oncol 1999;26(3): 316–23.

24. Matsuzuka F, Miyauchi A, Katayama S, et al. Clinical aspects of primary thyroid lymphoma: diagnosis and treatment based on our experience of 119 cases. Thyroid 1993;3(2):93–9.

25. King AD, Yuen EH, Lei KI, et al. Non-Hodgkin lymphoma of the larynx: CT and MR imaging findings. AJNR Am J Neuroradiol 2004;25(1):12–5.

26. LaCasce AS. Post-transplant lymphoproliferative disorders. Oncologist 2006;11(6):674–80.

27. Loevner LA, Karpati RL, Kumar P, et al. Posttransplantation lymphoproliferative disorder of the head and neck: imaging features in seven adults. Radiology 2000;216(2):363–9.

28. Zapater E, Bagan JV, Campos A, et al. Non-Hodgkin's lymphoma of the head and neck in association with HIV infection. Ann Otolaryngol Chir Cervicofac 1996;113(2):69–72.

29. Carbone A, Gloghini A. AIDS-related lymphomas: from pathogenesis to pathology. Br J Haematol 2005;130(5):662–70.

30. Marsot-Dupuch K, Quillard J, Meyohas MC. Head and neck lesions in the immunocompromised host. Eur Radiol 2004;14(Suppl 3):E155–67.

31. Schoder H, Meta J, Yap C, et al. Effect of whole-body (18)F-FDG PET imaging on clinical staging and management of patients with malignant lymphoma. J Nucl Med 2001;42(8):1139–43.

32. Jhanwar YS, Straus DJ. The role of PET in lymphoma. J Nucl Med 2006;47(8):1326–34.

33. Cremerius U, Fabry U, Neuerburg J, et al. Positron emission tomography with 18F-FDG to detect residual disease after therapy for malignant lymphoma. Nucl Med Commun 1998;19(11):1055–63.

34. Kostakoglu L, Coleman M, Leonard JP, et al. PET predicts prognosis after 1 cycle of chemotherapy in aggressive lymphoma and Hodgkin's disease. J Nucl Med 2002;43(8):1018–27.

# Imaging of Lymphoma of the Musculoskeletal System

Sinchun Hwang, MD

**KEYWORDS**

- Lymphoma • Bone muscle • Cutaneous
- Radiography • CT • MR imaging • PET

Musculoskeletal involvement by lymphoma may occur as a part of disseminated disease or an isolated manifestation (ie, primary lymphoma of bone or muscle). Clinical features, prognosis, and treatment of lymphoma differ for isolated, primary lymphoma and disseminated disease, but their imaging features are similar. This article reviews imaging features of lymphoma of bone, muscles, and subcutaneous tissue. Evaluation of bone marrow changes with MR imaging and positron emission tomography (PET) will be discussed as well as post-treatment changes.

The evaluation of musculoskeletal lymphoma often requires more than one imaging modality and may include radiography, bone scintigraphy, CT, MR imaging, and/or PET. Lymphoma is a heterogenous disease, and thus its imaging features vary among the different modalities. Radiography, bone scintigraphy, CT, PET, and MR imaging each provide different information about the disease process. Radiography and CT depict bone destruction. Bone scintigraphy depicts the osteoblastic reaction and bone formation. PET depicts 2-(18F) fluoro-2-deoxy-D-glucose (FDG)-avid lesions in the bone marrow, and MR imaging detects changes by tumor and treatment in the bone marrow composition. For example, marrow involvement of lymphomas is detected better with PET and MR imaging, whereas cortical bone destruction and pathologic fractures are visualized easily with radiography and CT. Plasma cell myeloma and plasmocytoma are included in the 2001 World Health Organization (WHO) Classification Scheme for Lymphoma but will not be discussed explicitly in this article.

## LYMPHOMA OF THE BONE

Primary lymphoma of bone (PLB) is rare, comprising less than 1% of all lymphomas,[1] 5% of extranodal non-Hodgkin lymphoma (NHL) and 3% to 5% of all primary bone tumors.[2,3] PLB initially was described as reticulum cell sarcoma by Oberling in 1928,[4] to distinguish it from other primary malignant bone tumors. Parker and Jackson[5] reported the first case series of NHL in adults in 1939. The term PLB was introduced by Ivins and Dahlin in 1963.[6] The diagnostic criteria for PLB include lymphoma within a single bone with or without regional nodal metastases and the absence of distal lesions within 6 months following the diagnosis.[7] When PLB involves more than one bone without distal metastases, it is recognized as a subgroup of PLB and termed primary multifocal osseous lymphoma or multifocal primary lymphoma of bone.[2,8,9] PLB has a predilection for the pelvis and appendicular skeleton, with the femur and tibia being the most common sites. Multifocal PLB also tends to involve vertebrae more often than PLB.[2,3] Within long bones, diaphyses and metaphyses commonly are involved. The location of the involved bone does not appear to have a statistically significant effect on the overall survival rate of PLB.[10]

Multiorgan involvement with involvement of the bone or relapsed lymphoma with involvement of the bone has imaging and immunocytologic features similar to those of PLB and will not be discussed separately.

Department of Radiology, Memorial Sloan-Kettering Cancer Center, 1275 York Avenue, New York, NY 10065, USA
*E-mail address:* hwangs1@mskcc.org

Radiol Clin N Am 46 (2008) 379–396
doi:10.1016/j.rcl.2008.03.008
0033-8389/08/$ – see front matter

## Clinical Features

The most common symptom is bone pain (61%), but B symptoms (fever, night sweat, and weight loss) are rare (13%) in PLB.[11] Palpable masses and an elevated level of lactate dehydrogenase (LDH) (31%)[11] may be present. Most cases of PLB and multifocal osseous lymphoma involvement result from NHL. PLB is more common in males (male-to-female ratio 1.5-2.3:1).[2,3,12] The median age is 42 to 54 years.[2,3,11–13] PBL is rare in children younger than 10 years of age.[14] The overall survival rate for PLB is better than the survival rates for other primary bone tumors. For example, in a study of 82 patients who had PLB, Beal and colleagues[11] reported that the 5-year survival rate (with combined radiation and chemotherapy, radiation alone or chemotherapy alone) was 88%, and in a study of 77 patients who had PLB, Barbieri and colleagues[13] reported that the 15-year survival rate (with radiation, with or without chemotherapy) was 88.3%. In contrast, a study of 1702 patients who had osteosarcoma by Bielack and colleagues[15] found 5-year and 15-year survival rates of 65% and 57%, respectively. In adults, favorable prognostic factors for overall survival include age younger than 40 years, lack of B symptoms, normal LDH level, and female gender.[11]

## Imaging

Lymphoma can occur in bone marrow, cortical bone, or both, and also may extend outside of bone. When tumor is confined only to bone marrow, infiltration of the bone marrow with lymphoma cells may have no imaging correlate on MR imaging or PET and often is diagnosed by bone marrow biopsy. When a cortical lesion is associated with an extraosseous soft tissue mass, it may be difficult to distinguish lymphoma of bone with extraosseous extension from soft tissue lymphoma invading the bone. This distinction, however, does not influence staging or treatment significantly.

## Radiography

Radiographic manifestation of osseous lymphoma is variable and nonspecific and tends to underrepresent the extent of osseous lesions, especially when lesions are confined to the marrow cavity. Therefore, additional imaging such as MR imaging or PET usually is obtained for further evaluation. The radiographic pattern can be normal, predominantly lytic, sclerotic, or mixed lytic–sclerotic. In particular, osseous lymphoma is known for having a deceivingly normal appearance on radiography while displaying extensive abnormality on

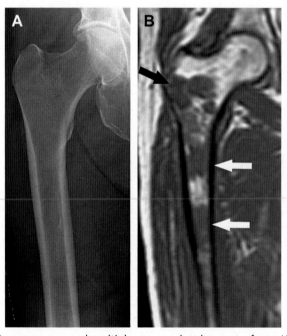

**Fig. 1.** Normal radiographic appearance and multiple marrow involvement of non-Hodgkin lymphoma at MR imaging. (*A*) Frontal radiograph of the right proximal femur is normal. (*B*) Coronal T1 weighted image reveals multiple low-signal-intensity lesions (*arrows*) in the medullary canal of the proximal femur.

cross-sectional modalities and bone scintigraphy (**Figs. 1–3**).[12] When it is visible on radiography, it most often displays a lytic pattern.[12,14] Lytic osseous lymphoma may be well circumscribed, or it may be characterized by a wide zone of transition (permeative or moth-eaten). Cortical destruction, extraosseous soft-tissue masses, and periosteal reaction indicate advanced local disease (**Fig. 4**).[2] Periosteal reactions are usually aggressive patterns, including linear, lamellated, or disrupted, and disrupted periosteal bone formation is considered to be an indicator of poor prognosis.[2] Pathologic fractures are not rare at the time of diagnosis (17% to 22%).[12,14] Differential diagnostic considerations of lytic osseous lymphoma include both malignant and benign categories. In adults, they may include metastases, chondroblastic osteosarcoma, multiple myeloma, plasmacytoma, osteomyelitis, and giant cell tumor (especially in the end of long bones). In children, differential diagnostic considerations may include Ewing sarcoma, primitive neuroectodermal tumor (PNET), infection, and eosinophilic granuloma.

A sclerotic pattern of osseous lymphoma was reported in 2% of PLB in a study of 237 patients[12]; it is seen more frequently in Hodgkin lymphoma (HL) (**Fig. 5**) and reported in 24% of 15 patients whose radiography was performed in one study.[16] Diffuse sclerosis may be related to fibrosis, with dense ivory vertebrae being a classic presentation,[17] and sclerosis can develop following chemotherapy or radiation.[2] Diffuse sclerotic osseous lesions also have been associated with other neoplastic and non-neoplastic processes such as primary bone tumor (osteosarcoma), metastases (from prostate or breast cancer), Paget's disease, and sarcoidosis.

## Bone Scan

Bone scintigraphy is superior to radiography in the detection of multifocal osseous involvement (**Fig. 6**), but it is less effective than MR imaging and PET in the detection of marrow involvement and lesions without bone remodeling. At bone scintigraphy, increased radiotracer uptake is the most common finding.[12] Bone scintigraphy, however, is not specific for tumor, because radiotracer uptake also is seen in benign processes such as fractures. The results of bone scintigraphy do not correlate with clinical outcomes.[8]

## CT

CT is an excellent imaging modality for assessing osseous involvement of lymphoma, including cortical and trabecular destruction, periosteal reaction, sequestra, and extraosseous extension. (**Figs. 7, 8**) Contrast-enhanced CT is also

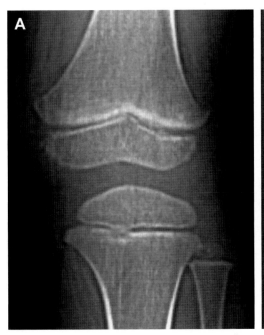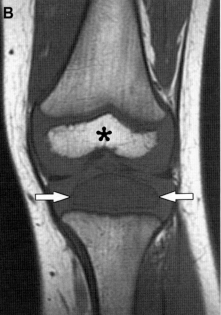

Fig. 2. Normal radiographic appearance and epiphyseal involvement of non-Hodgkin lymphoma at MR imaging. (*A*) Frontal radiograph of a 7-year-old patient with knee pain is normal. (*B*) Coronal T1 weighted image shows diffuse marrow involvement of the proximal epiphysis of the tibia (*arrows*). Note that the normal marrow of the distal femoral epiphysis is fatty (*) after physiologic conversion from red to yellow marrow.

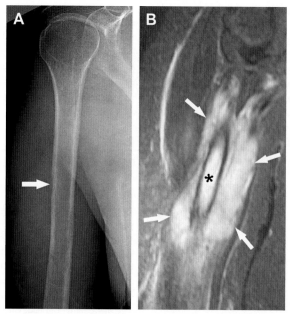

Fig. 3. A large mass on MR imaging without osseous destruction on radiograph. (A) Frontal radiograph of the humerus shows a subtle lucent focus (*arrow*) at the deltoid attachment. Otherwise, no osseous destruction is evident. (B) Coronal STIR image demonstrates a humeral lesion (*) and a large extraosseous mass (*arrows*) encasing the humerus.

occasionally useful in studying marrow involvement and planning targeted biopsy (**Fig. 9**). Osseous destruction is variable on CT, and the relative absence of cortical destruction is an imaging feature favoring lymphoma over other malignant and benign tumors that destroy the cortex, such as osteosarcoma and eosinophilic granuloma. Intramedullary lesions and extraosseous masses with a lack of cortical destruction suggest tumor spread by means of vascular channels of the cortex.[18] Extraosseous tumor growth of lymphoma with relative preservation of the cortex is known in lymphoma and best seen on CT and MR imaging (**Fig. 10**). This feature, however, also is observed in other malignancies such as Ewing sarcoma and PNET.

Sequestra, fragments of dead bone, are also features noted in osseous lymphoma at CT.[18] Although sequestra most are often associated with osteomyelitis, they also are seen in nonmatrix forming bone tumors such as fibrosarcoma, malignant fibrous histiocytoma, and eosinophilic granuloma.[12] CT is also superior to radiography and MR imaging in detecting and characterizing periosteal reactions.

### MR Imaging

Normal bone marrow consists largely of lipids and water. Because MR imaging is remarkably effective in detecting lipids and free mobile protons (ie, water), it offers major advantages in the evaluation of changes in bone marrow affected by lymphoma. The signal intensity of tumor within bone marrow is low to slightly high (relative to that of

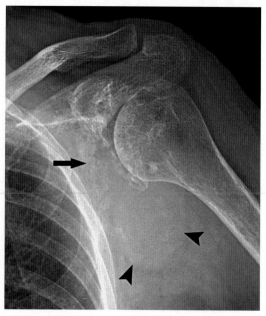

Fig. 4. Lytic radiographic appearance of non-Hodgkin lymphoma. Frontal view of the shoulder shows a permeative lytic lesion in the glenoid (*arrow*) and an extraosseous mass in the axilla (*arrowheads*).

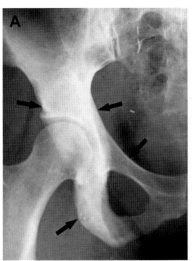
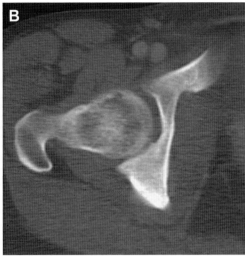

**Fig. 5.** Sclerotic radiographic appearance of Hodgkin lymphoma. (*A*) Frontal radiograph and (*B*) CT axial image of the right hip demonstrate diffuse sclerosis in the acetabulum, pubis, and ischium (*arrows in A*).

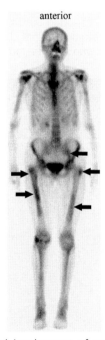

muscle) on T1 weighted images and high on T2 weighted images (**Fig. 11**). Although this imaging feature is helpful in detecting tumor, it is not specific for lymphoma. A T1 weighted sequence is best for evaluating the extent of tumor in terms of size and multifocal marrow involvement. Short tau inversion recovery or T2 weighted fat suppression images are also sensitive in detecting marrow lesions, but peri-lesional edema may not be distinguishable from tumor and may result in

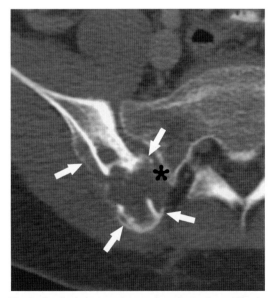

**Fig. 6.** Multifocal involvement of non-Hodgkin lymphoma on bone scan. Anterior whole-body bone scan demonstrates multiple areas of increased radiotracer uptake in the femora and left ilium (*arrows*). A pathologic compression fracture of T6 vertebra was also present in the posterior view (not shown). Subsequent MR imaging and positron emission tomography (not shown) confirmed multifocal osseous involvement. Foci of increased uptake in the shoulders, sternomanubrial region, and right knee are degenerative in origin.

**Fig. 7.** Cortical destruction and periosteal reaction in Hodgkin lymphoma. Axial CT image of the right pelvis reveals a destructive lesion in the right posterior ilium, extending into the sacroiliac joint (*). Periosteal reaction (*arrows*) is evident at the edge of the cortical destruction.

overestimation of osseous lesions. The signal intensity of osseous lymphoma on STIR and T2 weighted images is more variable (intermediate to high) (**Fig. 12**). Low signal intensity of lymphoma on T2 weighted images also has been reported in a few studies.[3,19] Extraosseous soft tissue masses are of low signal intensity on T1 weighted images and of high signal intensity on T2 weighted images, and contrast enhancement of extraosseous masses is predominantly diffuse and homogenous (see **Fig. 11**).[19] Extraosseous extension of tumor without cortical destruction is visualized well on MR imaging (**Fig. 13**). Involvement of lymphoma in bone marrow often can be multifocal or diffuse. Although bone marrow biopsy is a well-established method for diagnosing bone marrow involvement in lymphoma, MR imaging, as a noninvasive imaging tool, allows evaluation of larger areas of marrow and can guide biopsies to focal regions of involvement (**Fig. 14**).

MR imaging is less specific than histologic analysis in distinguishing viable tumor from post-treatment changes. In attempts to increase the accuracy of MR imaging in identifying treatment response and post-treatment changes, various complementary techniques have been evaluated, including the use of a quantitative T1 relaxation time, quantitative chemical-shift imaging, diffusion-weighted echo–planar imaging, and dynamic contrast-enhanced imaging.[20–23] Studies, however, have been limited by numbers of patients and technical complexities. With recent technical advances in MR imaging allowing faster scanning, whole-body MR imaging is becoming a promising tool for the diagnosis and staging of osseous involvement of lymphoma. The potential role of whole-body MR imaging is pending the results of larger studies.[24] Few detailed studies have been performed comparing PET and MR imaging for the evaluation of bone marrow disease in lymphoma.

## LYMPHOMA OF MUSCLES

Skeletal muscle involvement of lymphoma usually occurs as a part of disseminated disease. Although it is rare, lymphoma can occur in skeletal muscle as primary lymphoma of muscle (PLM). Samuel and colleagues[25] found eight cases of PLM in a database of over 6000 patients who had NHL, and Komatsuda and colleagues[26] reported 31 cases (both HL and NHL) among 2147 patients who had lymphoma. PLM usually occurs in patients over 60 years of age and is predominantly NHL (large B-cell type); thighs, chests, and arms are the most commonly reported sites.[25,27,28] B symptoms and elevation of LDH can be seen. Samuel and colleagues[25] reported that three of eight patients had B symptoms and that LDH was elevated in all six patients who were tested.

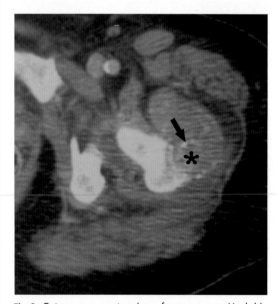

Fig. 8. Extraosseous extension of osseous non-Hodgkin lymphoma. Axial CT image of left proximal femur demonstrates a destructive lesion arising from the greater trochanter. Extraosseous soft tissue mass (*) contains bony fragments (*arrow*).

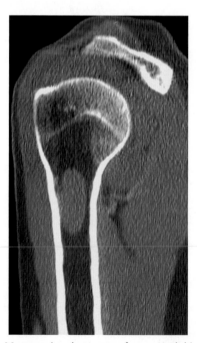

Fig. 9. Marrow involvement of non-Hodgkin lymphoma on contrast-enhanced CT. A coronal reformatted contrast-enhanced CT image shows an enhancing marrow lesion in the proximal humerus. It may be difficult to differentiate lymphoma in bone marrow from enhancing red marrow on CT.

## Imaging

On imaging, the appearance of lymphoma in muscle is variable. It can appear as muscle enlargement (diffuse or focal), infiltration, or a focal mass, and it may involve more than one muscle. When it is multifocal, lymphomatous involvement may or may not be contiguous.[27] The tumor may extend beyond the muscular compartment and fascial planes.

## MR Imaging

MR imaging is superior to other imaging modalities in delineating anatomic borders and the internal architecture of soft tissue. In particular, MR imaging has advantages for evaluating concurrent cortical marrow involvement. The signal intensity of lymphoma in muscle is intermediate (relative to muscle) on T1 weighted images and high on T2 weighted images (**Fig. 15**). Muscle enlargement, however, may not be apparent despite signal abnormality (**Fig. 16**).[29] Infiltration of adjacent subcutaneous tissue and fascial planes is not uncommon (see **Fig. 16**).[27,30] Contrast enhancement can be homogeneous or heterogeneous.

## CT

CT is used for evaluating soft-tissue masses as an alternative modality when MR imaging is not available or MR imaging is limited because of patient compliance issues such as claustrophobia and motion. CT also serves as a tool to guide biopsy of soft-tissue masses. Lymphoma in muscle can be homogeneously iso-dense to muscle on non-contrast CT (**Fig. 17**), and it may be difficult to detect lesions even with intravenous contrast administration (see **Fig. 17**).[29] The calcifications are usually absent.[30]

## Ultrasound

Ultrasound (US) has a minor role in the staging of malignant soft tissue masses. Because it is readily available and non-invasive, however, without

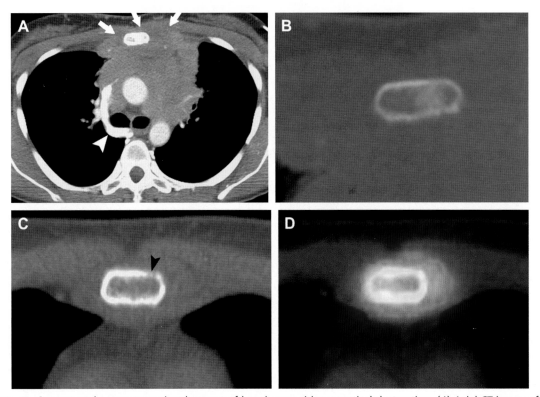

**Fig. 10.** Osseous and extraosseous involvement of lymphoma without cortical destruction. (*A*) Axial CT image of a patient with Hodgkin lymphoma shows a large mediastinal mass. The mass obstructs the superior vena cava, causing reflux of intravenous contrast into the azygous vein (*arrowhead*). The mass also infiltrates the anterior chest wall *(arrows)* and encases the sternum. (*B*) Magnified axial CT image of the sternum reveals a sclerotic lesion within the sternum without cortical destruction. (*C*) Axial CT image of a different patient with non-Hodgkin lymphoma shows a parasternal mass. Except for a subtle lucency in the anterior sternum (*arrowhead*), the cortex is intact. (*D*) Axial fused positron emission tomography–CT image of the sternum shows diffuse FDG uptake within the sternum and parasternal mass.

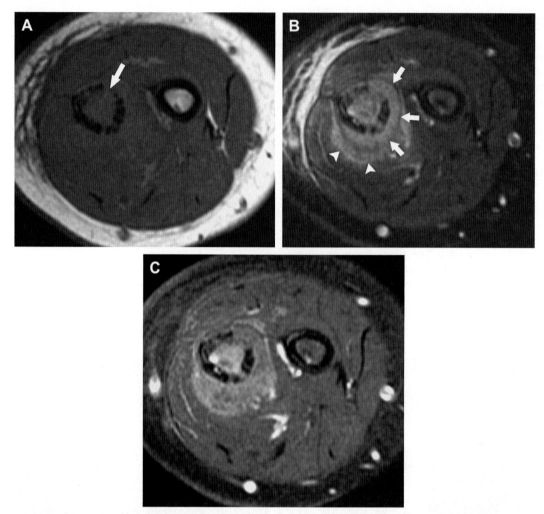

**Fig. 11.** Signal intensity of lymphoma on MR imaging. (*A*) On axial T1 weighted image of non-Hodgkin lymphoma in the forearm, the signal intensity of tumor within the ulna is intermediate to slightly high relative to the signal intensity of muscle. Cortical destruction (*arrow*) may be present as it is in this patient. (*B*) On axial T2 weighted image with fat suppression, the signal intensity of tumor is high. The extraosseous mass (*arrowheads*) also extends beyond the periosteum (*arrows*). (*C*) On axial T1 weighted MR image, diffuse contrast enhancement is seen within the tumor.

requiring intravenous contrast and ionizing radiation, US often is used as the initial imaging modality for a symptomatic mass. In addition, US provides real-time guidance during biopsies, allowing safe and accurate tissue sampling with avoidance of neurovascular structures and necrotic areas. The sonographic appearance of soft tissue lymphoma is solid, heterogeneous, and hypoechoic, and the borders of lesions may be defined well or poorly (**Fig. 18**).[27] Hypervascularity on color and power Doppler US is variable and not specific for malignancy.[31]

### Differential Diagnosis

Imaging features of lymphoma in skeletal muscle are nonspecific, and it can be difficult to differentiate lymphoma from various neoplastic and

non-neoplastic conditions such as primary soft tissue sarcoma, metastases, trauma, and myositis. When muscle involvement is diffuse, it can mimic muscle edema from deep vein thrombosis, infectious myositis, and inflammatory myositis. In contrast, when tumor is focal, primary soft tissue sarcoma, hematoma, and metastases are important differential considerations. Primary soft tissue sarcoma tends to be more heterogeneous in density than lymphoma on CT.

### LYMPHOMA OF CUTANEOUS AND SUBCUTANEOUS TISSUE

Primary cutaneous lymphoma refers to lymphoma in the skin without extracutaneous involvement of

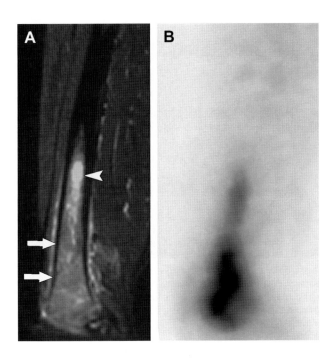

Fig. 12. Signal heterogeneity of osseous non-Hodgkin lymphoma on MR imaging. (*A*) Sagittal STIR image of the thigh demonstrates heterogeneous signal intensity within marrow of the distal femur. Signal intensity in the distal metadiaphysis (*arrows*) is lower than signal intensity in the distal diaphysis (*arrowhead*). (*B*) Sagittal positron emission tomography image also shows heterogenous uptake in the distal femur.

lymphoma at the time of diagnosis.[32,33] The skin is the second most common site of extranodal involvement of NHL after the gastrointestinal tract.[32] Depending on cellular origin, primary cutaneous lymphoma is classified as either cutaneous T cell lymphoma (CTCL) or cutaneous B cell lymphoma (CBCL). Mycosis fungoides is the most common type of CTCL.[32] CTCL generally appears as eczema-like skin rashes or plaque-like lesions affecting any part of the body, with or without localized or diffuse lymphadenopathy. CBCL often produces nodule-like lesions. Imaging

features of cutaneous lymphoma are nonspecific and include soft tissue thickening, infiltration, or a mass (**Figs. 19, 20**).[33,34] The Ann Arbor staging classification for lymphoma is of limited value for most primary cutaneous lymphomas, and specialized staging criteria, including the TMN classification, were introduced for these entities.[35] Imaging is important for identifying extracutaneous manifestations of lymphoma, and it usually includes CT of the chest, abdomen, and pelvis with contrast, alone, or with whole-body PET, or, alternatively, integrated whole-body PET CT.[35]

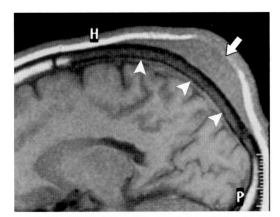

Fig. 13. Non-Hodgkin lymphoma involving the parietal bone and adjacent scalp without cortical destruction. Sagittal T1 weighted image of the head demonstrates low signal intensity in the parietal bone (*arrowheads*) and adjacent scalp mass (*arrow*) compatible with tumor involvement. There is no cortical destruction.

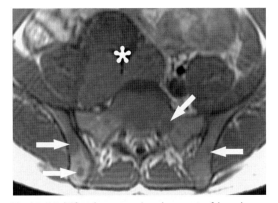

Fig. 14. Multifocal osseous involvement of lymphoma on MR imaging. Axial T weighted image of the pelvis demonstrates multiple marrow lesions in the iliac bones and sacrum (*arrows*). Right common iliac adenopathy (*) is also evident.

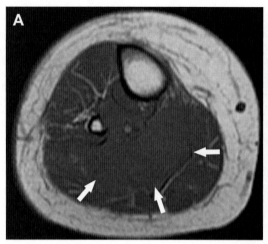
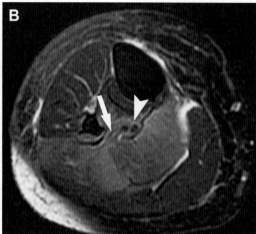

Fig. 15. Muscle lymphoma of the calf on MR imaging. (A) Axial T1 weighted image shows a mass (arrows) in the posterior compartment. The signal intensity of the mass is intermediate relative to that of muscle. (B) Axial STIR image demonstrates high signal intensity within the mass, which increases the lesion conspicuity. The mass extends through deep fascia (arrow) of the posterior compartment and encases the posterior tibial vessels (arrowhead). (Courtesy of Robert A. Lefkowitz, MD, New York, NY.)

## MUSCULOSKELETAL LYMPHOMA AND AIDS

In patients who have HIV and AIDS, lymphoma is a common neoplastic complication. For example, NHL is the second most common type of tumor in patients who have AIDS after Kaposi's sarcoma.[36] The risk of NHL is reported to be 60 times greater in patients who have AIDS than in the general population,[37] and lymphoma is considered one of the diagnostic criteria for AIDS. NHL in AIDS tends to be highly aggressive and widely disseminated in bones and muscles, and bone marrow involvement is seen in almost one third of affected patients.[38] The imaging appearance of NHL in AIDS is similar to that of lymphoma in the general population.

## Staging of Musculoskeletal Lymphoma

Lymphoma of bone or muscle without regional nodal involvement and without disseminated disease is classified as stage 1E, whereas lymphoma of bone or muscle with regional nodal involvement and without disseminated disease is classified as stage 2E, according to the Cotswolds modification of the Ann Arbor staging classification.[39]

## RESPONSE TO TREATMENT AND TREATMENT-RELATED CHANGES

Although CT remains the most commonly used imaging modality for the initial evaluation of lymphoma, it has obvious limitations in differentiating

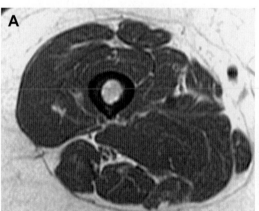
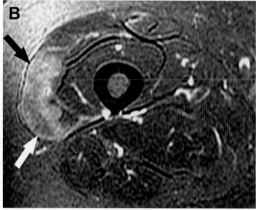

Fig. 16. Subtle muscle lymphoma of the thigh on MR imaging. (A) Axial T1 weighted image of the right thigh shows no obvious muscle enlargement or mass. (B) Axial STIR image at the same level shows a high signal intensity mass (arrows) involving the vastus lateralis muscle. (Courtesy of Robert A. Lefkowitz, MD, New York, NY.)

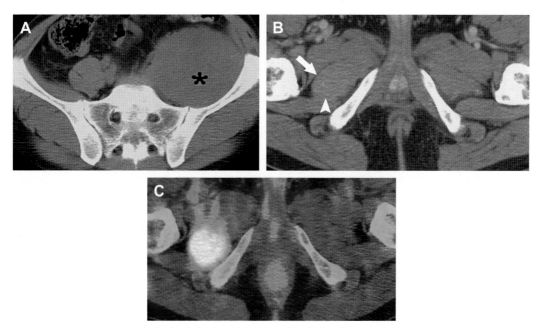

**Fig. 17.** Muscle involvement of non-Hodgkin lymphoma on CT. (*A*) Axial noncontrast CT shows a large mass involving the left iliopsoas muscle (*). The mass is iso-dense to the normal muscles. (*B*) Axial contrast-enhanced CT of a different patient shows a subtle bulging of the right adductor muscle (*arrow*) and loss of the fat plane (*arrowhead*) with the adjacent quadratus femoris muscle. Note that the enhanced bulged muscle is iso-dense to enhanced normal muscles. (*C*) Axial-fused CT–positron emission tomography image shows intense FDG uptake within the muscles, confirming tumor involvement.

viable tumor from post-treatment changes or in assessing bone marrow. PET and MR imaging offer advantages for monitoring treatment response in patients who have musculoskeletal lymphoma.

### Monitoring Treatment Response with FDG–Positron Emission Tomography and MR Imaging

In patients who have FDG PET-avid disease at initial staging, FDG PET allows the assessment of treatment response,[40,41] and it has been incorporated into the revised International Working Group Response Criteria.[42] Response to treatment is defined by a decrease in uptake as identified both on a semiquantitative standardized uptake value scale and by visual inspection. FDG PET shows tumor response earlier than do other imaging modalities, as a decrease in tracer uptake may be detected even before a decrease in tumor volume can be seen. Studies have shown that early response in the course of chemotherapy (as early as the second cycle of chemotherapy) on FDG PET is predictive of event-free and overall survival,[40,41] and FDG PET has potential for identifying

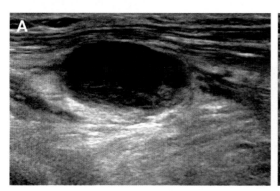
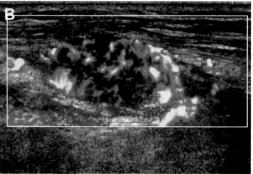

**Fig. 18.** Muscle lymphoma on ultrasound. (*A*) Longitudinal gray scale image demonstrates a well-circumscribed heterogeneously hypoechoic mass within the flexor compartment of the forearm. (*B*) On power Doppler image, the mass is hypervascular. (*Courtesy of* Ronald S. Adler, PhD, MD, New York, NY.)

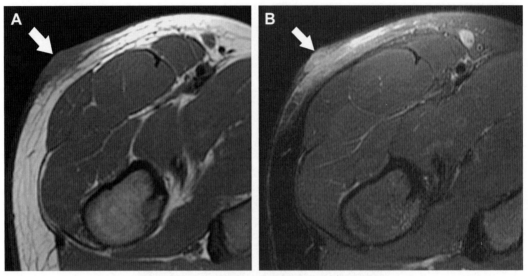

**Fig. 19.** Cutaneous non-Hodgkin lymphoma on MR imaging. (*A*) Axial T1 weighted image and (*B*) axial T2 weighted image with fat suppression demonstrate nodular thickening of the cutaneous and subcutaneous tissue (*arrows*) in the anterior right groin.

patients who may benefit from more aggressive therapies early in the course of treatment.

On MR imaging, a decrease in tumor size, a decrease in signal intensity on T2 weighted images, and a decrease in tumor contrast enhancement may be encountered after treatment (**Fig. 21**). Only the change in size of a mass like lesion is incorporated in the response criteria.[42,43] Residual lesions from necrosis, inflammation, and/or fibrosis of treated tumor are difficult to distinguish from viable tumor.[44,45] On CT, a decrease in size and a decrease in contrast enhancement of tumors indicates clinical response. They are not necessarily specific for residual tumor viability, however. In the author's experience, post-treatment changes may persist for anywhere from a few months to years on MR imaging or CT.

## Evaluation of Bone Marrow with MR Imaging After Treatment

Post-treatment changes in marrow may be encountered on MR imaging examinations obtained for reasons other than response assessment, such as evaluation of newly developed back pain. Post-treatment changes reflect changes in marrow composition during and after the course of treatments such as chemotherapy, administration of granulocyte-colony stimulating factor (G-CSF), stem cell transplantation, and radiation therapy. Occasionally, they may be related to post-treatment complications such as infarct and fractures. Knowledge of the marrow signal changes of red marrow hyperplasia and post-treatment effects on MR imaging are crucial for avoiding misdiagnosis of tumor at staging and follow-up.

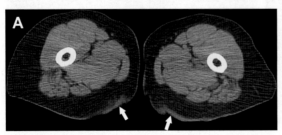
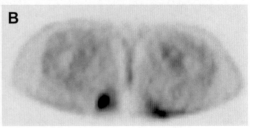

**Fig. 20.** Mycosis fungoides on CT and positron emission tomography (PET). (*A*) Axial CT image demonstrates mild skin thickening and subcutaneous infiltration of the posterior thighs (*arrows*). (*B*) Axial PET image reveals intense FDG uptake within the thickened skin and subcutaneous infiltration.

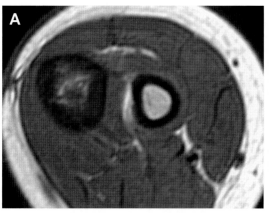
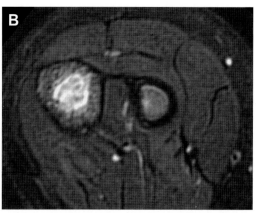

Fig. 21. Post-treatment changes of osseous lymphoma (the same patient in Fig. 11) on MR imaging. (A) Axial T1 weighted image and (B) axial fat-suppressed T2 weighted image show resolution of the extraosseous mass and cortical destruction (see Fig. 11). There is new diffuse cortical thickening. Given residual signal abnormality in the ulna, viable tumor is difficult to exclude. There was no FDG-avid disease in the positron emission tomography study (not shown).

After initiation of chemotherapy, the signal intensity of marrow becomes low on T1 weighted images and high on T2 weighted images, reflecting edema.[46] After chemotherapy, conversion from yellow to red marrow occurs in the reverse sequence of physiologic conversion from red to yellow marrow. Throughout the body, red marrow regenerates from the central skeleton to the peripheral, usually in a bilateral and symmetric fashion. In long bones, regeneration of red marrow occurs from metaphysis to diaphysis. The signal intensity of red marrow tends to be higher than that of muscle on T1 weighted images and intermediate to slightly high on fat-suppressed T2 weighted images and STIR sequences (Fig. 22). Contrast enhancement of red marrow is mild. Reconversion of yellow to red marrow

also can be stimulated by injection of G-CSF or profound chemotherapy-induced anemia. When it is diffuse, red marrow may be difficult to differentiate from tumor.

During and after chemotherapy, G-CSF often is administered to increase the number of neutrophil counts in the setting of chemotherapy-induced neutropenia, and the drug stimulates the bone marrow to produce granulocytes and stem cells. On MR imaging, multiple areas of red marrow develop in a discrete or diffuse pattern (Fig. 23), and the marrow signal intensity is identical to the signal of physiologic red marrow. The dose of G-CSF does not appear related to the extent of red marrow reconversion.[47] Awareness of marrow-stimulating therapy in the course of chemotherapy and the clinical status of individual

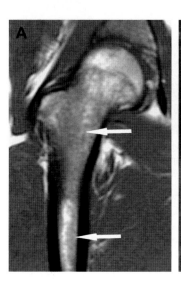
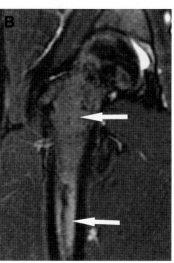

Fig. 22. Signal intensity of red marrow on MR imaging. (A) On coronal T1 weighted image of the proximal femur, the signal intensity of red marrow (arrows) in the proximal femur is high to intermediate relative to that of muscle. (B) On coronal fat-suppressed T2 weighted image, the signal intensity of red marrow (arrows) is intermediate to slightly high.

patients (such as decreased tumor burden in other parts of body) can help to diagnose red marrow reconversion.

Radiation therapy (RT) often is used to treat localized disease such as PLB and to offer palliative relief and local control of multifocal disease such as an impending or pathologic fracture. Radiation-induced changes can be acute or chronic. Immediately following RT, vascular congestion, hemorrhage, and edema ensue within irradiated marrow. An increase in signal intensity on T2 weighted and STIR sequences within a few days after RT is considered to represent marrow edema and hemorrhage, and yellow marrow is seen as early as 8 days after the start of RT.[48] Chronic changes include fatty replacement of marrow, which is evidenced by high-signal intensity within irradiated marrow on T1 weighted images (Fig. 24). In a study of 31 patients, complete conversion to yellow marrow within the radiation field

was seen 6 to 8 weeks after the start of pelvic RT in 90% of patients.[48] The ability of marrow to regenerate depends greatly on many factors, however, including patient age and radiation dose.[49]

## Evaluation of Bone Marrow with FDG-Positron Emission Tomography

The introduction of FDG PET imaging contributed significantly to the evaluation and staging of lymphoma, and at the author's hospital PET replaced gallium scans entirely. Focal or diffuse marrow uptake may be encountered in patients who have lymphoma (Fig. 25). In untreated patients, FDG uptake in marrow greater than FDG uptake in the liver is suggestive of bone marrow involvement.

In the post-treatment setting, diffuse FDG uptake in marrow after chemotherapy usually indicates rebound of normal marrow, and in patients treated with G-CSF, intense FDG uptake in marrow is accompanied by increased FDG uptake in the spleen. Clinical response of tumor at other sites is also helpful to support a diagnosis of rebound marrow. For example, after treatment, it would be very unusual to see a worsening of marrow disease (and hence an increase in SUV relative to the baseline scan SUV) when tumor in other organs had decreased.

Bone marrow evaluation with FDG PET raises two concerns, however. First, it is difficult to identify low-level disease in marrow at the time of staging on FDG PET. It is recognized that the sensitivity of FDG PET is insufficient and that PET cannot

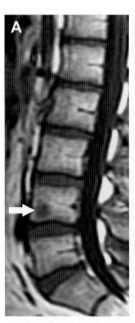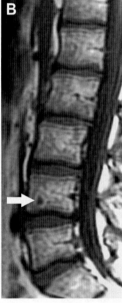

Fig. 23. Red marrow conversion in a 19-year-old patient with lymphoma after granulocyte-colony stimulating factor (G-CSF) treatment. (A) Sagittal T1 weighted image of the lumbar spine before G-CSF treatment demonstrates mildly fatty marrow and a focal lesion in the L4 vertebra (arrow). The focal lesion was also FDG-avid on positron emission tomography (not shown), compatible with tumor. (B) Sagittal T1 weighted image after G-CSF treatment shows diffuse decrease in signal intensity throughout bone marrow. The focal lesion in the L4 vertebra (arrow) is smaller, and pelvic adenopathy (not shown) also has resolved. Given improved disease at different sites, this decrease in signal intensity likely represents red marrow hyperplasia resulting from G-CSF treatment.

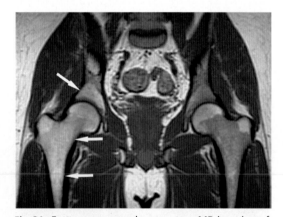

Fig. 24. Fatty marrow replacement on MR imaging after radiation therapy for a right pelvic tumor (patient does not have lymphoma). Coronal T1 weighted image of the pelvis demonstrates diffuse high signal intensity within the irradiated field of the right ilium, right acetabulum, and right proximal femur, compatible with fatty marrow replacement (arrows). Note the high-to-intermediate signal intensity of normal red marrow in the contralateral pelvis and left proximal femur.

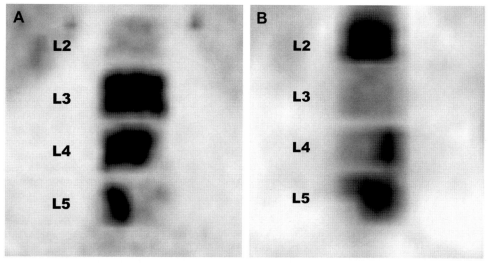

**Fig. 25.** Multifocal lymphoma on PET before (*A*) and after (*B*) chemotherapy and growth factor treatment. The L2 vertebra was not involved by lymphoma in the pretreatment PET scan (*A*), and after chemotherapy and growth factor treatment (*B*), there is new diffuse FDG uptake reflecting red marrow proliferation. The L3 vertebra showed diffuse FDG uptake in the pretreatment scan (*A*), and the uptake is resolved after treatment (*B*). The L4 and L5 vertebrae showed partial uptake in the right side of the vertebral bodies in the pretreatment scan (*A*). After treatment (*B*), the FDG uptake is decreased in the right side of L4 and L5 vertebrae, while it is increased in the left side, reflecting treatment response to the growth factor.

replace bone marrow biopsy.[50] The second concern is more theoretic and relates to the question of whether residual disease may be present in bone marrow that rebounds after chemotherapy. The author's current approach in complicated cases is to wait until rebound activity normalizes and perform a repeat PET scan to see if there is persistent focal uptake. In cases of strong clinical suspicion, a repeat bone marrow biopsy should be considered.

## COMPLICATIONS OF CHEMOTHERAPY AND RADIATION

Chemotherapy and radiation impair the ability of marrow and bone to regenerate and to heal,

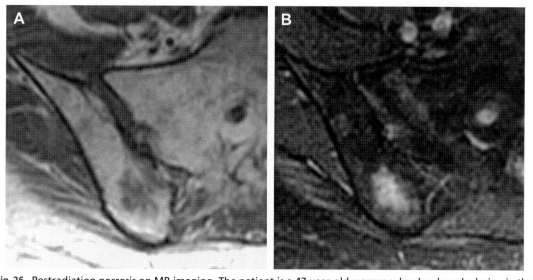

**Fig. 26.** Postradiation necrosis on MR imaging. The patient is a 47-year-old woman who developed a lesion in the right posterior ilium a few years after radiation therapy for sarcoma. (*A*) Axial T1 weighted image demonstrates a lesion of slightly high-to-intermediate signal intensity in the right posterior ilium, and the border of the lesion is irregular and feathery. (*B*) Axial T2 weighted image demonstrates high T2 signal in the lesion. Open biopsy showed fat necrosis and osteoporosis.

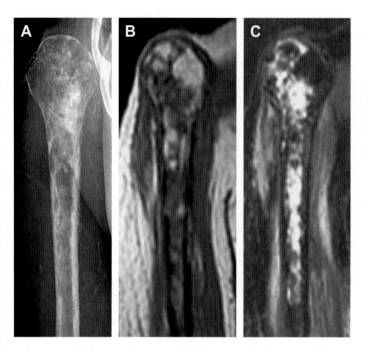

Fig. 27. Radiation osteitis in a 28-year-old woman treated with radiation therapy (RT) for soft tissue sarcoma of the right shoulder. (*A*) Frontal radiograph of the right humerus demonstrates diffuse mixed radiolucent and sclerotic appearance of the irradiated bone caused by areas of osteopenia and trabecular thickening (ie, radiation osteitis). The scapula also was resected in this patient because of RT-induced osteosarcoma (not shown). (*B*) Coronal T1 weighted image and (*C*) coronal fat-suppressed T2 weighted image demonstrate mixed areas of varied T1 and T2 signal intensity within the irradiated bone. The radiographic appearance had been stable for years, and no mass was identified on MR imaging.

causing various complications. Chemotherapy can induce anemia, leukopenia, and osteoporosis (by means of premature gonadal failure or directly interfering with bone formation and repair). In adults and children, avascular necrosis, osteoporosis, and fractures may occur during and after prolonged administration of steroids. RT is known for its risks of growth impairment in children, insufficiency fractures, osteonecrosis, and radiation osteitis (**Figs. 26, 27**).[51,52] RT-induced tumors are

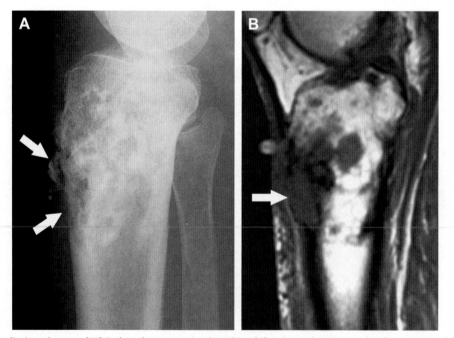

Fig. 28. Radiation therapy (RT)-induced sarcoma in the tibia. (*A*) A lateral radiograph of a 48-year-old woman shows a lytic lesion with cortical destruction (*arrows*) arising from the tibia. The patient received RT to the same area 26 years ago for treatment of osseous lymphoma. A patchy area of mixed lucency and sclerosis in the proximal tibia reflects RT-related treatment changes within the previous lymphoma. (*B*) Sagittal T1 weighted image confirms a tumor (*arrow*) arising from the tibia. Biopsy showed undifferentiated high-grade sarcoma.

a rare but well-known complication,[53] and they can be benign osteochondroma or sarcoma (Fig. 28). The most common histologic types of RT-induced sarcoma of bone include high-grade osteosarcoma, fibrosarcoma, and malignant fibrous histiocytoma, and they are known to be radioresistant.

## SUMMARY

Imaging plays a crucial role in staging and in the assessment of treatment response in patients who have lymphoma of the musculoskeletal system. On radiography, lymphoma of the bone is most commonly lytic, but the affected bone also can appear deceivingly normal, even when a large tumor is present. On CT and MR imaging, osseous destruction is variable. Relative preservation of the cortex in the presence of a large extraosseous tumor is not specific for lymphoma, but it is a helpful finding for differential diagnostic consideration of lymphoma at initial presentation. On CT, lymphoma of muscle can be homogeneous in attenuation, and it may not show contrast enhancement, making tumor detection more difficult. MR imaging and PET are the most effective imaging modalities in detecting multifocal lesions, including marrow lesions. Post-treatment changes often are encountered on MR imaging and PET, and when considered in light of the patient's therapy regimen (eg, radiation therapy and G-CSF) they usually can be differentiated from tumor. Post-treatment changes include diffuse FDG uptake in marrow after chemotherapy, indicating rebound of normal marrow, and MR imaging signal abnormalities that may persist for anywhere from a few months to years after treatment.

## REFERENCES

1. Fairbanks RK, Bonner JA, Inwards CY, et al. Treatment of stage IE primary lymphoma of bone. Int J Radiat Oncol Biol Phys 1994;28:363–72.
2. Krishnan A, Shirkhoda A, Tehranzadeh J, et al. Primary bone lymphoma: radiographic MR imaging correlation. Radiographics 2003;23(6):1371–83.
3. Hermann G, Klein MJ, Abdelwahab IF, et al. MRI appearance of primary non-Hodgkin's lymphoma of bone. Skeletal Radiol 1997;26(11):629–32.
4. Oberling C. Les reticulosarcomes et les reticuloendotheliosarcomes de la moelle osseuse (sarcomas d'Ewing). Bulletin de l'Association francaise pour l'etude du cancer 1928;17:259–96.
5. Parker F Jr, Jackson JH Jr. Primary reticulum cell sarcoma of bone. Surg Gynecol Obstet 1939;68:45–53.
6. Ivins JC, Dahlin DC. Malignant lymphoma (reticulum cell sarcoma) of bone. Proc Staff Meet Mayo Clin 1963;28(38):375–85.
7. Coley BL, Higinbotham NL, Groesbeck HP. Primary reticulum cell sarcoma of bone; summary of 37 cases. Radiology 1950;55(5):641–58.
8. Melamed JW, Martinez S, Hoffman CJ. Imaging of primary multifocal osseous lymphoma. Skeletal Radiol 1997;26(1):35–41.
9. Ostrowski ML, Unni KK, Banks PM, et al. Malignant lymphoma of bone. Cancer 1986;58(12):2646–55.
10. Mankin HJ, Hornicek FJ, Harmon DC, et al. Lymphoma of bone: a review of 140 patients. Therapy 2006;3(4):499–507.
11. Beal K, Allen L, Yahalom J. Primary bone lymphoma: treatment results and prognostic factors with long-term follow-up of 82 patients. Cancer 2006; 106(12):2652–6.
12. Mulligan ME, McRae GA, Murphey MD. Imaging features of primary lymphoma of bone. AJR Am J Roentgenol 1999;173(6):1691–7.
13. Barbieri E, Cammelli S, Mauro F, et al. Primary non-Hodgkin's lymphoma of the bone: treatment and analysis of prognostic factors for stage I and stage II. Int J Radiat Oncol Biol Phys 2004;59(3):760–4.
14. Glotzbecker MP, Kersun LS, Choi JK, et al. Primary non-Hodgkin's lymphoma of bone in children. J Bone Joint Surg Am 2006;88(3):583–94.
15. Bielack SS, Kempf-Bielack B, Delling G, et al. Prognostic factors in high-grade osteosarcoma of the extremities or trunk: an analysis of 1702 patients treated on neoadjuvant cooperative osteosarcoma study group protocols. J Clin Oncol 2002;20(3): 776–90.
16. Ostrowski ML, Inwards CY, Strickler JG, et al. Osseous Hodgkin disease. Cancer 1999;85(5):1166–78.
17. Bullough P. Hodgkin's lymphoma. In: Orthopedic pathology. New York: Mosby; 2004. p. 477.
18. Mulligan ME, Kransdorf MJ. Sequestra in primary lymphoma of bone: prevalence and radiologic features. AJR Am J Roentgenol 1993;160(6): 1245–8.
19. Heyning FH, Kroon HM, Hogendoorn PC, et al. MR imaging characteristics in primary lymphoma of bone with emphasis on nonaggressive appearance. Skeletal Radiol 2007;36(10):937–44.
20. Vande Berg BC, Michaux L, Scheiff JM, et al. Sequential quantitative MR analysis of bone marrow: differences during treatment of lymphoid versus myeloid leukemia. Radiology 1996;201:519–23.
21. Gerard EL, Ferry JA, Amrein PC, et al. Compositional changes in vertebral bone marrow during treatment for acute leukemia: assessment with quantitative chemical shift imaging. Radiology 1992;183:39–46.
22. Yasumoto M, Nonomura Y, Yoshimura R, et al. MR detection of iliac bone marrow involvement by malignant lymphoma with various MR sequences including diffusion-weighted echo–planar imaging. Skeletal Radiol 2002;31:263–9.

23. Dyke JP, Panicek DM, Healey JH, et al. Osteogenic and Ewing sarcomas: estimation of necrotic fraction during induction chemotherapy with dynamic contrast-enhanced MR imaging. Radiology 2003; 228:271–8.

24. Johnston C, Brennan S, Ford S, et al. Whole-body MR imaging: applications in oncology. Eur J Surg Oncol 2006;32:239–46.

25. Samuel LM, White J, Lessells AM, et al. Primary non-Hodgkin's lymphoma of muscle. Clin Oncol 1999;11(1):49–51.

26. Komatsuda M, Nagao T, Arimori S. An autopsy case of malignant lymphoma associated with remarkable infiltration in skeletal muscles. Rinsho Ketsueki 1981; 22(6):891–5.

27. Beggs I. Primary muscle lymphoma. Clin Radiol 1997;52(3):203–12.

28. Lanham GR, Weiss SW, Enzinger FM. Malignant lymphoma. A study of 75 cases presenting in soft tissue. Am J Surg Pathol 1989;13(1):1–10.

29. Panicek DM, Lautin JL, Schwartz LH, et al. Non-Hodgkin lymphoma in skeletal muscle manifesting as homogeneous masses with CT attenuation similar to muscle. Skeletal Radiol 1997;26(11):633–5.

30. Lee VS, Martinez S, Coleman RE. Primary muscle lymphoma: clinical and imaging findings. Radiology 1997;203(1):237–44.

31. Kaushik S, Miller TT, Nazarian LN, et al. Spectral Doppler sonography of musculoskeletal soft tissue masses. J Ultrasound Med 2003;22(12):1333–6.

32. Willemze R, Jaffe ES, Burg G, et al. WHO-EORTC classification for cutaneous lymphomas. Blood 2005;105(10):3768–85.

33. Lee HJ, Im JG, Goo JM, et al. Peripheral T-cell lymphoma: spectrum of imaging findings with clinical and pathologic features. Radiographics 2003; 23(1):7–26.

34. Malloy PC, Fishman EK, Magid D. Lymphoma of bone, muscle, and skin: CT findings. AJR Am J Roentgenol 1992;159(4):805–9.

35. Kim YH, Willemze R, Pimpinelli N, et al. TNM classification system for primary cutaneous lymphomas other than mycosis fungoides and Sezary syndrome: a proposal of the International Society for Cutaneous Lymphomas (ISCL) and the Cutaneous Lymphoma Task Force of the European Organization of Research and Treatment of Cancer (EORTC). Blood 2007;110(2):479–84.

36. Restrepo CS, Lemos DF, Gordillo H, et al. Imaging findings in musculoskeletal complications of AIDS. Radiographics 2004;24(4):1029–49.

37. Beral V, Peterman T, Berkelman R, et al. AIDS-associated non-Hodgkin lymphoma. Lancet 1991; 337:805–9.

38. Haskal ZJ, Lindan CE, Goodman PC. Lymphoma in the immunocompromised patient. Radiol Clin North Am 1990;28:885–99.

39. Lister TA, Crowther DM, Sutcliffe SB, et al. Report of a committee convened to discuss the evaluation and staging of patients with Hodgkin's disease; Cotwolds meeting. J Clin Oncol 1989;7:1630–6.

40. Lin C, Itti E, Haioun C, et al. Early 18F-FDG PET for prediction of prognosis in patients with diffuse large B cell lymphoma: SUV-based assessment versus visual analysis. J Nucl Med 2007;48(10):1626–32.

41. Hutchings M, Loft A, Hansen M, et al. FDG PET after two cycles of chemotherapy predicts treatment failure and progression-free survival in Hodgkin lymphoma. Blood 2006;107(1):52–9.

42. Cheson BD, Pfistner B, Juweid ME, et al. Revised response criteria for malignant lymphoma. J Clin Oncol 2007;25:579–86.

43. Rahmouni A, Luciani A, Itti E. MRI and PET in monitoring response in lymphoma. Cancer Imaging 2005;5 Spec No A:S106–12.

44. Lin C, Luciani A, Itti E, et al. Whole-body MRI and PET/CT in haematological malignancies. Cancer Imaging 2007;7 Spec No A:S88–93.

45. Yuki M, Narabayashi I, Yamamoto K, et al. Multifocal primary lymphoma of bone: scintigraphy and MR findings before and after treatment. Radiat Med 2000;18(5):305–10.

46. Altehoefer C, Laubenberger J, Lange W, et al. Prospective evaluation of bone marrow signal changes on magnetic resonance tomography during high-dose chemotherapy and peripheral blood stem cell transplantation in patients with breast cancer. Invest Radiol 1997;32(10):613–20.

47. Fletcher BD, Wall JE, Hanna SL. Effect of hematopoietic growth factors on MR images of bone marrow in children undergoing chemotherapy. Radiology 1993;189(3):745–51.

48. Blomlie V, Rofstad EK, Skjonsberg A, et al. Female pelvic bone marrow: serial MR imaging before, during, and after radiation therapy. Radiology 1995; 194(2):537–43.

49. Sacks EL, Goris ML, Glatstein E, et al. Bone marrow regeneration following large-field radiation: influence of volume, age, dose, and time. Cancer 1978;42: 1057–65.

50. Pakos EE, Fotopoulos AD, Ioannidis JP. 18F-FDG PET for evaluation of bone marrow infiltration in staging of lymphoma: a meta-analysis. J Nucl Med 2005;46:958–63.

51. Mammone JF, Schweitzer ME. MRI of occult sacral insufficiency fractures following radiotherapy. Skeletal Radiol 1995;24:101–4.

52. Mitchell DG, Rao VM, Dalinka MK, et al. Femoral head avascular necrosis: correlation of MR imaging, radiographic staging, radionuclide imaging, and clinical findings. Radiology 1987;162:709–15.

53. Weatherby RP, Dahlin DC, Ivins JC. Postradiation sarcoma of bone: review of 78 Mayo Clinic cases. Mayo Clin Proc 1981;56:294–306.

# Imaging of Complications of Hematopoietic Stem Cell Transplantation

Jyothi P. Jagannathan, MD[a,b], Nikhil Ramaiya, MD[c,d,*],
Ritu R. Gill, MBBS[b], Edwin Pascal Alyea III MD[c,d],
Pablo Ros, MD, MPH[a,b,e]

**KEYWORDS**
- Hematopoietic stem cell transplantation
- Complications • Imaging • CT

Hematopoietic stem cell transplantation (HSCT) is increasingly used for treatment of malignant and nonmalignant hematologic disorders, genetic and immunologic disorders, and solid tumors[1] (**Box 1**). Although advances in immunosuppressive therapy and management of infections have improved long-term survival, transplant recipients remain at risk for a multitude of complications, many of which are serious and life threatening. Post-transplant complications may be classified either according to the organ system or according to the time frame following transplantation. Complications may involve the chest, abdominopelvic organs, the central nervous system, or musculoskeletal tissues. This article reviews the various clinical and radiologic findings of key complications following HSCT and the pertinent differentiating factors.

## OVERVIEW AND GENERAL PRINCIPLES

Hematopoietic transplantation refers to any procedure where hematopoietic cells are given to the recipient with the intention of repopulating or replacing the existing system in part or in total.

Traditionally, HSCT is performed after conditioning regimen of high-dose chemotherapy with or without total body irradiation to ablate the bone marrow and tumor cells. Harvested pluripotent stem cells are then transfused to repopulate the marrow, and restore hematologic and immunologic competence. HSCT has replaced the previously used term "bone marrow transplantation" to indicate the range of donor cell sources now available: bone marrow, peripheral stem cells, and fetal cord blood. The source of stem cells can be from the patient themselves (autologous), an identical twin (syngenic), or related or unrelated donor (allogenic) (**Table 1**). The spectrum of complications differs: allogenic transplant recipients are at risk for developing graft-versus-host-disease (GVHD), not seen with autologous or syngenic transplantation; autologous transplant recipients have higher risk of relapse, although infections are less common.

The outcome following transplantation is dependent on multiple factors including the age of patient, type of transplant, the underlying disease process, and presence of residual disease at the time of transplantation. In general, relapse rates of tumor are higher in adults, in patients with

a Department of Radiology, Dana Farber Cancer Institute, 44 Binney Street, Boston, MA 02115, USA
b Department of Radiology, Brigham and Women's Hospital, Harvard Medical School, 75 Francis Street, Boston, MA 02115, USA
c Division of Medical Oncology, Dana Farber Cancer Institute, 44 Binney Street, Boston, MA 02115, USA
d Department of Medicine, Brigham and Womens Hospital, Harvard Medical School, 75 Francis Street, Boston, MA 02115, USA
e Department of Radiology, Hospital De Sant Pau, Universitat Autonoma De Barcelona, Barcelona, Spain 08025
* Corresponding author.
*E-mail address:* nramaiya@partners.org (N. Ramaiya).

Radiol Clin N Am 46 (2008) 397–417
doi:10.1016/j.rcl.2008.04.004

Box 1
Indications for hematopoietic stem cell transplantation

Malignant diseases

Acute myeloid leukemia

Myelodysplastic syndrome

Acute lymphoblastic leukemia

Chronic myelogenous leukemia

Chronic lymphocytic leukemia

Non-Hodgkin lymphoma

Hodgkin lymphoma

Multiple myeloma

Neuroblastoma, germ cell tumors, and other solid malignancies

Nonmalignant diseases

Thalassemia

Sickle cell anemia

Aplastic anemia

Miscellaneous genetic and immunologic disorders

residual disease, and following autologous transplantation.

Following HSCT, there is a predictable temporal sequence of immunosuppression and recovery, which helps in focusing on the most probable complication at different time points in the post-transplantation period (**Fig. 1**).[2] The time course after HSCT is divided into three phases, based on the immune status.

- The pre-engraftment phase, which typically lasts for 15 to 30 days following transplantation, is characterized by pancytopenia and disruption of host defense barriers.
- The early posttransplantation phase begins after successful engraftment of the donor stem cells and spans from 30 to 100 days after transplant. There is recovery of neutrophil count, but because of delay in lymphocyte recovery there is persistent cellular and humoral deficiency.
- The late posttransplantation phase begins 100 days after transplantation. Lymphocyte counts return to normal, but recovery of cellular and humoral immune function does not occur for approximately 1 year or later depending on clinical circumstances.

## PULMONARY COMPLICATIONS

Pulmonary complications occur in 40% to 60% of stem cell transplant recipients and account for significant morbidity and mortality.[2] The framework of timeline following transplantation is especially useful in the context of pulmonary complications. With increasing use of prophylactic antibiotics, the spectrum of pulmonary complications has shifted from infectious to noninfectious causes.[3] High-resolution CT (HRCT) is considered to be the primary imaging modality in early diagnosis of pulmonary infections following transplantation because it enables early detection of abnormalities, helps narrow the differential diagnosis, decides the technique and site to obtain tissue diagnosis, and monitors response to treatment.[4–7]

### Pre-engraftment Phase (0–30 Days)

Both infectious and noninfectious complications are common, resulting from toxicity of the pre-transplantation conditioning regimen and secondary to the effects of pancytopenia. Noninfectious pulmonary complications include pulmonary edema, engraftment syndrome, diffuse alveolar hemorrhage, and drug-induced pulmonary toxicity. Profound neutropenia and impairment of host mucosal defenses predispose to both bacterial and fungal infections. Radiographically evident bacterial pneumonia is rare in the bone marrow transplant recipients in the pre-engraftment phase, because of prompt use of empiric antibiotic therapy in febrile neutropenic patients. Fungal infections dominate, accounting for 25% to 50% of

Table 1
Types of transplantation

|  | Autologous | Allogenic |
|---|---|---|
| Donor source | Patient themselves | Unrelated donor, matched or mismatched |
| Indications | Lymphoma | Acute leukemias, chronic leukemias |
|  | Myeloma | Myeloproliferative disorders |
| Complications | ++ | +++ |
| Risk of relapse | +++ | ++ |

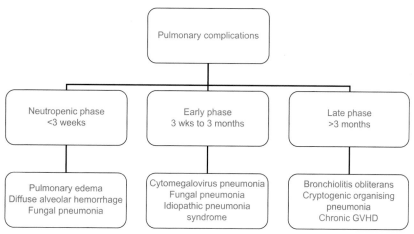

Fig. 1. Pulmonary complications following hematopoietic stem cell transplantation.

all pneumonias in allogenic transplant recipients. The most frequent fungal pathogen is *Aspergillus*, followed by *Candida*.

## Fungal pneumonia

*Aspergillus* pneumonia occurs principally but not exclusively in allogenic recipients, with prevalence of 10% to 15%.[8] It can occur at any time following transplantation. Neutropenia is the principal risk factor in the early stages, whereas steroid treatment for GVHD is a strong risk factor in the post-transplantation phase.[8,9] Two forms have been described: angioinvasive and tracheobronchial aspergillosis.[10,11] Radiologically, angioinvasive aspergillosis manifests as large pulmonary nodules, masses, parenchymal opacification, or combination of these.[11] Lesions are multiple and show upper lobe predominance. On CT, especially on HRCT, the nodules may be surrounded by a haze of ground-glass attenuation (halo sign), which is a common but not specific sign, also seen in infection by *Candida*, *Pseudomonas*, cytomegalovirus (CMV), and actinomycosis (**Fig. 2A**). The halo is thought to represent hemorrhage around a central zone of infarction and coagulative necrosis, secondary to invasion and blockage of the venules by the fungus. Cavitation producing the air-crescent sign coincides with neutrophil recovery and is a good prognostic sign (**Fig. 2B**).[12] Pleural effusions and lymphadenopathy are uncommon. ELISA done on blood or bronchoalveolar lavage (BAL) fluids to detect galactomannan, a cell wall antigen, is highly sensitive and specific (>90%) for invasive pulmonary aspergillosis.[13] Tracheobronchial aspergillosis presents with cough, wheeze, and stridor, secondary to invasion of the central and peripheral airways as the name suggests. On CT, findings include thickened airway walls; debris-filled lumina; small (<5 mm) centrilobular nodules; and patchy peribronchial consolidation (**Fig. 3**).

Candidial infection is becoming a frequent source of fungemia in posttransplant recipients.[14] The portal of entry is thought to be indwelling venous catheters or the gastrointestinal tract. Patients present with rapid onset of clinical symptoms including fever, respiratory distress, productive cough, and chest pain. The tracheobronchial form results in an acute bronchopneumonia-like picture or multiple poorly marginated nodules, whereas hematogenous dissemination results in miliary or multiple nodules with or without surrounding ground-glass halo (**Fig. 4**).[5,15] The Zygomycetes, *Mucor* and *Rhizopus*, are uncommon causes of invasive fungal pneumonia, with prevalence of 1% to 2%.[14] Pulmonary zygomyces are angioinvasive similar to *Aspergillus*, and produce pulmonary infarction, halo sign, and cavitation (**Fig. 5**). With the increasing use of newer antifungals, such as voriconazole, which is highly efficacious against invasive *Aspergillus*, these may become more common. *Nocardia* presents with multiple nodular infiltrates or pleural-based masses that frequently cross fissures and can cavitate. *Cryptococcus* is seen as solitary or multiple nodules with or without cavitation. There may be associated neurologic symptoms.

## Pulmonary edema

Pulmonary edema is a common complication during the first few weeks and is of multifactorial etiology. It can be secondary to increased hydrostatic pressure from intravenous fluids, chemotherapy, and radiation-induced cardiac or renal

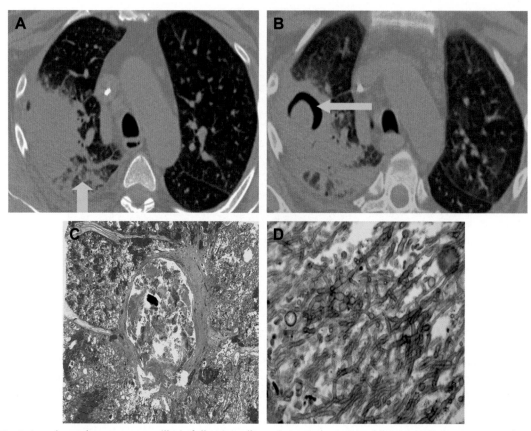

Fig. 2. Invasive pulmonary aspergillosis following allogenic transplantation. (*A*) Initial CT demonstrates dense consolidation with surrounding hazy ground-glass attenuation (halo sign) (*arrow*). (*B*) CT scan 2 weeks later shows cavitation with air-crescent sign (*arrow*). (*C*) Low-power and (*D*) high-power photomicrograph demonstrates fungal hyphae.

dysfunction, or abnormal capillary permeability from drug-induced pulmonary toxicity, sepsis, or transfusion reactions.[2] Radiographic abnormalities include Kerley's B lines, indistinctness of the pulmonary vessels, rapid-onset pulmonary infiltrates, and pleural effusions. Diffuse ground-glass attenuation, especially in the dependent regions, engorgement of the pulmonary vessels,

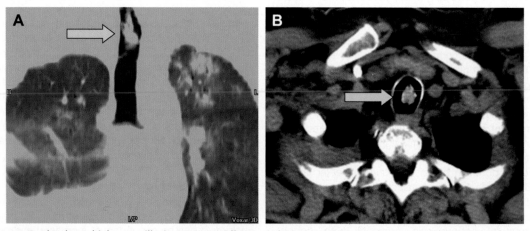

Fig. 3. Tracheobronchial aspergillosis status postallogeneic bone marrow transplantation. (*A*) Coronal reformatted images show irregular intraluminal mass in the trachea (*arrow*). (*B*) Axial CT image through the proximal trachea showing tracheal plaques in addition to the hyperdense aspergilloma (*arrow*).

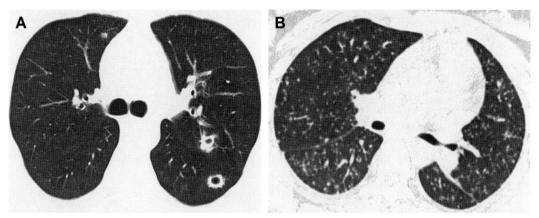

Fig. 4. CT scans in two different patients with pulmonary candidiasis. (*A*) Axial CT demonstrates nodules with cavitation. (*B*) CT scan in another patient with fever and violaceous skin papules demonstrates multiple randomly distributed micronodules.

peribronchial cuffing, and smooth interlobular septal thickening can be seen at CT,[12] although pulmonary edema is almost always diagnosed clinically and with chest radiography rather than with HRCT.

### Engraftment syndrome

Engraftment syndrome is a clinical entity characterized by fever, erythematous rash, and noncardiogenic pulmonary edema occurring at the time of neutrophil recovery.[15] It can occur following both allogenic and autologous transplantation, with reported incidence as high as 7% to 11%[16] Clinically, it can mimic pulmonary infections and acute GVHD. Imaging findings are nonspecific ranging from normal to bilateral ground-glass opacification, airspace consolidation predominantly distributed in the hilar and peribronchial regions, smooth interlobular septal thickening, and small

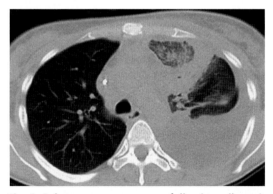

Fig. 5. Pulmonary zygomycoses following allogenic transplantation. Axial CT shows consolidative opacity with surrounding ground-glass attenuation and moderate volume pleural effusion. Patient underwent wedge resection and pathology was consistent with Zygomycetes pneumonia.

pleural effusions (**Fig. 6**).[17,18] Treatment with corticosteroids has been reported to be beneficial.[19]

### Diffuse alveolar hemorrhage

Diffuse alveolar hemorrhage is a serious and potentially life-threatening complication in the early posttransplant period. It has a prevalence of 2% to 20%, with greater frequency following allogenic transplantation. Diffuse alveolar hemorrhage is commonly observed within 1 month of transplantation, often during the periengraftment phase. Patients present with acute-onset fever, dyspnea, and nonproductive cough. Hemoptysis is rare. At radiography, there is diffuse air-space disease resembling pulmonary edema.[20] CT demonstrates bilateral consolidation or ground-glass attenuation with superimposed reticular opacities, predominantly perihilar and in the lower lung zones (**Fig. 7**).[18] There may be rapid deterioration in the radiographic appearances, despite minimal change in clinical signs. Definitive diagnosis is made by BAL, which demonstrates progressively bloodier return with each successive lavage or presence of hemosiderin-laden macrophages. The mortality rate has been reported to be variable ranging from 20% to 70% in different studies. Late-onset hemorrhage, allogenic transplantation, and isolation of microorganism at BAL are associated with poor outcome.[3,21]

### Drug-induced lung toxicity

This occurs in up to 10% of the patients, and is frequently seen after chemotherapeutic agents, such as bleomycin, methotrexate, and busulfan. Concomitant radiotherapy increases the risk, with incidence up to 30%.[22] There is a wide range of radiologic appearances, reflecting different histologic patterns, the most common being diffuse alveolar damage, hypersensitivity pneumonitis, and

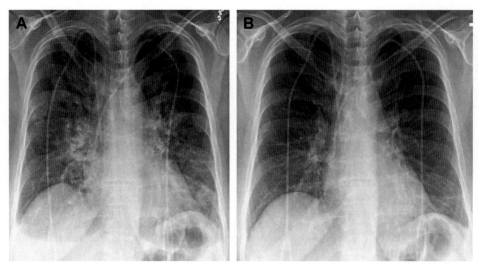

Fig. 6. Engraftment syndrome in 43-year-old woman with fever and diffuse skin rash, 8 days postallogenic transplantation. (A) Initial radiograph reveals bilateral central air-space opacities and small pleural effusions, without vascular congestion. (B) Follow-up chest radiograph after a short course of steroids shows complete interval resolution.

organizing pneumonia.[23] HRCT findings include bilateral ground-glass attenuation, intralobular and interlobular interstitial thickening, centrilobular nodules, peribronchial or subpleural areas of consolidation, and linear opacities.[23,24] The imaging findings are nonspecific and diagnosis is often made by exclusion.

### Early Posttransplantation Phase (Days 31–100)

The most important pathogens causing pneumonia in this phase are CMV and *Aspergillus*. *Pneumocystis jiroveci* pneumonia is rare in the presence of effective prophylaxis. Idiopathic pneumonia syndrome and acute GVHD are important noninfectious complications.

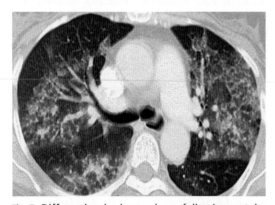

Fig. 7. Diffuse alveolar hemorrhage following autologous transplantation. Axial CT reveals extensive bilateral ground-glass opacification with superimposed reticular pattern.

### Cytomegalovirus

Allogenic transplant recipients are at increased risk of CMV pneumonia because of delayed reconstitution of cellular immunity and need for immunosuppression for GVHD prophylaxis. Most CMV infections result from reactivation of the latent virus in seropositive recipients. The use of CMV-negative marrow and blood products, and early aggressive use of antivirals, have significantly decreased the incidence of CMV pneumonia.[25] Definitive diagnosis is established by detection of virus using rapid culture in the BAL fluid, in the presence of appropriate clinical and radiologic findings. The chest radiograph may reveal bilateral interstitial opacities, focal or diffuse consolidation, and nodular opacities (**Fig. 8**).[7,11] The abnormalities are distributed in the mid and lower zones, likely related to hematogenous dissemination. Isolated involvement of the upper zone is very uncommon. HRCT usually demonstrates mixed pattern of ground-glass opacities, small centrilobular nodules, and air-space consolidation.[5,26] Other viral infections, including respiratory syncytial virus pneumonia, have a similar radiographic picture.[27]

### Pneumocystis jiroveci

The incidence of *P Jiroveci* (previously called *Pneumocystis carinii*) pneumonia has reduced dramatically since the introduction of routine prophylaxis with trimethoprim-sulphmethoxazole. Currently, it is seen in patients who are unable to tolerate trimethoprim-sulphmethoxazole prophylaxis or in patients on other prophylactic agents,

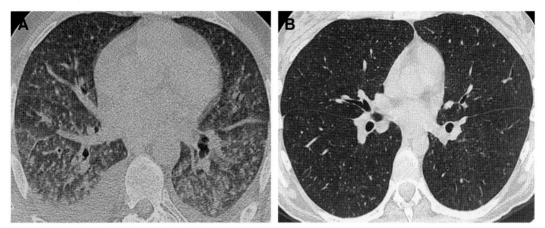

Fig. 8. Cytomegalovirus pneumonia following allogenic transplantation. (A) Axial HRCT shows diffuse ground-glass attenuation and small nodules. (B) In another patient axial HRCT image shows diffuse bilateral tiny centrilobular nodules.

such as aerosolized pentamidine and atovaquone. The median onset of *Pneumocystis* pneumonia is 60 days after transplantation. Chest radiographs may be normal or reveal reticulonodular infiltrates progressing to air-space consolidation. The most characteristic finding on CT is ground-glass attenuation, diffuse or perihilar in distribution, or mosaic pattern with sparing of secondary pulmonary lobules (**Fig. 9**).[7,11] Pneumatoceles, cavitation, and air cysts may develop, but rare. BAL is diagnostic in 90%, obviating open lung biopsy. Elevated lactate hydrogenase and positive testing for glucan are also helpful.

### Idiopathic pneumonia syndrome
Idiopathic pneumonia syndrome is a diagnosis of exclusion, defined as "diffuse lung injury occurring after marrow transplantation for which infectious etiology is not identified"[28] (**Box 2**). It is the most common cause of diffuse radiographic abnormalities between 30 and 180 days after transplantation, although it can occur at any time point.[29] The pathogenesis of diffuse alveolar damage is unclear and could result from drug toxicity, undiagnosed infection, or GVHD. Radiographic findings are nonspecific and include bilateral air-space opacification. HRCT shows progressive air-space consolidation with bibasilar prominence similar to noncardiogenic pulmonary edema (**Fig. 10**). Pleural effusions may be present. No definite treatment exists and mortality is high.[30]

### Pulmonary cytolytic thrombi
Pulmonary cytolytic thrombi is a recently reported rare complication in children following allogenic HSCT, often associated with active GVHD.[31] Patients present with fever and small pulmonary nodules. Pathologically, it consists of basophilic thrombi resulting in small infarcts, and is likely a manifestation of acute GVHD.

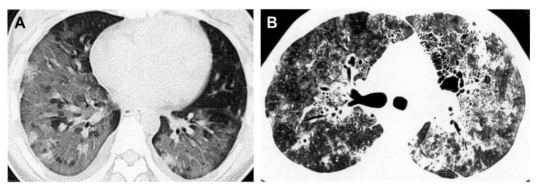

Fig. 9. *Pneumocystis jiroveci* pneumonia. (A) Axial CT demonstrates diffuse geographic pattern of ground-glass attenuation with sparing of the adjacent lobules. (B) In another patient axial HRCT shows patchy ground-glass and air space opacification with interspersed cavitation.

## Late Posttransplantation Phase (After 100 Days)

Chronic GVHD is the most common complication affecting long-term survivors of allogenic stem cell transplantation. Pulmonary manifestations of chronic GVHD are bronchiolitis obliterans and cryptogenic organizing pneumonia. Infection in the absence of chronic GVHD is uncommon in this phase, because of near complete recovery of immunologic function.

### Bronchiolitis obliterans

Bronchiolitis obliterans is an obstructive pulmonary disorder secondary to injury to the small airways. It is characterized clinically by nonreversible airflow obstruction and histologically by intraluminal fibrosis. It has strong association with chronic GVHD and has reported prevalence of 6% to 20% following allogenic transplantation.[32] Patients present with increasing nonproductive cough, dyspnea, and wheezing or asymptomatic deterioration of pulmonary function. Absence of fever and pulmonary infiltrates helps to distinguish it from cryptogenic organizing pneumonia and infections. Pulmonary function tests show obstructive pattern with reduction in forced expiratory volume in 1 second, and is considered the gold standard for the diagnosis. Chest radiograph maybe normal or may show hyperinflation. HRCT, especially paired inspiratory and expiratory scans, may show bronchial dilatation, bronchiolectasis, mosaic attenuation, and expiratory air-trapping (**Fig. 11**).[11,33]

### Cryptogenic organizing pneumonia

Cryptogenic organizing pneumonia, previously referred to as "bronchiolitis obliterans organizing pneumonia," is characterized by polypoid granulation tissue in the lumina of bronchioles and alveolar ducts associated with a variable amount of interstitial and air-space mononuclear cell infiltration. Acute and chronic GVHD are strong risk factors for the development of cryptogenic organizing pneumonia.[32] HRCT demonstrates

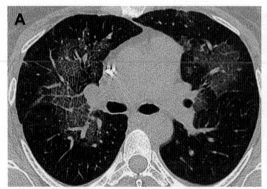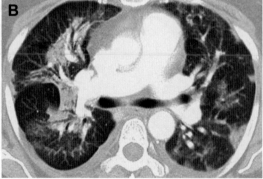

Fig. 10. Idiopathic pneumonia syndrome in the early transplantation period. (*A*) Initial CT scan showed bilateral patchy ground-glass opacities. Infectious screen was negative and patient deteriorated despite empiric antibiotic therapy. (*B*) Follow-up CT shows multifocal consolidative opacities.

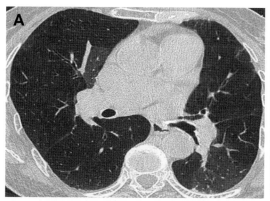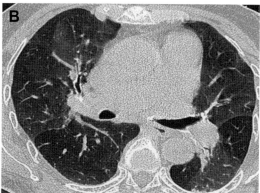

Fig. 11. Bronchiolitis obliterans 2 years postallogenic transplantation. Paired (*A*) inspiratory and (*B*) expiratory images shows air trapping with mosaic attenuation, more evident on the expiratory images.

bilateral patchy areas of air-space consolidation, ground-glass opacities, and nodules or masses with open bronchus sign (**Fig. 12**).[11,18] Consolidation is seen predominantly in subpleural or peribronchial location, whereas ground-glass opacification is randomly distributed. Less frequent findings include irregular linear or reticulonodular opacities. About 80% of patients respond to corticosteroid therapy.

## ABDOMINOPELVIC COMPLICATIONS
### Periengraftment Period (Days 0–100)

Toxicity of the pretransplantation conditioning regimen and pancytopenia result in both infectious and noninfectious complications in the period. Common complications include hepatic veno-occlusive disease, acute GVHD, neutropenic typhlitis, infections, pneumatosis intestinalis, and hemorrhagic cystitis.[34] Bacterial pathogens are the predominant cause of infection during the first month following transplantation. Empiric antibiotics also lead to overgrowth of normal bowel

flora, such as *Clostridium difficile*, resulting in pseudomembranous enterocolitis. Fungal infections, most commonly *Aspergillus* and *Candida* species, can cause gastrointestinal ulcers, and in disseminated cases may form microabscesses in the liver, spleen, and kidneys. CMV is the most important pathogen during the early posttransplantation period (31–100 days), causing gastroenteritis and hepatitis, apart from pneumonia.[35]

### Hepatic complications
Hepatic complications contribute to significant morbidity and mortality in the posttransplant period.[36] Common causes of hepatic dysfunction in the posttransplant period are drug toxicity, hepatic veno-occlusive disease, acute hepatic GVHD, cholestasis, and infections.[36]

### Hepatic veno-oclusive disease
Hepatic veno-occlusive disease is among the spectrum of organ injury syndromes occurring after stem cell transplantation, occurring in approximately 10% of allogenic transplant recipients

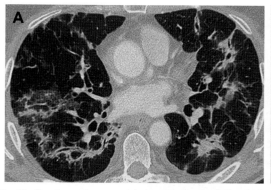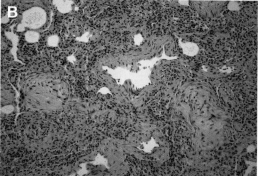

Fig. 12. Cryptogenic organizing pneumonia following allogenic stem cell transplantation. Axial HRCT shows consolidation in a peribronchial and subpleural location with traction bronchiectasis, bronchial wall thickening, and ill-defined centrilobular nodules. Microscopy (x100) with H-E stain demonstrates plugs of fibroblast-rich connective tissue filling terminal bronchioles and alveolar airspaces with associated chronic inflammation. (*Courtesy of* Lynnette Sholl, MD, Boston, MA.)

with myeloablative conditioning regimen.[37] The incidence of veno-occlusive disease is lower after autologous transplantation and reduced intensity conditioning regimen.[37,38] The proposed mechanism of injury is metabolite-induced endothelial damage of the hepatic sinusoids, with subsequent fibrosis and occlusion of hepatic outflow.[39] Veno-occlusive disease typically occurs in the first 4 weeks following transplantation, often within the first 20 days.[40] Clinical criteria for diagnosis are painful hepatomegaly, jaundice and ascites, or unexplained weight gain.[37,40,41] The most

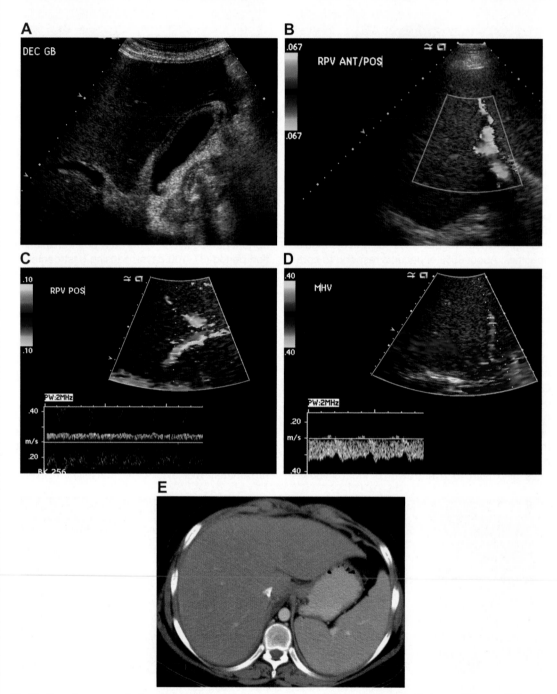

**Fig. 13.** Hepatic veno-occlusive disease following allogenic transplantation. Ultrasound shows diffuse gallbladder wall thickening and ascites (A), reversal of flow in the main and right portal vein (B, C), and monophasic flow in the middle hepatic vein (D). (E) Axial contrast-enhanced CT in a second patient shows narrowing of the hepatic inferior vena cava. Hepatic veins not visualized because of nonopacification and compression.

common ultrasound findings are ascites and marked gallbladder wall thickening (>6–8 mm). Doppler findings are more specific and may demonstrate portal venous pulsatility, hepatofugal portal venous flow, increased hepatic artery resistive index (>0.8), and loss of triphasic flow pattern in the hepatic veins (**Fig. 13, Table 2**).[42] Doppler examinations may also have prognostic significance, with splenomegaly, ascites, and flow in the paraumbilical vein shown to correlate with the severity of veno-occlusive disease.[43] A recent study reported that periportal edema, ascites, and narrowed right hepatic vein were useful CT signs to distinguish from hepatic GVHD[44] (**Box 3**). The distinction between the two cannot be reliably made on the imaging findings alone, however, and biopsy is frequently performed to establish the diagnosis. Prompt recognition of veno-occlusive disease is essential, because untreated disease is associated with significant mortality and morbidity. Heparin has not proved to be beneficial. Most patients are treated symptomatically with sodium and fluid restriction along with diuretic therapy.

## Infections

Liver abscesses, both bacterial and fungal, can occur in the posttransplantation setting. Five patterns of ultrasound findings in fungal infections of the liver have been described, corresponding to different stages in evolution.[45,46] During the active phase "wheel in wheel," "wagon wheel," or the "bull's eye" lesions are seen. Echogenic foci in the late stages are said to correspond with healing. CT and MR imaging have been shown to be superior in the detection of fungal microabscesses.[47] Lesions are seen on arterial phase CT as uniformly hyperattenuating or hypoattenuating with hyperattenuating rim.[48] MR imaging may also distinguish

the different stages (acute, subacute, and chronic healed) (**Fig. 14, Table 3**).[47] Fungal lesions in the liver or spleen may not be visible until the patient recovers from the neutropenic stage of disease and may become invisible if neutropenia recurs.[47,49] Repeat imaging within 2 weeks may be prudent if initial scans were negative in patients with strong clinical suspicion of hepatosplenic fungal infection, especially if imaging was done in the neutropenic phase. Focal liver lesions in children following HSCT may also be secondary to post-transplant lymphoproliferative disorder (PTLD) or regenerative hepatic nodules.

### Bowel complications

GVHD is a significant cause of morbidity following allogenic transplantation. GVHD occurs when donor T lymphocytes damage the epithelium of the recipients.[50] The degree of histocompatibility between the donor and recipient influences the development of GVHD, with recipients of mismatched transplants having the highest risk. Moderate to severe GVHD occurs in 30% to 50% of matched allogenic transplants.[50] Although graft-versus-host response is generally detrimental, graft-versus-malignancy effect is thought to be beneficial in patients with hematologic malignancies, such as leukemias and lymphomas.[51,52] GVHD is divided into two distinct forms (acute and chronic) based on the time of occurrence and clinical manifestations.

Acute GVHD usually presents within 2 to 10 weeks following transplantation,[50] and most commonly affects the skin, gastrointestinal tract, and the liver. Maculopapular rash and pruritis are the usual presenting symptoms, and almost always precedes gastrointestinal involvement. Mucositis progressing to strictures is the usual course, and

**Table 2**
**Findings that help differentiate between hepatic veno-occlusive disease and acute graft-versus-host disease**

|  | Hepatic Veno-Occlusive Disease | Acute Graft Versus Host Disease |
|---|---|---|
| Time frame | Usually around day 20 (typically between 1 and 5 wk) | Usually around 2–10 wk |
| Periportal edema | ++ | −/+ |
| Ascites | +++ | −/+ |
| Narrowed hepatic vein (right hepatic vein <5 mm) | +++ | −/+ |
| Small bowel wall thickening | −/+ | +++ |
| Doppler examination | >6 criteria[a] | |

Final diagnosis requires biopsy.
[a] Doppler criteria outlined by Lassau N, Auperin A, Leclere J, et al. Prognostic value of Doppler-ultrasonography in hepatic veno-occlusive disease. Transplantation 2002;74:60; with permission.

findings in acute GVHD include fluid-filled and dilated bowel loops, bowel wall thickening and abnormal enhancement, and mesenteric fat stranding (**Fig. 15**).[53] The abnormalities involve the small bowel with or without involvement of the large bowel. Negative oral contrast agent on CT may be helpful in demonstrating mucosal hyperemia and the "halo sign." There may be associated gallbladder–biliary tract abnormalities and ascites. Imaging findings frequently overlap with infectious, inflammatory, and radiation enteritis and tissue sampling is often necessary to confirm diagnosis.

Neutropenic colitis or typhlitis (from the Greek word for cecum, *typhlon*) is an uncommon complication of stem cell transplant, more commonly seen in children. Patients present with clinical triad of fever, right lower quadrant pain, and bloody or watery diarrhea. CT demonstrates bowel wall thickening involving cecum, right colon, and occasionally terminal ileum, pericolonic fat stranding, and ascites (**Fig. 16**).[18,34,54] Bowel necrosis and perforation are feared complications. Treatment consists of bowel rest, antibiotics, and maintenance of fluid-electrolyte balance.

CT findings may help in the differentiation and characterization of the gastrointestinal abnormalities in posttransplant patients, especially in the neutropenic setting.[54] Neutropenic enterocolitis commonly involves the right-sided colon, especially cecum, but could occur anywhere in the small or large bowel. Pneumatosis, mesenteric stranding, and ascites are more frequent with neutropenic colitis than GVHD, which could also involve both the small and large bowel. Associated bowel dilatation and mucosal enhancement are frequent findings in acute GVHD. *C difficile* colitis causes extensive wall thickening and nodularity, mostly limited to the colon, frequently manifesting as pancolitis. Cytomegaloviral colitis shares many similar features with *C difficile* colitis, including marked wall thickening and nodularity in a pancolitis distribution (**Fig. 17**).

Pneumatosis intestinalis maybe seen in clinically well patients following transplantation, so-called "benign pneumatosis intestinalis."[55,56] The pathogenesis is unclear, and is thought to result from steroid-induced hypertrophy of Peyer's patches with resultant mucosal defects through which air can enter the gut wall. Associated gas in the mesenteric and portal venous system and pneumoperitoneum may be seen. The radiographic findings resolve after conservative management, and do not warrant surgical intervention.[57] Pneumatosis in the setting of neutropenic typhlitis or CMV enteritis is more concerning, however, because it implies imminent bowel perforation.

can involve any segment of the gastrointestinal tract from the esophagus to colon. Symptoms vary depending on the site of involvement. Esophageal and gastric GVHD are best demonstrated on fluoroscopic single- or double-contrast studies.

The most common imaging findings are seen with involvement of the small bowel and colon. CT

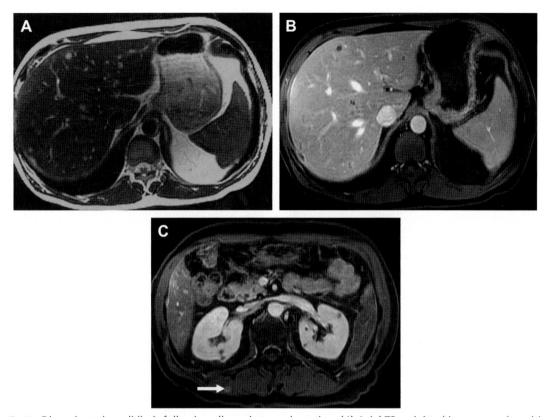

**Fig. 14.** Disseminated candidiasis following allogenic transplantation. (*A*) Axial T2-weighted image reveals multiple hyperintense lesions, measuring less than 1 cm. Transfusional hemosiderosis with diffuse low signal of the liver parenchyma is also appreciated. (*B, C*) Axial T1-weighted fat-suppressed gradient recalled echo images after gadolinium contrast show enhancing lesions in the liver, spleen, kidneys, and paraspinal muscles (*arrow*).

### Renal and urinary tract complications

Hemorrhagic cystitis is an uncommon complication following stem cell transplantation. Two forms have been reported, differing in time of occurrence, severity, and pathogenesis. Pre-engraftment cystitis occurring within the first few days of transplantation is mild, brief, and responds to supportive therapy, whereas postengraftment cystitis occurring 40 to 80 days following transplantation is protracted, associated with GVHD often grade 3, requiring surgical intervention.[58] In both forms, CT and ultrasound demonstrate focal or diffuse bladder wall thickening and in some cases, intraluminal hematoma or sloughed mucosa (**Fig. 18**).

**Table 3**
**MR imaging of hepatosplenic fungal infections**

|  | T1-weighted | T2-weighted | Enhancement Characteristics | Pathology |
|---|---|---|---|---|
| Acute | Isointense, hypointense | Hyperintense | Moderate enhancement | Microabscess |
| Subacute | Isointense to hyperintense with perilesional hypointense rim (bull's eye) | Hyperintense with perilesional hypointense rim | Perilesional enhancement | Necrotizing granulomas |
| Chronic | Hypointense | Hypointense | No enhancement | Fibrous tissue |

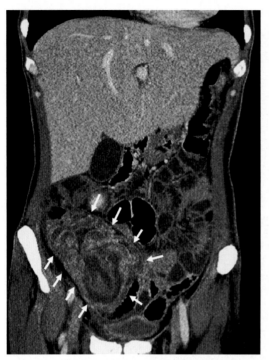

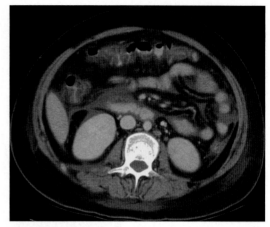

Fig. 17. Cytomegalovirus enterocolitis following stem cell transplantation. Axial CT shows marked wall thickening and nodularity involving the ascending and transverse colon.

Fig. 15. Neutropenic colitis in periengraftment period. Coronal reformatted CT image shows marked thickening of the fluid-filled cecum and the ascending colon (*arrows*).

nephrolithiasis, and spontaneous subcapsular hemorrhage.

Renal abscesses secondary to bacterial and fungal infections are also common following transplantation, commonly occurring early in the transplant period. Other rarer complications are papillary necrosis, renal vein thrombosis,

## *Late Posttransplantation Phase (Beyond Day 100)*

The most common complication in this phase is chronic GVHD, with prevalence of 60% to 80% following allogenic transplantation.[59,60] Acute GVHD is often present in these transplant recipients, although not a prerequisite. Clinical manifestations of chronic GVHD resemble autoimmune collagen vascular disorders, such as lichen planus, xerostomia, keratoconjunctivitis sicca, polyserositis, esophagitis and stricture, scleroderma, and myositis.[60] Chronic hepatic GVHD frequently manifests as cholestasis and in severe cases can result in "vanishing bile duct syndrome," with multiple biliary strictures resembling sclerosing cholangitis.[61] Prolonged steroid therapy used to treat chronic GVHD could also cause secondary complications, such as osteoporosis, secondary diabetes, avascular necrosis, and opportunistic infections.

## HEAD AND NECK

Central nervous system complications include infection, ischemia, hemorrhage, toxicity from chemotherapy and radiation, and recurrent malignancy, of which infection is the most common.[62] GVHD has not been confirmed in the central nervous system, possibly because of lack of lymphatics in the brain.

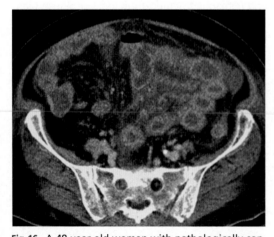

Fig. 16. A 48-year-old woman with pathologically confirmed acute graft-versus-host disease. Axial contrast-enhanced CT scan shows diffuse thickening of the small bowel with mural enhancement and ascites.

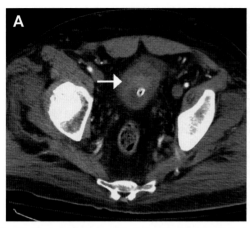
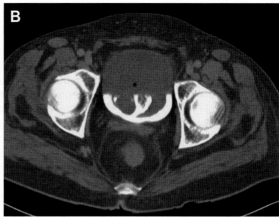

Fig. 18. Hemorrhagic cystitis following allogenic transplantation. (A) Axial CT image shows bladder wall thickening and high-density material in the urinary bladder (arrow). (B) In another patient, there is polypoidal filling defect within the partly opacified urinary bladder consistent with blood clot.

## Central Nervous System Infections

In the pre-engraftment period, there is profound neutropenia placing the patient at high risk for infections from gram-negative bacteria, viral, and fungal pathogens. In the early postengraftment period because of depressed cellular immunity, CMV, fungal, and gram-positive infections predominate, whereas during the late postengraftment period in which there is impaired humoral immunity, encapsulated bacteria and herpes zoster virus are commonly seen.

Aspergillus is the most common cause of focal infective brain lesions after stem cell transplantation. On CT and MR imaging, multiple low-attenuation lesions are seen with negligible mass effect or contrast enhancement, possibly reflecting intact blood brain barrier caused by inability to mount inflammatory response.[63] Mucor infection also causes large vessel occlusion and has more aggressive features. Bacterial infections and toxoplasmosis are rare because of routine prophylaxis. Herpes encephalitis may cause signal changes in the temporal lobe, best appreciated on MR imaging.[63]

## Noninfectious Central Nervous System Complications

Subdural hematoma, infarction, and intraparenchymal hemorrhage are the commonly reported cerebrovascular complications. Imaging appearances are similar to those seen in the general population. Toxicity from pretransplantation conditioning and GVHD prophylaxis increases the risk of a potentially reversible neurotoxic effect,

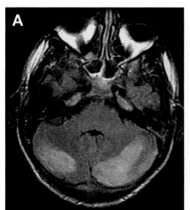
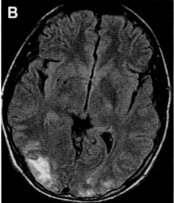
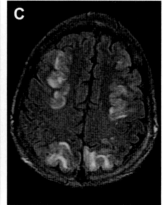

Fig. 19. Posterior reversible encephalopathy following allogenic transplantation. (A–C) Axial FLAIR images show symmetric cortical and subcortical hyperintensity in the cerebellar hemispheres, bilateral occipital, and frontoparietal regions.

termed "posterior reversible encephalopathy syn-drome".[64] Posterior reversible encephalopathy syndrome typically occurs within 1 month of initiation of therapy and is manifested as visual disturbances, cerebellar ataxia, confusion, and seizures. CT and MR imaging reveal abnormalities in the gray and white matter of occipital, parietal, posterior temporal, and frontal lobes (**Fig. 19**). Radiation therapy can also produce white matter changes and necrosis.

## Sinusitis

Sinusitis occurs in up to one third of posttransplant recipients, often within the first 2 years, and can be an underrecognized source of fever in the posttransplant period.[65,66] The usual pathogens are *Aspergillus*, *Streptococcus pneumoniae*, and *Haemophilus influenza*. Invasive fungal sinusitis, usually caused by *Aspergillus*, is a potentially fatal condition, and implies mucosal, submucosal, bone, or vascular invasion. The imaging findings of mucosal thickening, paranasal sinus opacification, and soft tissue inflammation overlap with bacterial sinusitis.[67] CT findings of periantral soft tissue invasion, bone erosion, and orbital invasion are rare and late signs. An early initial finding of invasive sinusitis may be marked unilateral thickening of a paranasal sinus.[67] Definitive diagnosis often requires histopathologic evidence of tissue invasion by fungal hyphae.

## MUSCULOSKELETAL COMPLICATIONS

Bone infarction and avascular necrosis may occur, secondary to total body irradiation used in the conditioning regimen to either GVHD or steroids used to treat GVHD. It has a prevalence of 5% to

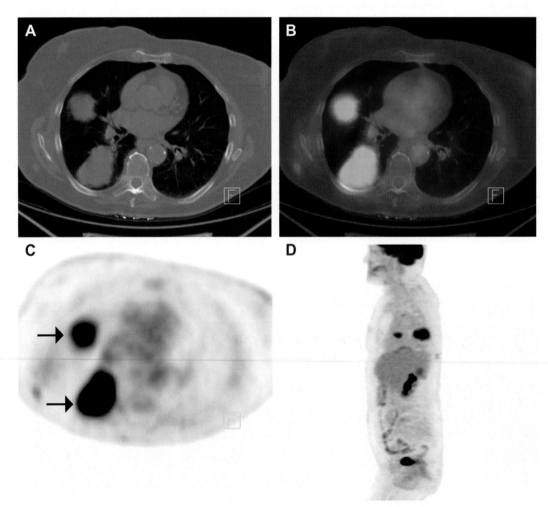

**Fig. 20.** Relapse of non-Hodgkin lymphoma following autologous transplantation. (*A–D*) Axial positron emission tomography–CT images shows intensely fluorodeoxyglucose-avid pulmonary masses (*arrows*).

20% following allogenic transplantation.[68,69] MR imaging findings are similar to those patients with avascular necrosis without history of bone marrow transplantation, and include serpingous areas of altered signal intensity with or without articular collapse.[70]

## NEW MALIGNANCIES FOLLOWING TRANSPLANTATION

New malignancies after HSCT have been classified into three categories: (1) solid tumors; (2) hematologic malignancies (most commonly myelodysplastic syndrome and acute myeloid leukemia); and (3) PTLD.[71] There is significantly higher risk (8.3 times) of new solid cancers than the general population,[72] especially melanoma, cancers of the buccal cavity, liver, brain, and thyroid. In patients who underwent transplantation for hematologic or solid malignancy, the possibility of recurrence of the primary tumor must also be considered. Recurrence of solid malignancies usually manifests within 2 years of transplantation, although late recurrences are not uncommon with hematologic malignancies. New lymphadenopathy, masses, or unexplained fever should be viewed with suspicion for recurrent lymphoma (**Fig. 20**).

### Posttransplant Lymphoproliferative Disorder

PTLD occurs almost exclusively following allogenic transplantation. It is a rare complication with a prevalence of 0.5% to 1.5%,[73] but is frequently fatal. PTLD results from uncontrolled Epstein-Barr virus–induced proliferation of engrafted donor B lymphocytes because of pharmacologic T-cell oversuppression. The spectrum can range from benign mononucleosis-like picture to fulminant lymphoma. PTLD following HSCT differs from that after solid organ transplantation, in that it occurs earlier (median onset 70–90 days) and behaves more aggressively.[74] Radiologically, it manifests as generalized lymphadenopathy, pulmonary nodules and masses, hepatosplenomegaly, diffuse organ infiltration, and ascites (**Fig. 21**).[75] The mainstay of therapy is reduction of immunosuppression, with cytotoxic chemotherapy and rituximab used in more aggressive forms. Localized disease may respond to definitive local therapy, such as surgery or radiation.

## SUMMARY

HSCT is an effective and promising therapy for a number of malignant and nonmalignant disorders, including lymphomas and leukemias. The success of the transplantation is, however, limited by high incidence of complications, especially involving the lungs. Allogenic transplant recipients are at risk for developing GVHD and complication thereof, not seen with autologous or syngenic transplantation. Autologous transplant recipients have higher risk of relapse, although infections and late transplantation complications are less common. Fungal pneumonias in all phases and CMV in early posttransplantation phase are the most important infectious pulmonary complications. In the abdomen, hepatic veno-occlusive disease and GVHD contribute to significant morbidity and mortality. Relapse of lymphoproliferative malignancy is very common following autologous transplantation, with rates as high as 50% in

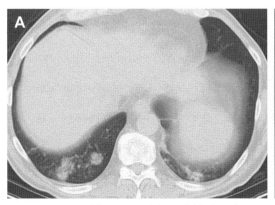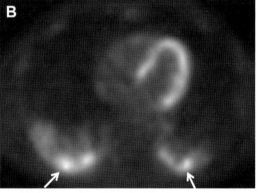

**Fig. 21.** A 44-year-old woman with Hodgkin lymphoma, 2 years postallogenic bone marrow transplantation with increasing shortness of breath. (*A*) CT scan shows peribronchovascular nodular opacities in lower lobes. (*B*) Positron emission tomography–CT demonstrates moderate fluorodeoxyglucose accumulation within the nodules (*arrows*). Subsequently, video-assisted thorascopic surgery and wedge resection revealed posttransplant lymphoproliferative disorder.

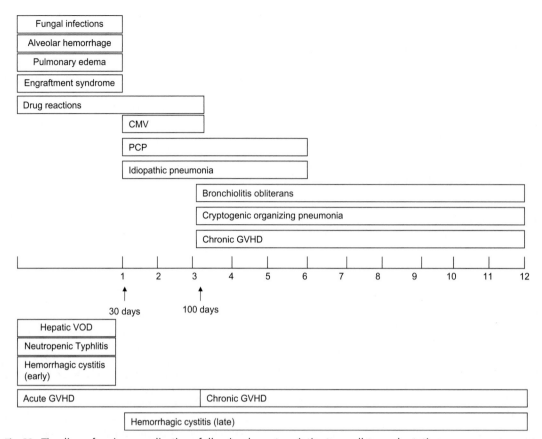

**Fig. 22.** Timeline of major complications following hematopoietic stem cell transplantation.

3 years. Combining clinical factors, such as type of transplant, conditioning regimen, and time course after transplantation, with key imaging findings often narrows the differential (**Fig. 22**).

## REFERENCES

1. Ljungman P, Urbano-Ispizua A, Cavazzana-Calvo M, et al. Allogeneic and autologous transplantation for haematological diseases, solid tumours and immune disorders: definitions and current practice in Europe. Bone Marrow Transplant 2006;37:439.
2. Soubani AO, Miller KB, Hassoun PM. Pulmonary complications of bone marrow transplantation. Chest 1996;109:1066.
3. Afessa B, Litzow MR, Tefferi A. Bronchiolitis obliterans and other late onset non-infectious pulmonary complications in hematopoietic stem cell transplantation. Bone Marrow Transplant 2001;28:425.
4. Choi YH, Leung AN. Radiologic findings: pulmonary infections after bone marrow transplantation. J Thorac Imaging 1999;14:201.
5. Escuissato DL, Gasparetto EL, Marchiori E, et al. Pulmonary infections after bone marrow transplantation: high-resolution CT findings in 111 patients. AJR Am J Roentgenol 2005;185:608.
6. Heussel CP, Kauczor HU, Heussel GE, et al. Pneumonia in febrile neutropenic patients and in bone marrow and blood stem-cell transplant recipients: use of high-resolution computed tomography. J Clin Oncol 1999;17:796.
7. Leung AN, Gosselin MV, Napper CH, et al. Pulmonary infections after bone marrow transplantation: clinical and radiographic findings. Radiology 1999; 210:699.
8. Marr KA, Carter RA, Crippa F, et al. Epidemiology and outcome of mould infections in hematopoietic stem cell transplant recipients. Clin Infect Dis 2002;34:909.
9. Barnes PD, Marr KA. Risks, diagnosis and outcomes of invasive fungal infections in haematopoietic stem cell transplant recipients. Br J Haematol 2007;139: 519.
10. Franquet T, Gimenez A, Hidalgo A. Imaging of opportunistic fungal infections in immunocompromised patient. Eur J Radiol 2004;51:130.
11. Worthy SA, Flint JD, Muller NL. Pulmonary complications after bone marrow transplantation: high-resolution CT and pathologic findings. Radiographics 1997;17:1359.
12. Kim MJ, Lee KS, Kim J, et al. Crescent sign in invasive pulmonary aspergillosis: frequency and related

CT and clinical factors. J Comput Assist Tomogr 2001;25:305.

13. Verweij PE, Meis JF. Microbiological diagnosis of invasive fungal infections in transplant recipients. Transpl Infect Dis 2000;2:80.

14. Jahagirdar BN, Morrison VA. Emerging fungal pathogens in patients with hematologic malignancies and marrow/stem-cell transplant recipients. Semin Respir Infect 2002;17:113.

15. Spitzer TR. Engraftment syndrome following hematopoietic stem cell transplantation. Bone Marrow Transplant 2001;27:893.

16. Maiolino A, Biasoli I, Lima J, et al. Engraftment syndrome following autologous hematopoietic stem cell transplantation: definition of diagnostic criteria. Bone Marrow Transplant 2003;31:393.

17. Evans A, Steward CG, Lyburn ID, et al. Imaging in haematopoietic stem cell transplantation. Clin Radiol 2003;58:201.

18. Wah TM, Moss HA, Robertson RJ, et al. Pulmonary complications following bone marrow transplantation. Br J Radiol 2003;76:373.

19. Capizzi SA, Kumar S, Huneke NE, et al. Peri-engraftment respiratory distress syndrome during autologous hematopoietic stem cell transplantation. Bone Marrow Transplant 2001;27:1299.

20. Witte RJ, Gurney JW, Robbins RA, et al. Diffuse pulmonary alveolar hemorrhage after bone marrow transplantation: radiographic findings in 39 patients. AJR Am J Roentgenol 1991;157:461.

21. Majhail NS, Parks K, Defor TE, et al. Diffuse alveolar hemorrhage and infection-associated alveolar hemorrhage following hematopoietic stem cell transplantation: related and high-risk clinical syndromes. Biol Blood Marrow Transplant 2006;12:1038.

22. Patz EF Jr, Peters WP, Goodman PC. Pulmonary drug toxicity following high-dose chemotherapy with autologous bone marrow transplantation: CT findings in 20 cases. J Thorac Imaging 1994;9:129.

23. Ellis SJ, Cleverley JR, Muller NL. Drug-induced lung disease: high-resolution CT findings. AJR Am J Roentgenol 2000;175:1019.

24. Akira M, Ishikawa H, Yamamoto S. Drug-induced pneumonitis: thin-section CT findings in 60 patients. Radiology 2002;224:852.

25. Konoplev S, Champlin RE, Giralt S, et al. Cytomegalovirus pneumonia in adult autologous blood and marrow transplant recipients. Bone Marrow Transplant 2001;27:877.

26. Gasparetto EL, Ono SE, Escuissato D, et al. Cytomegalovirus pneumonia after bone marrow transplantation: high resolution CT findings. Br J Radiol 2004;77:724.

27. Franquet T, Rodriguez S, Martino R, et al. Thin-section CT findings in hematopoietic stem cell transplantation recipients with respiratory virus pneumonia. AJR Am J Roentgenol 2006;187:1085.

28. Clark JG, Hansen JA, Hertz MI, et al. NHLBI workshop summary. Idiopathic pneumonia syndrome after bone marrow transplantation. Am Rev Respir Dis 1993;147:1601.

29. Kantrow SP, Hackman RC, Boeckh M, et al. Idiopathic pneumonia syndrome: changing spectrum of lung injury after marrow transplantation. Transplantation 1997;63:1079.

30. Fukuda T, Hackman RC, Guthrie KA, et al. Risks and outcomes of idiopathic pneumonia syndrome after nonmyeloablative and conventional conditioning regimens for allogeneic hematopoietic stem cell transplantation. Blood 2003;102:2777.

31. Woodard JP, Gulbahce E, Shreve M, et al. Pulmonary cytolytic thrombi: a newly recognized complication of stem cell transplantation. Bone Marrow Transplant 2000;25:293.

32. Freudenberger TD, Madtes DK, Curtis JR, et al. Association between acute and chronic graft-versus-host disease and bronchiolitis obliterans organizing pneumonia in recipients of hematopoietic stem cell transplants. Blood 2003;102:3822.

33. Sargent MA, Cairns RA, Murdoch MJ, et al. Obstructive lung disease in children after allogeneic bone marrow transplantation: evaluation with high-resolution CT. AJR Am J Roentgenol 1995;164:693.

34. Benya EC, Sivit CJ, Quinones RR. Abdominal complications after bone marrow transplantation in children: sonographic and CT findings. AJR Am J Roentgenol 1993;161:1023.

35. Einsele H, Bertz H, Beyer J, et al. Infectious complications after allogeneic stem cell transplantation: epidemiology and interventional therapy strategies. Guidelines of the Infectious Diseases Working Party (AGIHO) of the German Society of Hematology and Oncology (DGHO). Ann Hematol 2003;82(Suppl 2):S175.

36. Arai S, Lee LA, Vogelsang GB. A systematic approach to hepatic complications in hematopoietic stem cell transplantation. J Hematother Stem Cell Res 2002;11:215.

37. Carreras E, Bertz H, Arcese W, et al. Incidence and outcome of hepatic veno-occlusive disease after blood or marrow transplantation: a prospective cohort study of the European Group for Blood and Marrow Transplantation. European Group for Blood and Marrow Transplantation Chronic Leukemia Working Party. Blood 1998;92:3599.

38. Kusumi E, Kami M, Kanda Y, et al. Hepatic injury following reduced intensity unrelated cord blood transplantation for adult patients with hematological diseases. Biol Blood Marrow Transplant 2006;12:1302.

39. Wadleigh M, Ho V, Momtaz P, et al. Hepatic veno-occlusive disease: pathogenesis, diagnosis and treatment. Curr Opin Hematol 2003;10:451.

40. Kumar S, DeLeve LD, Kamath PS, et al. Hepatic veno-occlusive disease (sinusoidal obstruction syndrome) after hematopoietic stem cell transplantation. Mayo Clin Proc 2003;78:589.

41. McDonald GB, Hinds MS, Fisher LD, et al. Veno-occlusive disease of the liver and multiorgan failure after bone marrow transplantation: a cohort study of 355 patients. Ann Intern Med 1993;118:255.

42. Lassau N, Leclere J, Auperin A, et al. Hepatic veno-occlusive disease after myeloablative treatment and bone marrow transplantation: value of gray-scale and Doppler US in 100 patients. Radiology 1997; 204:545.

43. Lassau N, Auperin A, Leclere J, et al. Prognostic value of Doppler-ultrasonography in hepatic veno-occlusive disease. Transplantation 2002;74:60.

44. Erturk SM, Mortele KJ, Binkert CA, et al. CT features of hepatic venoocclusive disease and hepatic graft-versus-host disease in patients after hematopoietic stem cell transplantation. AJR Am J Roentgenol 2006;186:1497.

45. Gorg C, Weide R, Schwerk WB, et al. Ultrasound evaluation of hepatic and splenic microabscesses in the immunocompromised patient: sonographic patterns, differential diagnosis, and follow-up. J Clin Ultrasound 1994;22:525.

46. Grunebaum M, Ziv N, Kaplinsky C, et al. Liver candidiasis: the various sonographic patterns in the immunocompromised child. Pediatr Radiol 1991; 21:497.

47. Semelka RC, Kelekis NL, Sallah S, et al. Hepatosplenic fungal disease: diagnostic accuracy and spectrum of appearances on MR imaging. AJR Am J Roentgenol 1997;169:1311.

48. Metser U, Haider MA, Dill-Macky M, et al. Fungal liver infection in immunocompromised patients: depiction with multiphasic contrast-enhanced helical CT. Radiology 2005;235:97.

49. Pestalozzi BC, Krestin GP, Schanz U, et al. Hepatic lesions of chronic disseminated candidiasis may become invisible during neutropenia. Blood 1997; 90:3858.

50. Ferrara JL, Reddy P. Pathophysiology of graft-versus-host disease. Semin Hematol 2006;43:3.

51. Baron F, Maris MB, Sandmaier BM, et al. Graft-versus-tumor effects after allogeneic hematopoietic cell transplantation with nonmyeloablative conditioning. J Clin Oncol 1993;23:2005.

52. Slavin S, Nagler A, Naparstek E, et al. Nonmyeloablative stem cell transplantation and cell therapy as an alternative to conventional bone marrow transplantation with lethal cytoreduction for the treatment of malignant and nonmalignant hematologic diseases. Blood 1998;91:756.

53. Kalantari BN, Mortele KJ, Cantisani V, et al. CT features with pathologic correlation of acute gastrointestinal graft-versus-host disease after bone marrow transplantation in adults. AJR Am J Roentgenol 2003;181:1621.

54. Kirkpatrick ID, Greenberg HM. Gastrointestinal complications in the neutropenic patient: characterization and differentiation with abdominal CT. Radiology 2003;226:668.

55. Day DL, Ramsay NK, Letourneau JG. Pneumatosis intestinalis after bone marrow transplantation. AJR Am J Roentgenol 1988;151:85.

56. Yeager AM, Kanof ME, Kramer SS, et al. Pneumatosis intestinalis in children after allogeneic bone marrow transplantation. Pediatr Radiol 1987;17:18.

57. Ade-Ajayi N, Veys P, Stanton M, et al. Conservative management of pneumatosis intestinalis and pneumoperitoneum following bone-marrow transplantation. Pediatr Surg Int 2002;18:692.

58. Leung AY, Mak R, Lie AK, et al. Clinicopathological features and risk factors of clinically overt haemorrhagic cystitis complicating bone marrow transplantation. Bone Marrow Transplant 2002;29:509.

59. Martin PJ, Carpenter PA, Sanders JE, et al. Diagnosis and clinical management of chronic graft-versus-host disease. Int J Hematol 2004;79:221.

60. Ratanatharathorn V, Ayash L, Lazarus HM, et al. Chronic graft-versus-host disease: clinical manifestation and therapy. Bone Marrow Transplant 2001;28:121.

61. Geubel AP, Nudde A, Ferrant A, et al. Diffuse biliary tract involvement mimicking primary sclerosing cholangitis after bone marrow transplantation. J Hepatol 1990;10:23.

62. Sostak P, Padovan CS, Yousry TA, et al. Prospective evaluation of neurological complications after allogeneic bone marrow transplantation. Neurology 2003;60:842.

63. Coley SC, Jager HR, Szydlo RM, et al. CT and MRI manifestations of central nervous system infection following allogeneic bone marrow transplantation. Clin Radiol 1999;54:390.

64. Trullemans F, Grignard F, Van Camp B, et al. Clinical findings and magnetic resonance imaging in severe cyclosporine-related neurotoxicity after allogeneic bone marrow transplantation. Eur J Haematol 2001;67:94.

65. Drakos PE, Nagler A, Or R, et al. Invasive fungal sinusitis in patients undergoing bone marrow transplantation. Bone Marrow Transplant 1993;12: 203.

66. Savage DG, Taylor P, Blackwell J, et al. Paranasal sinusitis following allogeneic bone marrow transplant. Bone Marrow Transplant 1997;19:55.

67. DelGaudio JM, Swain RE Jr, Kingdom TT, et al. Computed tomographic findings in patients with invasive fungal sinusitis. Arch Otolaryngol Head Neck Surg 2003;129:236.

68. Socie G, Selimi F, Sedel L, et al. Avascular necrosis of bone after allogeneic bone marrow transplantation: clinical findings, incidence and risk factors. Br J Haematol 1994;86:624.

69. Torii Y, Hasegawa Y, Kubo T, et al. Osteonecrosis of the femoral head after allogeneic bone marrow transplantation. Clin Orthop Relat Res 2001;382:124.

70. Wiesmann A, Pereira P, Bohm P, et al. Avascular necrosis of bone following allogeneic stem cell transplantation: MR screening and therapeutic options. Bone Marrow Transplant 1998;22:565.

71. Baker KS, DeFor TE, Burns LJ, et al. New malignancies after blood or marrow stem-cell transplantation in children and adults: incidence and risk factors. J Clin Oncol 2003;21:1352.

72. Curtis RE, Rowlings PA, Deeg HJ, et al. Solid cancers after bone marrow transplantation. N Engl J Med 1997;336:897.

73. Loren AW, Porter DL, Stadtmauer EA, et al. Posttransplant lymphoproliferative disorder: a review. Bone Marrow Transplant 2003;31:145.

74. Burney K, Bradley M, Buckley A, et al. Posttransplant lymphoproliferative disorder: a pictorial review. Australas Radiol 2006;50:412.

75. Pickhardt PJ, Siegel MJ. Posttransplantation lymphoproliferative disorder of the abdomen: CT evaluation in 51 patients. Radiology 1999;213:73.

# Imaging of Late Complications from Mantle Field Radiation in Lymphoma Patients

Sandra Brennan, MD, FFR RCSI, FRCR (UK)[a,b,*], Lucy E. Hann, MD[a,b], Joachim Yahalom, MD[b,c], Kevin C. Oeffinger, MD[d], Jürgen Rademaker, MD[a,b]

**KEYWORDS**

- Hodgkin lymphoma • Radiotherapy • Mantle field
- Breast cancer • Thyroid cancer • Coronary calcifications
- Coronary CT angiography

For over three decades, Hodgkin lymphoma (HL) has been one of the most curable cancers, with 10-year survival rates now exceeding 90%. This high cure rate, even in the 1970s, was largely because of the radiosensitive nature of HL. Radiotherapy (RT) to all involved and uninvolved lymph nodes (total lymphoid irradiation) included the mantle field, which encompasses the primary lymph node regions of the neck, supraclavicular, infraclavicular, axillary, and mediastinal areas. Inverted Y field encompassing the para-aortic and pelvic nodes and the spleen provided curative therapy for most patients with localized disease and was the primary therapeutic modality for early stage disease in the 1960s to 1980s.

Included within the mantle field are critical structures, including the thyroid, carotid arteries, breast tissue, and the proximal coronary arteries, and the heart valves. Because of the toxic effect of radiation on these structures, HL survivors face an increased risk of serious morbidity and premature mortality that may not become clinically apparent until many years after the cancer. For example, Swerdlow and colleagues[1] reported that among a British cohort of 7003 HL survivors with average of 11.2 years of follow-up, the standardized mortality risk secondary to myocardial infarction was 3.2 for those who were treated with mediastinal irradiation. By 25 years after the HL diagnosis, the actuarial risk of developing a solid tumor was 21.9% in an international population-based analysis of 32,591 HL survivors.[2] HL survivors in general have an increased risk of chronic health conditions and subsequent cancers.[3,4]

Importantly, early detection of some of these conditions, including breast cancer and ischemic coronary artery disease, can lead to an improvement in long-term outcomes. In the following sections, the role of imaging studies to detect breast and thyroid cancer and cardiovascular disease is discussed. Pulmonary fibrosis, lung cancer, radiation-related bone lesions, and esophageal disorders are not discussed, because radiologic management issues in these entities are limited.

## CONCEPTS FOR RADIATION FIELDS IN LYMPHOMA

It should be emphasized that the patients who demonstrated the increased morbidity and

[a] Department of Radiology, Memorial Sloan-Kettering Cancer Center, 1275 York Avenue, New York, NY 10021, USA
[b] Weil Medical College of Cornell University, New York, NY, USA
[c] Department of Radiation Oncology, Memorial Sloan-Kettering Cancer Center, 1275 York Avenue, New York, NY 10021, USA
[d] Department of Pediatrics and Medicine, Memorial Sloan-Kettering Cancer Center, 1275 York Avenue, New York, NY 10021, USA
* Corresponding author.
*E-mail address:* brennans@mskcc.org (S. Brennan).

Radiol Clin N Am 46 (2008) 419–430
doi:10.1016/j.rcl.2008.04.005

radiologic.theclinics.com

mortality following the successful treatment of their HL were treated with radiation therapy fields, dose, and technology that no longer exist. Furthermore, the chemotherapy that has been prevalent more than 25 years ago and increased the risk of leukemia and solid tumors has also been replaced with less carcinogenic agents.

Until the 1990s, radiation therapy in early and even in advanced disease was used often as a single modality. This "radical RT" approach required maximizing the radiation field to include all involved and uninvolved lymph nodes areas and spleen, a field that was termed "total lymphoid irradiation". The radiation dose was elevated to near tolerance level of 4400 cGy, and poor imaging and targeting required maintaining generous margins around the original bulky tumors.

When chemotherapy became available, successful treatment of HL no longer depended on radiation alone, and RT followed effective chemotherapy as a consolidating component of a combined modality approach. Because of the reduction in disease volume accomplished by chemotherapy, the radiation field could be minimized to include only the involved lymph node site; this approach is termed "involved-field RT." More recently, the field has been further reduced to encompass only the originally involved lymph node (not site), called "involved node RT." Concomitantly, the radiation dose was reduced from 4400 to 3000 cGy or even lower to 2000 cGy.

New high-quality CT and positron emission tomography (PET) scans integrated with new planning and radiation delivery methods reduced the required "safety margins" and normal organ exposure. As a result of those changes, with current RT, breast tissue exposure is often completely avoided or markedly reduced, the left ventricle of the heart is commonly fully shielded, and the radiation dose to the coronary arteries is substantially reduced. The impact of these changes has already been reflected in decreased morbidity from breast cancer in more recently treated patients (even when accounting for length of follow-up) and is likely to alter positively the risk of coronary artery disease.

## BREAST CANCER

It is well known that radiation exposure increases the risk of cancers.[5] Breast cancer incidence is increased in women who were exposed to atomic bomb radiation and in those women with tuberculosis who underwent multiple chest fluoroscopies.[6] The increased risk of breast cancer in women treated for HL is not surprising given that a large mantle field was used to treat lymph nodes in the upper body.[7] Most of the breast exposure resulted from RT of the axillae. A large amount of breast tissue, particularly the upper outer quadrants, was exposed to either the full prescribed dose, at relatively high doses (>40 Gy), or to an attenuated dose. Mantle RT resulted in a more than 10-fold spectrum of RT dose delivered across the breast (3–42 Gy for tumor doses of 40 Gy) with lower doses delivered to the tissue beneath the lung block and the largest dose delivered to the unshielded upper outer quadrants.

In most studies, the increased risk of breast cancer begins 10 to 15 years after treatment and the excess risk persists for at least 20 years.[3,8,9] Cases have been reported, however, as early as 8 years after RT. The relative risk of breast cancer increases with younger age at first irradiation.[8,9] The relative risk ranges from 17 to 458 for those treated before age 16.[2,10] In contrast, no statistically significant increase in breast cancer risk has been reported in patients treated after age 40.[2,9]

In a study by Travis and colleagues[10] breast cancers developed a mean of 18 years after treatment. The mean age at diagnosis of breast cancer was 40 years or greater. Treatment of HL with RT alone (>4 Gy delivered to the area in which subsequent breast cancer developed) was associated with a significantly increased (3.2-fold) risk of breast cancer. The risk was dose related and was greatest at the site at which the breast was irradiated. Only a 1.4-fold increased risk was conveyed by treatment with both RT and alkylating agents. Risk of breast cancer decreased with increasing number of alkylating agent cycles. Women who became menopausal before age 40 years experienced significant reductions in risk of breast cancer.

In a study by van Leeuwen and colleagues[11], the risk of breast cancer increased significantly with increased radiation dose. Patients who received 38.5 Gy or more had a relative risk of 4.5 times that of patients who received less than 4 Gy. Patients who received both chemotherapy and RT had a significantly lower risk than those treated with RT alone. Reaching menopause before age 36 was associated with a strongly reduced risk of breast cancer.

Because the average age of breast cancer diagnosed after HL is 40 years, routine screening that starts at 40 could potentially miss cancers in this high-risk population. All agree that routine screening of women treated for HL in childhood or adolescence should be performed at a younger age than normally indicated.[12–15] Dershaw and colleagues[12] recommend routine screening before age 35, or 8 years after treatment. Diller and colleagues[13] also began mammographic screening at 8 years after radiation and recommended mammography every other year until age 30 and then annually. Yahalom and coworkers[14] recommended beginning annual mammograms no later than 8 years from treatment.

A study by Bloom and colleagues[16] found that regular mammography was uncommon in women under the age of 40 despite two thirds of the women being aware that breast cancer was a late effect of HL treatment. Being aware was associated with considering oneself at high risk but did not relate to getting regular screening. Diller and colleagues[13] found that 40% of patients did not seem to understand that they were at higher risk. Patients who were followed by an oncologist were more likely to understand that they were at higher risk but were not more likely to have had a mammogram in the previous 2 years.

Several studies have shown that most breast cancers in HL survivors are visible mammographically, likely because of the high prevalence of microcalcifications (62%–72%).[12,13,17] Dershaw and colleagues[12] reported a mammographic detection rate of breast cancer of 90% in women treated with mantle radiation for HL. This high rate was related to the development of microcalcifications in these tumors. In the study by Diller and colleagues[13] all cancers were evident on the mammogram. Kwong and colleagues[17] studied screening mammograms of patients treated for HL and found that high-density breast tissue was common and their recall (17.2%) and biopsy rates (7%) were unusually high. Because mammography has an overall false-negative rate of up to 15% in the general population, alternative screening methods should also be considered.

Because patients in this group tend to be younger and premenopausal with dense breasts, mammography is limited. Overall prior studies of women at increased risk of breast cancer have found a high sensitivity for MR imaging (71%–100%) versus mammography (16%–40%) (**Figs. 1–3**).[18–23] Studies that included ultrasound had a similar sensitivity to mammography. Although evidence of the efficacy of MR imaging screening is not yet available in the HL survivor group, it is believed that MR imaging screening might offer similar benefits as for women with a strong family history or BRCA1 or BRCA2 mutations. The sensitivity of MR imaging in detecting an invasive breast cancer approaches 100%. Specificity is lower than sensitivity and false-positives occur, which leads to higher callback rates and more benign biopsies.[24,25] The specificity of MR imaging (81%–99%) is significantly lower than mammography (93%–99%) in all studies to date. Callback rates ranged from 8% to 17% in the MR imaging screening studies, and biopsy rates ranged from 3% to 15%.

Kriege and colleagues[18] screened 1909 women with an estimated 15% or higher lifetime risk of breast cancer. MR imaging detected 80% of the invasive breast cancers compared with 33% by mammography. Mammography, however, outperformed MR imaging for detecting ductal carcinoma in situ. MR imaging does not currently have as high a negative predictive value for ductal carcinoma in situ as with invasive cancer. Although MR imaging can detect mammographically occult ductal carcinoma in situ, it cannot be used to exclude the need for biopsy of suspicious microcalcification. Mammographically suspicious findings warrant biopsy regardless of a negative MR imaging examination. The MR image should be interpreted in conjunction with the mammogram, not replace the mammogram. Many centers

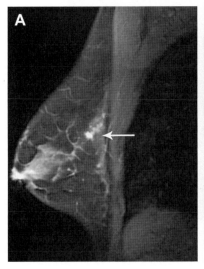 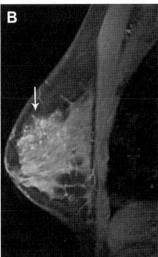

**Fig. 1.** A 55-year-old woman treated with mantle and abdominal radiation 25 years previously for stage 1A Hodgkin disease. Screening breast MR imaging recommended biopsy of two sites. Ductal carcinoma in situ was (DCIS) diagnosed at both. (*A*) Sagittal fat-suppressed T1-weighted postcontrast image of the right breast demonstrates an irregular enhancing mass in the 12:00 axis posterior third (*arrow*). (*B*) Sagittal fat-suppressed T1-weighted postcontrast image showing asymmetric nodular enhancement in the upper outer right breast (*arrow*).

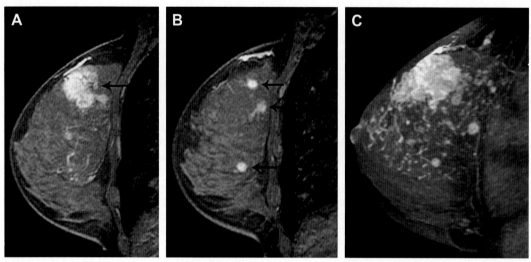

**Fig. 2.** A 31-year-old woman with dense breasts presented with a palpable mass in the right breast. Biopsy yielded invasive ductal carcinoma and DCIS. Breast MR imaging shows unsuspected multicentric disease, which was confirmed at mastectomy. (*A*) Sagittal fat-suppressed T1-weighted postcontrast images of the right breast showing a heterogenous mass, which was palpable in the upper outer quadrant (arrow) and (*B*) additional unsuspected satellite masses in the upper and lower quadrants (*arrows*) all seen on the (*C*) maximum intensity projection image.

recommend MR imaging and mammography at the same time; others recommend staggering them every 6 months. There is no evidence to support one approach over the other, except to ensure MR imaging be provided in addition to, not instead of, mammography.

Within the breast cancer recommendations, there is reasonable consensus. In 2007 the American Cancer Society updated the guidelines for the early detection of breast cancer.[26] Based on expert consensus opinion, annual screening

mammography with adjunct breast MR imaging is now recommended for women with an approximately 20% to 25% or greater lifetime risk of breast cancer. Included in this group are women with a strong family history of breast or ovarian cancer and women who were treated with radiation to the chest between the ages of 10 and 30 years. The new Children's Oncology Group (COG) Long-Term Follow-Up Guidelines are consistent with the American Cancer Society guidelines.[27] The COG recommends that women

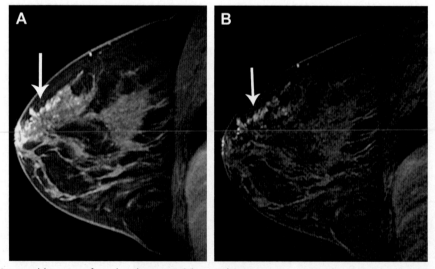

**Fig. 3.** A 44-year-old woman found to have suspicious enhancement on screening MR imaging. Biopsy yielded DCIS. (*A*) Sagittal fat-suppressed T1-weighted postcontrast image and (*B*) subtraction image showing nodular enhancement in the upper inner right breast (*arrow*) extending to the nipple in a ductal distribution.

who received radiation doses greater than or equal to 20 Gy should begin screening with mammography and adjunct breast MR imaging 8 years after radiation or at age 25, whichever occurs last.

## THYROID CANCER

Thyroid disease is common, occurring in up to 67% of patients who have received mantle irradiation for HL, and because the risk continues with long-term follow-up, continued surveillance of these patients is recommended.[28–32] Hypothyroidism, Graves' disease, thyroiditis, thyroid atrophy, and nodular thyroid disease are more frequent in this group.[28,30,33–35] In a study of survivors of childhood HL, the risk of thyroid nodules was 27 times greater and thyroid cancer rates were 18 times more frequent when compared with sibling controls.[30] Other reports have shown a relative risk of thyroid cancer following mantle RT in the range of 10% to 17%.[9,28] Increasing radiation dose, female gender, and younger age at the time of initial treatment have been shown to correlate with subsequent risk of developing thyroid carcinoma.[9,28,36–42] A plateau of risk may occur at higher radiation levels.[9,37–43] Sigurdson and colleagues[41] found highest risk of thyroid cancer at radiation doses between 20 and 29 Gy, with a fall in thyroid cancer rates at doses higher than 30 Gy. Thyroid cancers found in HL and non-HL survivors usually occur at least 5 to 10 years after initial lymphoma diagnosis[36,37], and the excess risk of thyroid cancer continues without a plateau even after more than 20-year follow-up.[8,33,44–46]

Radiation-induced thyroid cancers are papillary and follicular cell types, similar to thyroid cancers in the general population.[36] To date there are no specific cell mutations to differentiate these secondary treatment-related cancers on a molecular level.[47] Thyroid cancers that develop after radiation therapy are no more aggressive and 5-year survival is excellent, in the range of 95% to 100%.[32,41] Although thyroid cancer is one of the more frequent neoplasms consequent to RT, it does not contribute to excess mortality. Breast cancer, hematologic malignancies, and cardiovascular complications secondary to radiation therapy are more significant determinants for overall survival.[4]

Following mantle RT it is recommended that patients have an annual examination to monitor thyroid function; palpable abnormalities should be further evaluated with ultrasound.[37,48,49] In a study of ultrasound findings in 30 long-term HL survivors, Eftekhari and colleagues[50] described atrophy and thyroid nodularity that increased in size and number over time; no thyroid malignancies were reported in this small series. Crom and colleagues[51] studied 96 childhood cancer survivors who had received radiation and found that ultrasound had increased rate of detection of thyroid nodules compared with physical examination and nearly half of patients had thyroid nodules evident on sonography. One patient had papillary carcinoma.

Gray-scale sonographic features of typical papillary carcinoma are hypoechogenicity, microcalcification, irregular margins, and taller than wide shape (**Fig. 4**).[52–59] Microcalcifications are highly

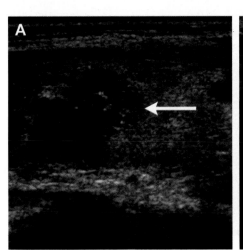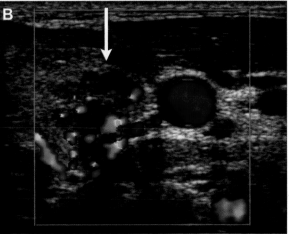

**Fig. 4.** Thyroid sonogram in a 47-year-old woman postchemotherapy and postradiation for Hodgkin disease has findings suspicious for malignancy. Papillary carcinoma was confirmed by fine-needle aspiration biopsy. (*A*) Longitudinal image reveals a hypoechoic irregular solid nodule (*arrow*) with microcalcification. (*B*) Transverse color Doppler images show increased vascularity within the nodule (*arrow*).

specific but they are seen in only half of papillary carcinomas.[53] Vascularity is increased in nearly 42% of thyroid cancers, but not all carcinomas are vascular and many benign thyroid nodules may have increased vascularity (**Fig. 5**).[60] Follicular carcinomas appear as oval masses with peripheral halo and vascularity, indistinguishable from benign adenomas. Cystic thyroid lesions are usually benign etiology.[61] Selection of patients for biopsy should be based on these established ultrasound criteria.[61,62] It is important to avoid unnecessary intervention given the increased incidence of benign thyroid nodules found after mantle radiation and the relatively indolent nature of thyroid carcinoma.[49]

Another criterion used for determining the need for biopsy is FDG-PET positivity (**Fig. 6**). It has been reported that 14% to 40% of focal FDG-PET avid thyroid lesions are malignant.[63–66] Are and colleagues[63] found that FDG-positive thyroid lesions were rare, occurring in only 3% of patients, but the rate of primary thyroid cancer was increased in this group. Standard uptake value was not useful to differentiate benign from malignant lesions. In another study, the rate of malignancy for PET-positive thyroid lesions compared with patients without PET was more than doubled.[65] This evidence supports the need to biopsy any FDG-PET avid focal thyroid lesion.

COG recommends annual clinical thyroid examinations in patients with prior mediastinal radiation.[27] If a thyroid nodule is palpated, ultrasound and potentially fine-needle aspiration are recommended for further evaluation.

## CARDIOVASCULAR COMPLICATIONS

Coronary calcifications are a common CT finding in lymphoma patients who were previously treated with mediastinal radiation and represent an important CT finding (**Fig. 7**). An increase in cardiovascular mortality and morbidity has been identified as a long-term risk following mediastinal radiation therapy[1,2,67–69], especially for patients, who have received more than 30 Gy of mantle radiation.[70] HL, for example, has a bimodal incidence curve and a significant number of patients receive radiation treatment in young adulthood (age 15–35).

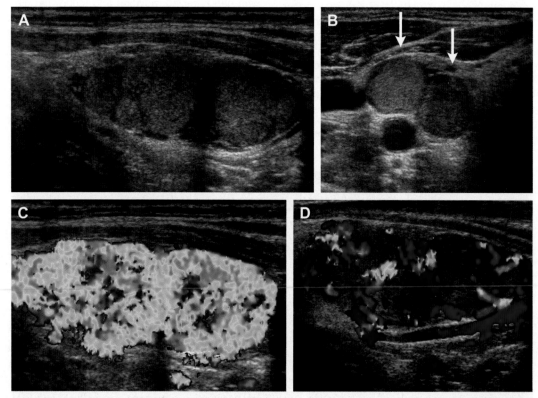

**Fig. 5.** A 30-year-old man with hypothyroidism after therapy for mediastinal large B cell–type lymphoma had nodules replacing the right lobe. Cytology results were consistent with benign nodular goiter. Longitudinal (*A*) and transverse (*B*) images reveal lobulated nodules (*arrows*) replacing the right lobe. (*C*) The right lobe nodules were markedly vascular on initial Doppler images. (*D*) Vascularity diminished 1 month after thyroid replacement therapy.

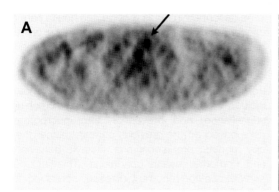

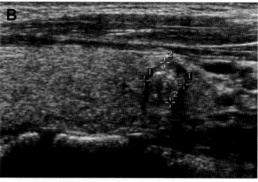

Fig. 6. A 37-year-old woman with history of mediastinal B-cell lymphoma treated with chemotherapy and radiation. Incidental left thyroid lobe papillary carcinoma was detected by PET scan. (A) FDG-PET scan reveals increased uptake (arrow) in the left thyroid lobe. (B) A small nodule (calipers) with calcification is seen on longitudinal sonogram.

Recent studies documented an increased incidence of cardiovascular events approximately 19 years after the radiation.[71] The relative risk for acute myocardial infarction was highest when patients were irradiated before 20 years of age and decreased with increasing age at treatment.[70] The risk of coronary artery disease in these patients may be reduced with aggressive intervention, medical management, and follow-up, and screening for asymptomatic coronary artery disease has been advocated in this population.[1,67–72]

Most patients are evaluated with stress echocardiography or nuclear scintigraphy to look for inducible ischemia. A recent study by Heidenreich and colleagues[73] evaluated the HL survivors treated with mediastinal irradiation. Sixty-three patients (21%) had an abnormal test; 22 of these

63 patients showed greater than or equal to 50% stenosis on angiography. By screening with stress echocardiography and nuclear scintigraphy, the authors found a 2.7% prevalence of severe, three-vessel, or left main coronary artery disease, and a 7.5% prevalence of coronary artery stenosis greater than 50% in patients treated with mediastinal irradiation in doses greater than or equal to 35 Gy for HL at a mean of 15 years following irradiation.[73] These numbers likely underestimate the prevalence of coronary artery disease because patients were not required to undergo angiography and were excluded if they had known coronary artery disease. It should be noted that this approach only identifies patients with a positive stress test and fails to identify patients with coronary artery disease and a negative stress test, who might also benefit from medical interventions, such as risk profile modification.

Combined coronary CT angiography[74] and calcium scores is also a promising tool for evaluation of radiation-related coronary artery disease.[75] Coronary CT angiography has significant advantages compared other tests, such as stress tests or cardiac catheterization, because it is noninvasive and has higher sensitivity in disease detection (see Fig. 7). CT angiography is often difficult to interpret when coronary calcifications are present because blooming artifact may obscure the adjacent vessel lumen. Patients in this category require additional testing, such as with a stress test or a cardiac angiogram. Measurement of calcium score alone would not allow identification of patients who need to undergo further functional testing. Both patients with low or moderate calcium scores (<400) and patients with higher scores (≥400) may have soft plaques and may be at risk for coronary events. Calcium scores allow assessment of plaque burden, but the use of coronary

Fig. 7. A 39-year-old man status post-45 Gy administered 25 years ago (Hodgkin lymphoma, mantle field radiation). Maximum intensity projection image shows extensive calcification in the coronaries. Note additional calcifications within the anulus fibrosis, aortic vessel wall, and anterior pericardium.

artery calcium scoring techniques as a screening tool for identification of individuals at risk for acute coronary events is hampered by several limitations, including insufficient scientific backing and statistical considerations.[76,77]

An increased incidence of noncoronary arteriosclerotic vascular disease after radiation therapy was also recognized.[68,78] In one surgical study with patients who received irradiation for lymphoma, breast cancer, and head and neck malignancies, the mean interval between irradiation and arterial revascularization was 15.2 years.[78] Most patients (80%) had symptomatic disease. In another study of patients who were treated with radiation therapy from 1962 to 1998, the actual incidence of noncoronary arteriosclerotic disease was 2% at 5 years, 3% at 10 years, and 7% at 20 years. For all patients in the study who developed noncoronary vascular disease, the median age at the time of radiation therapy was 34, and the median time from therapy to event was 17 years. In the study, the median low-cervical radiation doses for patients who developed subclavian stenosis and carotid artery disease were 44 Gy (range, 37–48 Gy) and 38 Gy (range, 30–57 Gy), respectively.

COG recommends periodic evaluation with yearly history and physical examinations for signs or symptoms of cardiac complications.[27] Cardiology consultation to evaluate risk for coronary artery disease (5–10 years after radiation) should be considered in a patient who received more than 40 Gy chest radiation alone or more than 30 Gy chest radiation plus anthracycline therapy. Doppler ultrasound of carotid or subclavian vessels should be performed in symptomatic patients. Color Doppler 10 years after completion of radiation therapy to the neck should be considered as a baseline.

## RISK-BASED HEALTH CARE AND SCREENING GUIDELINES

HL survivors who were treated with mantle RT are at an increased risk of several types of serious morbidity, and the risk for some of these conditions can be reduced by preventive strategies. Highlighting this principle, the Institute of Medicine released two seminal reports on cancer survivorship.[79,80] In the 2003 report, *Childhood Cancer Survivorship: Improving Care and Quality of Life*, the Institute of Medicine strongly recommended lifelong follow-up health care for all childhood cancer survivors.[79] This recommendation was echoed in the 2006 report focused on survivors of adult cancer, *From Cancer Patient to Cancer Survivor: Lost in Transition*.[80]

As described in these reports, the health care of cancer survivors should be based on their unique health risks following chemotherapy, surgery, and radiation. Content, intensity, and frequency of health care that addresses these risks vary from survivor to survivor.[81] Such care should include a systematic plan for lifelong screening, surveillance, and prevention that incorporates risks based on the previous cancer, cancer therapy, genetic predispositions, lifestyle behaviors, and comorbid health conditions. This includes surveillance for recurrent disease, screening for late effects and subsequent cancers, promotion of risk-reducing healthy lifestyles, and targeted counseling and education.

To assist clinicians in delivering risk-based health care to long-term survivors of pediatric and young adult cancers, including HL, COG developed the *COG Long-Term Follow-Up Guidelines for Survivors of Childhood, Adolescent, and Young Adult Cancers*, released in 2003.[27] The guidelines can be found on the following Web site: www.survivorshipguidelines.org. The COG guidelines include screening recommendations for men and women who were treated with mantle radiation as described in the previous sections.

Evidence-based recommendations for screening of childhood cancer survivors have also been developed by several European groups, including the Scottish Intercollegiate Guidelines Network[82] and United Kingdom Children's Cancer Study Group Late Effects Group.[83] In contrast, the literature base of late effects following therapy for adult cancers has not yet evolved to the depth and breadth of that available for those following pediatric cancer.[84] Recently, the American Society of Clinical Oncologists Cancer Survivorship Expert Panel reviewed the literature and determined that there was not adequate evidence yet to develop a set of screening recommendations for survivors of adult cancer.[85]

## SUMMARY

HL is one of the most curable cancers because of its sensitivity to both radiation and several chemotherapy agents. Radical RT alone provided curative therapy for patients with HL as early as six decades ago. Yet, the radiation field included normal organs, such as breast tissue, thyroid, and coronary arteries, that were at risk for long-term complications. Dedicated imaging approaches have been developed to evaluate late radiation effects on these structures. In addition, new treatment approaches have been developed to reduce radiation fields and dose and decrease exposure of critical organs.

The increased risk of breast cancer usually begins 10 to 15 years after treatment, but cases have been reported as early as 8 years. Women who received radiation doses greater than or equal to 20 Gy should begin screening with mammography 8 years after radiation or at age 25, whichever occurs last. Recently, MR imaging of the breast is also recommended because it shows advantage for evaluation of dense breasts and diagnosis of invasive cancers in this high-risk population. Thyroid cancer and benign thyroid nodules are more frequent postirradiation. Thyroid nodules that have suspicious sonographic features, such as microcalcification, hypoechogenicity, irregular margins, and taller than wide shape, should be biopsied. Biopsy is also recommended for any FDG-PET avid nodule. An increase in cardiovascular mortality and morbidity has been identified and screening for asymptomatic coronary artery disease has been advocated. Most patients are evaluated with stress echo or nuclear scintigraphy. Symptomatic patients should be evaluated for noncoronary arteriosclerotic vascular disease.

## REFERENCES

1. Swerdlow AJ, Higgins CD, Smith P, et al. Myocardial infarction mortality risk after treatment for Hodgkin disease: a collaborative British cohort study. J Natl Cancer Inst 2007;99:206–14.

2. Dores GM, Metayer C, Curtis RE, et al. Second malignant neoplasms among long-term survivors of Hodgkin's disease: a population-based evaluation over 25 years. J Clin Oncol 2002;20(16):3484–94.

3. Oeffinger KC, Mertens AC, Sklar CA, et al. Chronic health conditions in adult survivors of childhood cancer. N Engl J Med 2006;355(15):1572–82.

4. Mertens AC, Yasui Y, Neglia JP, et al. Late mortality experience in five-year survivors of childhood and adolescent cancer: the Childhood Cancer Survivor Study. J Clin Oncol 2001;19(13):3163–72.

5. Moysich KB, Menezes RJ, Michalek AM. Chernobyl-related ionizing radiation exposure and cancer risk: an epidemiological review. Lancet Oncol 2002;3(5):269–79.

6. Little MP, Boice JD Jr. Comparison of breast cancer incidence in the Massachusetts tuberculosis fluoroscopy cohort and in the Japanese atomic bomb survivors. Radiat Res 1999;151(2):218–24.

7. Ng AK, Mauch PM. Controversies in early-stage Hodgkin's disease. Oncology (Williston Park) 2002;16:588–95, 598.

8. van Leeuwen FE, Klokman WJ, et al. Long-term risk of second malignancy in survivors of Hodgkin's disease treated during adolescence or young adulthood. J Clin Oncol 2000;18(3):487–97.

9. Swerdlow AJ, Barber JA, et al. Risk of second malignancy after Hodgkin's disease in a collaborative British cohort: the relation to age at treatment. J Clin Oncol 2000;18:498–509.

10. Travis LB, Hill D, Dores GM, et al. Breast cancer following radiotherapy and chemotherapy among young women with Hodgkin disease. JAMA 2003;290:465–75.

11. van Leeuwen FE, Klokman WJ, Stovall M, et al. Roles of radiation dose, chemotherapy, and hormonal factors in breast cancer following Hodgkin's disease. J Natl Cancer Inst 2003;95(13):971–80.

12. Dershaw DD, Yahalom J, Petrek J. Breast carcinoma in women previously treated for Hodgkin disease: mammographic evaluation. Radiology 1992;184:421–3.

13. Diller L, Nancarrow CM, Shaffer K, et al. Breast cancer screening in women previously treated for Hodgkin's disease: a prospective cohort study. J Clin Oncol 2002;20:2085–91.

14. Yahalom J, Petrek JA, Biddinger PW, et al. Breast cancer in patients irradiated for Hodgkin's disease: a clinical and pathologic analysis of 45 events in 37 patients. J Clin Oncol 1992;10:1674–81.

15. Hudson MM, Poquette CA, Lee J, et al. Increased mortality after successful treatment for Hodgkin's disease. J Clin Oncol 1998;16:3592–600.

16. Bloom JR, Stewart SL, Hancock SL. Breast cancer screening in women surviving Hodgkin disease. Am J Clin Oncol 2006;29:258–66.

17. Kwong A, Hancock S, Bloom J, et al. Mammographic screening in women at increased risk of breast cancer after treatment of Hodgkin's disease. Breast J 2008;14(1):39–48.

18. Kriege M, Brekelmans CT, Boetes C, et al. Efficacy of MRI and mammography for breast cancer screening in women with a familial or genetic predisposition. N Engl J Med 2004;351:427–37.

19. Kuhl CK, Schrading S, Leutner CC, et al. Mammography, breast ultrasound, and magnetic resonance imaging for surveillance of women at high familial risk for breast cancer. J Clin Oncol 2005;23:8469–76.

20. Leach MO, Boggis CR, Dixon AK, et al. Screening with magnetic resonance imaging and mammography of a UK population at high familial risk of breast cancer: a prospective multicentre cohort study (MARIBS). Lancet 2005;365:1769–78.

21. Lehman CD, Blume JD, Weatherall P, et al. Screening women at high risk for breast cancer with mammography and magnetic resonance imaging. Cancer 2005;103:1898–905.

22. Sardanelli F. Breast MR imaging in women at high risk of breast cancer. Is something changing in early breast cancer detection? Eur Radiol 2007;17(4):873–87.

23. Warner E, Plewes DB, Hill KA, et al. Surveillance of BRCA1 and BRCA2 mutation carriers with magnetic resonance imaging, ultrasound mammography, and clinical breast examination. JAMA 2004;292: 1317–25.

24. Morris EA, Liberman L, Ballon DJ, et al. MRI of occult breast carcinoma in a high-risk population. AJR Am J Roentgenol 2003;181:619–26.

25. Morris EA. Diagnostic breast MR imaging: current status and future directions. Radiol Clin North Am 2007;45:863–80.

26. Saslow D, Boetes C, Burke W, et al. American Cancer Society guidelines for breast screening with MRI as an adjucnt to mammography. CA Cancer J Clin 2007;57:75–89.

27. Landier W, Bhatia S, Eshelman DA, et al. Development of risk-based guidelines for pediatric cancer survivors: the Children's Oncology Group Long-Term Follow-Up Guidelines from the Children's Oncology Group Late Effects Committee and Nursing Discipline. J Clin Oncol 2004;22(24):4979–90.

28. Hancock SL, Cox RS, McDougall IR. Thyroid diseases after treatment of Hodgkin's disease. N Engl J Med 1991;325(9):599–605.

29. Shafford EA, Kingston JE, Healy JC, et al. Thyroid nodular disease after radiotherapy to the neck for childhood Hodgkin's disease. BR J Cancer 1999; 80(5–6):808–14.

30. Sklar C, Whitton J, Mertens A, et al. Abnormalities of the thyroid in survivors of Hodgkin's disease: data from the Childhood Cancer Survivor Study. J Clin Endocrinol Metab 2000;85(9):3227–32.

31. Stewart RR, David CL, Eftekhari F, et al. Thyroid gland: US in patients with Hodgkin disease treated with radiation therapy in childhood. Radiology 1989;172(1):159–63.

32. Acharya S, Sarafoglou K, LaQuaglia M, et al. Thyroid neoplasms after therapeutic radiation for malignancies during childhood or adolescence. Cancer 2003;97(10):2397–403.

33. Alemann BM, van Leeuwen F. Are we improving the long-term burden of Hodgkin's lymphoma patients with modern treatment? Hematol Oncol Clin North Am 2007;21(5):961–75.

34. Illes A, Biro E, Miltenyi Z, et al. Hypothyroidism and thyroiditis after therapy for Hodgkin's disease. Acta Haematol 2003;109(1):11–7.

35. Bethge W, Guggenberger D, Bamberg M, et al. Thyroid toxicity of treatment for Hodgkin's disease. Ann Hematol 2000;79(3):114–8.

36. Inskip PD. Thyroid cancer after radiotherapy for childhood cancer. Med Pediatr Oncol 2001;36(5): 568–73.

37. Maule M, Scelo G, Pastore G, et al. Risk of second malignant neoplasms after childhood leukemia and lymphoma: an international study. J Natl Cancer Inst 2007;99(10):790–800.

38. Tward JD, Wendland MM, Shrieve DC, et al. The risk of secondary malignancies over 30 years after the treatment of non-Hodgkin lymphoma. Cancer 2006; 107(1):108–15.

39. Tucker MA, Morris Jones PH, Boice JD, et al. Therapeutic radiation at a young age is linked to secondary thyroid cancer. Cancer Res 1991;51:2885–8.

40. Ronckers CM, Sigurdson AJ, Stovall M, et al. Thyroid cancer in childhood cancer survivors: a detailed evaluation of radiation dose response and its modifiers. Radiat Res 2006;166(4):618–28.

41. Sigurdson AJ, Ronckers CM, Mertens AC, et al. Primary thyroid cancer after a first tumour in childhood (the Childhood Cancer Survivor Study): a nested case-control study. Lancet 2005;365:2014–23.

42. Lee CKK, Aeppli D, Nierengarten ME. The need for long-term surveillance for patients treated with curative radiotherapy for Hodgkin's disease: University of Minnesota experience. Int J Radiat Oncol Biol Phys 2000;48(1):169–79.

43. Hancock SL, McDougall IR, Constine LS. Thyroid abnormalities after therapeutic external radiation. Int J Radiat Oncol Biol Phys 1995;31(5):1165–70.

44. Ng AK, Bernardo VP, Weller E, et al. Second malignancy after Hodgkin disease treated with radiation therapy with or without chemotherapy: long-term risks and risk factors. Blood 2002; 100(6):1989–96.

45. Lin HMJ, Teitell MA. Second malignancy after treatment of pediatric Hodgkin disease. J Pediatr Hematol Oncol 2005;27(1):28–36.

46. Bhatia S, Robison LL, Oberlin O, et al. Breast cancer and other second neoplasms after childhood Hodgkin's disease. N Engl J Med 1996;334(12):745–51.

47. Thomas GA. Solid cancers after therapeutic radiation: can we predict which patients are most at risk? Clin Oncol 2004;16:429–34.

48. Landier W. Establishing and enhancing services for childhood cancer survivors: long-term follow-up program resource guide. Children's Oncology Group. 2007. Available at: www.survivorshipguidelines.org. Accessed January 9, 2008.

49. Metzger ML, Howard SC, Hudson MM, et al. Natural history of thyroid nodules in survivors of pediatric Hodgkin lymphoma. Pediatr Blood Cancer 2006; 46:314–9.

50. Eftekhari F, Nader S, Libshitz HI. Imaging findings in postradiation changes of the thyroid and parathyroid glands. Semin Roentgenol 1993;28(4):333–43.

51. Crom DB, Kaste SC, Tubergen DG, et al. Ultrasonography for thyroid screening after head and neck irradiation in childhood cancer survivors. Med Pediatr Oncol 1997;28(1):15–21.

52. Solbiati L, Charboneau JW, Osti V, et al. The thyroid gland. In: Rumack CM, Wilson SR, Charboneau JW, editors. 3rd edition, Diagnostic ultrasound, vol. 1. St. Louis (MO): Elsevier Mosby; 2005. p. 735–70.

53. Peccin S, deCastsro JA, Furlanetto TW, et al. Ultra-sonography: is it useful in the diagnosis of cancer in thyroid nodules? J Endocrinol Invest 2002;25(1):39–43.

54. Chan BK, Desser TS, McDougall IR, et al. Common and uncommon sonographic features of papillary thyroid carcinoma. J Ultrasound Med 2003;22(10):1083–90.

55. Kim EK, Park CS, Chung WY, et al. New sonographic criteria for recommending fine-needle aspiration biopsy of nonpalpable solid nodules of the thyroid. AJR Am J Roentgenol 2002;178:687–91.

56. Alexander EK, Marqusee E, Orcutt J, et al. Thyroid nodule shape and prediction of malignancy. Thyroid 2004;14(11):953–8.

57. Cappelli C, Castellano M, Pirola I, et al. Thyroid nodule shape suggests malignancy. Eur J Endocrinol 2006;155(1):27–31.

58. Lyshchik A, Drozd V, Demidchik Y, et al. Diagnosis of thyroid cancer in children: value of gray-scale and power Doppler US. Radiology 2005;235(2):604–13.

59. Hoang JK, Lee WK, Lee M, et al. US features of thyroid malignancy: pearls and pitfalls. Radiographics 2007;27:847–65.

60. Frates MC, Benson CB, Doubilet PM, et al. Can color Doppler sonography aid in the prediction of malignancy of thyroid nodules? J Ultrasound Med 2003;22(2):127–31 [quiz: 132–4].

61. Reading CC, Charboneau JW, Hay ID, et al. Sonography of thyroid nodules: a classic pattern diagnostic approach. Ultrasound Q 2005;21:157–65.

62. Frates MC, Benson CB, Charboneau JW, et al. Management of thyroid nodules detected at US: Society of Radiologists in Ultrasound consensus conference statement. Radiology 2005;237:794–800.

63. Are C, Hsu JF, Schoder H, et al. FDG-PET detected thyroid incidentalomas: need for further investigation? Ann Surg Oncol 2007;14(1):239–47.

64. Chen YK, Ding HJ, Chen KT, et al. Prevalence and risk of cancer of focal thyroid incidentaloma identified by 18F-fluorodeoxyglucose positron emission tomography fro cancer screening in healthy subjects. Anticancer Res 2005;25(2B):1421–6.

65. Berger DM, Akhurst T, Zakowski MF, et al. Incidental FDG-PET positive thyroid lesions in cancer patients: correlation with ultrasound biopsy and surgical pathology [abstract 156]. In: American Roentgen Ray Society 105th Annual Meeting Abstract Book. New Orleans (LA): American Roentgen Ray Society; 2005. p. 40.

66. Kim TY, Kim WB, Ryu JS, et al. 18F-fluorodeoxyglucose uptake in thyroid from positron emission tomogram (PET) for evaluation in cancer patients: high prevalence of malignancy in thyroid PET incidentaloma. Laryngoscope 2005;115(6):1074–8.

67. Patel DA, Kochanski J, Suen AW, et al. Clinical manifestations of noncoronary atherosclerotic vascular disease after moderate dose irradiation. Cancer 2006;106:718–25.

68. Hull MC, Morris CG, Pepine CJ, et al. Valvular dysfunction and carotid, subclavian, and coronary artery disease in survivors of Hodgkin lymphoma treated with radiation therapy. JAMA 2003;290:2831–7.

69. Hancock SL, Donaldson SS, Hoppe RT. Cardiac disease following treatment of Hodgkin's disease in children and adolescents. J Clin Oncol 1993;11:1199–203.

70. Hancock SL, Tucker MA, Hoppe RT. Factors affecting late mortality from heart disease after treatment of Hodgkin's disease. JAMA 1993;270:1949–55.

71. Aleman BM, van den Belt-Dusebout AW, De Bruin ML, et al. Late cardiotoxicity after treatment for Hodgkin lymphoma. Blood 2007;109:1878–86.

72. Adams MJ, Lipsitz SR, Colan SD, et al. Cardiovascular status in long-term survivors of Hodgkin's disease treated with chest radiotherapy. J Clin Oncol 2004;22:3139–48.

73. Heidenreich PA, Schnittger I, Strauss HW, et al. Screening for coronary artery disease after mediastinal irradiation for Hodgkin's disease. J Clin Oncol 2007;25:43–9.

74. Hoffmann MH, Shi H, Schmitz BL, et al. Noninvasive coronary angiography with multislice computed tomography. JAMA 2005;293:2471–8.

75. Rademaker J, Schoeder H, Ariaratnam NS, et al. Coronary artery disease following radiation therapy for Hodgkin lymphoma: coronary CT angiography findings and Ca scores in 9 asymptomatic patients. AJR Am J Roentgenol 2008;191:32–7.

76. Cheng GC, Loree HM, Kamm RD, et al. Distribution of circumferential stress in ruptured and stable atherosclerotic lesions: a structural analysis with histopathological correlation. Circulation 1993;87:1179–87.

77. Leontiev O, Dubinsky TJ. CT-based calcium scoring to screen for coronary artery disease: why aren't we there yet? AJR Am J Roentgenol 2007;189:1061–3.

78. Hassen-Khodja R, Kieffer E. Radiotherapy induced supra-aortic trunk disease: early and long term results of surgical and endovascular reconstruction. J Vasc Surg 2004;40:254–61.

79. Hewitt M, Weiner SL, Simone JV, editors. Childhood cancer survivorship: improving care and quality of life. Washington, DC: The National Academies Press; 2003.

80. Hewitt M, Greenfield S, Stovall E. From cancer patient to cancer survivor: lost in transition. Washington, DC: The National Academies Press; 2006.

81. Oeffinger KC. Longitudinal risk-based health care for adult survivors of childhood cancer. Curr Probl Cancer 2003;27:143–67.

82. Scottish Intercollegiate Guidelines Network (SIGN). Long term follow up of survivors of childhood cancer. Guideline no. 76. Available at: www.sign.ac.uk/pdf/sign76.pdf. Accessed May 2008.

83. Skinner R, Wallace WH, Levitt G. Therapy based long-term follow up: a practice statement. United Kingdom Children's Cancer Study Group Late Effects Group. Available at: www.ukccsg.org. Accessed May 2008.

84. Earle CC. Cancer survivorship research and guidelines: maybe the cart should be beside the horse. J Clin Oncol 2007;25:3800–1.

85. Carver JR, Shapiro CL, Ng A, et al. American Society of Clinical Oncology clinical evidence review on the ongoing care of adult cancer survivors: cardiac and pulmonary late effects. J Clin Oncol 2007;25:3991–4008.

# Index

*Note:* Page numbers of article titles are in **boldface** type.

Radiol Clin N Am 46 (2008) 431–436
doi:10.1016/S0033-8389(08)00077-8

# Erratum

In the article "Sonographic Evaluation of First-trimester Bleeding" by Raj Mohan Paspulati, Shweta Bhatt, and Sherif Nour, which was published in the March 2004 issue of *Radiologic Clinics of North America*, an author's name was printed incorrectly. Dr. Nour's name should have been published as Sherif Gamal Nour, MD.

Radiol Clin N Am 46 (2008) 437
doi:10.1016/j.rcl.2008.05.001

# *Moving?*

## *Make sure your subscription moves with you!*

To notify us of your new address, find your **Clinics Account Number** (located on your mailing label above your name), and contact customer service at:

**E-mail: elspcs@elsevier.com**

**800-654-2452 (subscribers in the U.S. & Canada)**
**1-407-563-6020 (subscribers outside of the U.S. & Canada)**

**Fax number: 407-363-9661**

**Elsevier Periodicals Customer Service**
6277 Sea Harbor Drive
Orlando, FL  32887-4800

*To ensure uninterrupted delivery of your subscription, please notify us at least 4 weeks in advance of move.